Single Session Therapies

This volume presents the latest information from international leaders as well as emerging experts on how to make Single Session Therapy (SST) efficient and effective.

Key topics involve different productive mindsets and multi-theoretical clinical methods with different problems and populations (including individuals, families, adolescents, children, and couples), as well as walk-in and by-appointment access, digital services, implementation and training, the structure and aesthetics of a single session, and connections to sports coaching.

It is an essential book for practicing professionals, such as psychologists, social workers, psychiatrists, counselors, case workers, and behavioral healthcare specialists, as well as graduate students and healthcare administrators and policymakers.

Flavio Cannistrà, Psy. D, is the Co-Director of the Italian Center for Single Session Therapy, the author/editor of *Single Session Therapy: Principles and Practice* and *Brief Therapy Conversations*, and was the co-organizer of the 4th International Symposium on SST, held in Rome in November 2023.

Michael F. Hoyt, Ph.D., is in independent practice in Mill Valley, CA. He is the author/editor of *Brief Therapy and Beyond* and *Single Session Therapy: A Clinical Introduction to Principles and Practices* and is the recipient of various professional awards.

Single Session Therapies

Why and How One-at-a-Time Mindsets
Are Effective

Edited by
Flavio Cannistrà and Michael F. Hoyt

Routledge
Taylor & Francis Group

NEW YORK AND LONDON

Designed cover image: Michael F. Hoyt & Phillip B. Ziegler

First published 2025
by Routledge
605 Third Avenue, New York, NY 10158

and by Routledge
4 Park Square, Milton Park, Abingdon, Oxon, OX14 4RN

Routledge is an imprint of the Taylor & Francis Group, an informa business

ISBN: 978-1-032-69381-1 (hbk)
ISBN: 978-1-032-69693-5 (pbk)
ISBN: 978-1-032-69382-8 (ebk)

DOI: 10.4324/9781032693828

Typeset in Sabon
by Apex CoVantage, LLC

To my mother, who taught me thinking.
To my father, who taught me goodness.
—F.C.

To my dear friend, Clem, who lived every moment.
"Hey, amigo!"
—M.F.H.

Contents

Figures

Tables

About the Contributors

Editors

Flavio Cannistrà, Psy. D, is Co-Founder of the Italian Center for Single Session Therapy and the School of Specialization in Brief Systemic-Strategic Psychotherapies (the ICNOS Institute), based in Rome. He was also Co-Director of the Fourth International SST Symposium, the first to be held in Europe. He has been a speaker at Brief Therapy conferences in Europe, the United States, Australia, and Japan. Along-side his clinical work, he is an active researcher studying the processes and methods that make brief therapies effective and accessible, and has published in various international journals. Among his books are *Single-Session Therapy: Principles and Practices* (with F. Piccirilli; first published in Italian, translated into English and Japanese) and *Brief Therapy Conversations: Exploring Efficient Intervention in Psychotherapy* (with M.F. Hoyt; first published in English, translated into Italian).

Michael F. Hoyt, Ph.D, is a psychologist based in Mill Valley, California. He was one of the originators (with M. Talmon and R. Rosenbaum) of the Single Session Therapy (SST) approach and is the author of *Brief Therapy and Beyond: Stories, Language, Love, Hope, and Time* and *Single Session Therapy: A Clinical Introduction to Principles and Practices*; the co-author of *Brief Therapy Conversations: Exploring Efficient Intervention in Psychotherapy* (with F. Cannistrà); and the co-editor of *Capturing the Moment: Single Session Therapy and Walk-In Services* (with M. Talmon), *Single-Session Therapy by Walk-In or Appointment: Administrative, Clinical, and Supervisory Aspects of One-at-a-Time Services* (with M. Bobele, A. Slive, J. Young, and M. Talmon), and *Single Session Thinking and Practice in Global, Cultural, and Familial Contexts: Expanding Applications* (with J. Young and P. Rycroft).

Chapter Authors

Keigo Asai, Ph.D., is an associate professor at Hokkaido University of Education, Japan. He is a clinical psychologist and member of the National Foundation of Brief Therapy Japan, providing brief therapy and SST training and supervision to psychologists and teachers. He is also a school counselor at public primary and junior high schools in Japan.

Rubin Battino, M.S., has a private practice in Yellow Springs, Ohio. He is an adjunct professor for the Department of Human Services at Wright State University and is the author of numerous books on psychotherapy, including *Using Guided Imagery and Hypnosis in Brief Therapy and Palliative Care*; *Expectation: The Very Brief Therapy Book*; *When All Else Fails: Some New and Some Old Tools for Doing Brief Therapy*; and *Ericksonian Approaches: A Comprehensive Manual* (with T.L. Smith). He is also a professor emeritus of chemistry.

Monte Bobele, Ph.D., is Emeritus Professor of Psychology at Our Lady of the Lake University in San Antonio, Texas; an AAMFT clinical fellow and approved supervisor; and cofounder with A. Slive of Single-Session Solutions for Consulting and Training. He is the co-editor of *When One Hour Is All You Have: Effective Counseling for Walk-In Clients* and *Implementing Single-Session Therapy in Open Access Services* (with A. Slive); *Single-Session Therapy by Walk-In or Appointment* (with M.F. Hoyt, A. Slive, J. Young, and M. Talmon); and *Creative Therapy in Challenging Situations: Unusual Interventions to Help Clients* (with M.F. Hoyt).

Valeria Campinoti, Psy.D., is a member of the ICNOS Institute and the Italian Center for Single Session Therapy. She has held various roles, including Co-Director of the 4th International SST Symposium. A specialist in addiction psychology, she has collaborated with several communities for addicted patients and conducted research-intervention activities on youth distress and the relationship between adolescents and crime. She has long dealt with emotional addiction issues, helping women overcome the end of dysfunctional relationships.

Scot J. Cooper, RP, is a registered psychotherapist, international trainer, and consultant in brief narrative therapy. He is a manager of the Child and Youth Mental Health Services at H-N REACH, the lead children's mental health center for Haldimand-Norfolk counties in rural Ontario, Canada, where he practices, supervises students, and oversees the walk-in clinic. He is also the lead for Brief Narrative Practices, a portal to personalized post-graduate specialty training and consultation in brief therapy. He is the author of *Brief Narrative Practice in Single-Session Therapy*.

Windy Dryden, Ph.D., is Emeritus Professor of Psychotherapeutic Studies at Goldsmiths University of London and is a fellow of the British Psychological Society. His many publications include *Single-Session Integrated CBT (SSI-CBT)*; *Single-Session Therapy: 100 Key Points and Techniques*; *Single-Session One-at-a-Time Therapy: A Rational Emotive Behavior Approach*; and *Single-Session Counseling: Principles and Practice*.

Suzanne Fuzzard, BAppSc (OT), is an occupational therapist and family therapist who, since 1989, has worked across the adult, youth, domestic violence, and mental health fields in Australia and the United Kingdom. She is the center manager for headspace Murray Bridge and Victor Harbor, South Australia. Her special interest is innovation to provide the best possible service to young people and their families.

Angelica Giannetti, Psy.D., is a member and lecturer of the ICNOS Institute and part of the core team of the Italian Center for Single Session Therapy. She has deepened the study and clinical practice of brief therapies applied to disability and families. She contributed to the books *Single Session Therapy: Principles and Practices* and *Solution-Focused Brief Therapy* (both edited by F. Cannistrà & F. Piccirilli) as well as to scientific articles such as "Examining the Incidence and Clients' Experiences of Single Session Therapy in Italy: A Feasibility Study."

Sarah Lewis, RN(MH), is CEO at Normal Magic Under 18's Mental Health Service, based in Devon, UK. She is a registered mental health nurse with over 20 years of experience working with children, young people, and adults. She and her team are passionate about early intervention and prevention care.

Nancy McElheran, RN, MN, RMFT, is a licensed clinical nurse specialist and an approved supervisor with the Canadian Association of Marriage and Family Therapy (CAMFT). She was the Director and clinical supervisor of the Eastside Family Centre in Calgary, Canada, and was involved in its development and operation for many years. She maintains her consultation, supervisory, and teaching role at the Eastside Community Mental Health Service.

John K. Miller, Ph.D., LMFT, is a former full professor in the School of Social Development and Public Policy at Fudan University in Shanghai, China; an adjunct professor in the Department of Psychology at the Royal University of Phnom Penh (RUPP) in Cambodia; and the director of the Sino-American Family Therapy Institute (SAFTI).

Francesca Moccia, Psy.D., is a core team member of the ICNOS Institute and the Italian Center for Single Session Therapy. She has held positions as a counselor and trainer in major corporations. Her interest in developmental psychology led her to create the master's program in Brief Therapies for the Developmental Age, of which she is the director. She is, in addition, a lecturer at ICNOS in constructivist epistemology and strategic therapy.

Giorgio Nardone, Ph.D., is Director of Centro di Terapia Strategica (Strategic Therapy Center) in Arezzo, Italy. He is also Professor of Brief Psychotherapy at the Post Graduate School of Clinical Psychology, University of Siena, Italy. He is the author of many publications, including *The Art of Change: Strategic Therapy and Hypnotherapy Without Trance* (with P. Watzlawick); *The Strategic Dialogue: Rendering the Diagnostic Interview a Real Therapeutic Intervention* (with A. Salvini); *Knowing Through Changing: The Evolution of Brief Strategic Therapy* (with C. Portelli); and *Advanced Brief Strategic Therapy for Young People with Anorexia Nervosa: An Effective Guide for Clinicians* (with E. Vanteroni).

Beatrice Pavoni, Psy.D., is a member of the ICNOS Institute and the Italian Center for Single Session Therapy. Over time she has held various roles, including Communication Director of the 4th International SST Symposium. Her clinical focus includes anxiety disorders and eating disorders, and she is a lecturer in the ICNOS Institute's Master of Brief Therapies in Developmental Age for Eating Disorders.

Vanessa Pergher, Psy.D., is a member of the Italian Center for Single Session Therapy. She manages the ICNOS Institute's walk-in center, One Session, which she described for the book *Open Access/One-at-a-Time Single-Session Psychotherapy* (edited by M. Bobele and A. Slive). Her clinical specialty involves work with individuals, mainly those with anxiety disorders.

Federico Piccirilli, Psy.D., is a psychologist and psychotherapist. He is a founding member and Director of the ICNOS Institute, and a cofounder of the Italian Center for Single Session Therapy. His publications include *Single-Session Therapy: Principles and Practice* (with F. Cannistrà, first published in Italian in 2018) and *Terapia breve centrata sulla soluzione: Principi e pratiche* (*Solution-Focused Brief Therapy: Principles and Practices*, with F. Cannnistrà).

Giada Pietrabissa, Ph.D., Psy.D., is a psychologist and research fellow in clinical psychology in the Department of Psychology at Catholic

University of Milan and a member of the Clinical Psychology Research Laboratory at IRCCS Istituto Auxologico Italiano in Milan.

Tim Pitt, Ph.D., is a sport and performance psychologist based in Hathersage, England. He is a Director at Mindflick, a high-performance coaching company that blends technology and coaching to deliver rapid and impactful change to unlock the potential of individuals and teams. He is the author of numerous publications on the philosophy of language, brief methodologies, and single session thinking in elite sport contexts.

Sam Porter, MSc, is a trainee sport and performance psychologist based in Hathersage, England. He consults for Mindflick, a high-performance coaching company that blends technology and coaching to deliver rapid and impactful change to unlock the potential of individuals and teams. His doctoral research has explored the single session mindset and understanding how the world's most successful sports coaches get the best out of those they lead.

Svetlana Prokasheva, Ph.D., is an educational psychologist and director of an educational psychological service in Omer, Israel. She cooperates with the Martin Springer Center for Conflict Studies, Ben-Gurion University of the Negev, and coordinates a research program in Ukraine that is interested in the Salutogenic question "How can people cope with stressful situations and stay well?"

Robert Rosenbaum, Ph.D., is a psychotherapist, neuropsychologist, and international teacher of Dayan (Wild Goose) qigong and Zen meditation. He was a co-originator (with M. Talmon and M.F. Hoyt) of the Single Session Therapy approach. His books include *Zen and the Heart of Psychotherapy*; *Walking the Way: 81 Zen Encounters with the Tao Te Ching*; *What's Wrong with Mindfulness (and What's Not): Zen Perspectives* (co-edited with B. Magid); and *That Is Not Your Mind! Zen Reflections on the Surangama Sutra*. He is based in Sacramento, California.

Pam Rycroft, MPsych., is a psychologist and family therapist at The Bouverie Centre in Melbourne, Australia. She is a co-editor (with M.F. Hoyt and J. Young) of *Single Session Thinking and Practice in Global, Cultural, and Familial Contents: Expanding Applications* and has published numerous papers in the field of Single Session Therapy, has contributed to the training of hundreds of professionals, and was co-convenor of the First and Third SST International Symposia.

Jessica L. Schleider, Ph.D., is an associate professor of medical social sciences, pediatrics, and psychology at Northwestern University in

Chicago, Illinois, where she is the Director of the Lab for Scalable Mental Health, developing digital, self-guided single session interventions (SSIs) for adolescents and others. She is the author of *Little Treatments, Big Effects: How to Build Meaningful Moments That Can Transform Your Mental Health*; co-author (with M.L. Dobias and M.C. Mullarkey) of *The Growth Mindset Workbook for Teens*; and co-editor (with S.D. Bennett, P. Myles-Hooton, and R. Shafran) of *Oxford Guide to Brief and Low Intensity Interventions for Children and Young People*.

Arnold Slive, Ph.D., is a licensed psychologist (Texas) and AAMFT Clinical Fellow and Approved Supervisor. His interests are in brief, strength-based, systemic psychotherapy, program development, supervision, and teaching. He has worked in hospital mental health, residential treatment, children's mental health, and private practice. In Calgary, he was a founder of the Eastside Family Centre, a walk-in single-session counseling center, and was Clinical Director of Wood's Homes. He has a career interest in developing strategies to make mental health increasingly accessible. He is a past president of the Alberta Association of Marriage and Family Therapy and was a Fulbright specialist teaching walk-in/single-session services in Canada. He is the co-editor (with M. Bobele) of *When One Hour Is All You Have: Effective Counseling for Walk-In Clients* and *Implementing Single-Session Therapy in Open Access Services*; and of *Single-Session Therapy by Walk-In or Appointment* (with M.F. Hoyt, M. Bobele, J. Young, and M. Talmon). He was a visiting professor at Our Lady of the Lake University, San Antonio, Texas. He is a consultant to Stepped Care Solutions as well as to One Stop Talk in Ontario, Canada.

Martin Söderquist, Ph.D., is a psychologist and family and couple therapist based in Malmö, Sweden. He has more than 40 years of experience in therapeutic work, training, and supervision in different contexts. He has published six books in Swedish and several articles in international journals. *Single Session One at a Time Counselling with Couples: Challenge and Possibility* was published by Routledge in 2023.

Katy Stephenson, MSC., is a family and systemic psychotherapist (family therapist) who has worked in the health and social care sector for over 20 years, predominantly in youth mental health services in CAMHS (UK) and headspace (Australia). She is passionate about responding to the needs of young people in ways that prevent over-pathologizing and instead instill and upskill the system to support young people in compassionate, conducive ways. She hopes to continue her research in different contexts to support how services respond to the evolving needs of young people's well-being, providing better access when needed.

Moshe Talmon, Ph.D., was one of the originators (with R. Rosenbaum and M.F. Hoyt) of the Single Session Therapy (SST) approach. He is the author of *Single-Session Therapy: Maximizing the Effect of the First (and Often Only) Therapeutic Encounter* and *Single Session Solutions: A Guide to Practical, Effective, and Affordable Therapy*; the co-editor (with M.F. Hoyt) of *Capturing the Moment: Single Session Therapy and Walk-In Services*; and co-editor (with M.F. Hoyt, M. Bobele, A. Slive, and J. Young) of *Single-Session Therapy by Walk-In or Appointment: Administrative, Clinical, and Supervisory Aspects of One-at-a-Time Services*.

Owen Thomas, Ph.D., is a professor of performance psychology at Cardiff School of Sport and Health Sciences, Cardiff Metropolitan University, UK. He is a chartered sport and exercise psychologist with the British Psychological Society and a registered practitioner psychologist with the Health and Care Professions Council. He supervised and co-designed Dr. Tim Pitt's program of PhD research, which was the first systematic exploration of single-session therapy within the sport psychology community. His expertise and empirical research centers on understanding and evaluating performance and/or psychological well-being across a range of performance domains.

Helen van Empel, MSc., is a psychologist and entrepreneur who is dedicated to making mental health care more accessible to all. In 2012, she cofounded an addiction care company called Kick Your Habits; in 2020 she launched One Session; and she is the Co-Director of Yet, a start-up that offers online Single Session Therapy (SST). She is the author of the first book in Dutch about SST, *Single Session Therapy: Help je Cliënt Korte en Krachtig Voorut (Single Session Therapy: Help Your Client Move Forward Briefly and Powerfully)*. She is based in Amsterdam, the Netherlands.

Jeff Young, Ph.D., is a clinical psychologist and emeritus professor of family therapy and systemic practice at La Trobe University in Melbourne, Australia, where he served for many years as Director of The Bouverie Centre. He was a co-convenor of the First and Third International Symposia on Single Session Therapies and Walk-In Services. He is a co-editor (with M.F. Hoyt, M. Bobele, A. Slive, and M. Talmon) of *Single Session Therapy by Walk-In or Appointment*; and co-editor (with M.F. Hoyt and P. Rycroft) of *Single Session Thinking and Practice in Global, Cultural, and Familial Contexts: Expanding Applications*; and is the author of *No Bullshit Therapy: How to Engage People Who Don't Want to Work with You*.

Rita Zijlstra, Ph.D., is a clinical neuropsychologist with an MBA in business administration. She works in a strategic partnership with Tilburg University at the academic collaborative center Digital Health and Mental Wellbeing. She has been working for four years as a CIO at Zorg van de Zaak Network where she contributes to the mission "Everyone stronger at work." She is also pursuing an MBA in business and IT at Nyenrode University to take mental health and digital wellness a step further.

Acknowledgments

Many, many thanks:

- To the authors who wrote the chapters, the clients whose stories are told herein, and to the agencies and organizations that were contexts for the services described.
- To our teachers and students, who have taught us so much.
- To the Italian Center for Single Session Therapy for hosting the 4th International Symposium in Rome, November 10–12, 2023, upon which many of the chapters are based.
- To Sarah Rae and the editorial staff at Routledge Publishers, for embracing this project; to Pragati Sharma for her excellent attention to a myriad of details; to Adhilakshmi Parasuraman and Apex CoVantage India for their fine production; and to all those (printing, sales, delivery, and others) whose labor has brought this project to fruition.
- To our respective professional partners. For Cannistrà: to Federico Piccirilli for joining me in the making of the ICSST; to Matteo Fusco and Michela Spagnolo from Beople for helping us in designing the company; and to Giada Pietrabissa and Gianluca Castelnuovo at Università Cattolica for their continuing support and research guidance. For Hoyt: to Moshe Talmon and Bob Rosenbaum for inviting me into the original SST project; to Kaiser Permanente and the Stanley Garfield Award for Clinical Innovation grant to study SST; and to the APF Dorothy and Nicholas Cummings Psyche Prize for its support of my writing.
- To Phillip Ziegler for photo and cover design assistance.
- To our families and friends for their love and support. For Cannistrà: My dear Flavia. For Hoyt: My dear Jennifer.
- To one another, for friendship, learning, and love.

Grazie mille!
—Flavio Cannistrà, Rome, Italy
—Michael F. Hoyt, Mill Valley, California, USA

Part I

Opening

Chapter 1

Editors' Introduction

Flavio Cannistrà and Michael F. Hoyt

The 4th International Single Session Therapy Symposium, titled *Single Session Therapies: What, How, and Why Single Session Mindsets and Practices are Effective, Efficient, and Excellent*, was held in Rome on November 10–12, 2023. Hosted by the Italian Center for Single Session Therapy under the co-directorship of Flavio Cannistrà and Valeria Campinoti, it brought together experts from around the world to describe and discuss the latest information. This book is based on those presentations, plus others that expand understanding of SST ideas, implementations, mindset, and methods. It is intended to give an updated overview of the state of SST, with special attention to three particular aspects:

1. theory and epistemology, recognizing that a single session mindset is one of the most important factors for this way of helping people;
2. implementation and findings, enlarging knowledge and visions about what we know that can be achieved in one session and in which fields; and
3. practices and techniques, continuing to offer therapists skills that enhance their ability to maximize every single session.

We recognize that this book cannot give expression to all who are involved in "Single Session Thinking and Practice" (as Hoyt, Young, & Rycroft, 2021 have called it), but we hope this contribution will share many of those voices and help to inform further SST developments.

What Is Single Session Therapy?

Single Session Therapy (SST) is therapy that is approached one session at a time (OAAT). Although the general term *single session therapy* had appeared previously (e.g., Sproel, 1975; Bloom, 1981; Rockwell & Pinkerton, 1982), in his watershed book *Single Session Therapy: Maximizing the Effect of the First (and Often Only) Therapeutic Encounter*, Moshe

DOI: 10.4324/9781032693828-2

Talmon (1990, p. xv) gave it a specific and somewhat arbitrary definition for research purposes:

> Single-session therapy is defined here as one face-to-face meeting between a therapist and a patient with no previous or subsequent sessions within one year.

In the *Encyclopedia of Psychotherapy*, Brett Steenbarger (2002, p. 669) wrote:

> Single-session therapy is a general term that is used to describe any form of psychotherapy that seeks to address the presenting problems of clients within a single visit.

The *APA Dictionary* (https://dictionary.apa.org/single-session-therapy; retrieved September 11, 2020) gives the following definition:

> *Single Session Therapy (SST)*: Therapy that ends after one session, usually by choice of the client but also as indicated by the type of treatment (e.g., Ericksonian psychotherapy, solution-focused brief therapy). Some clients claim enough success with one hour of therapy to stop treatment, although some therapists believe that this claim represents a flight into health or temporary relief from symptoms. Preparation for the session (e.g., by telephone) increases the likelihood of the single-session therapy being successful.

More generally, as Hymmen, Stalker, and Cait (2013, p. 61) put it:

> SST refers to a conscious approach to make the most of the first session knowing it may be the only session the client decides to attend—not to the situation where there is an expectation that the client will attend multiple sessions but chooses to attend just one.

SST is a deliberate approach to "capture the moment" (Young & Rycroft, 1997; Hoyt & Talmon, 2014), to make the most of the first (and often only) session. Whether sixty minutes (or more, or less), it is one session by intention (Bloom, 1992), "by design not by default" (Budman & Gurman, 1988), the one session being what Hurn (2005) calls "planned success" rather than "unplanned failure."

Thus, along similar lines, Hoyt et al. (2021, p. 3) articulated:

> The essence of single session thinking is to approach the first session as if it will be the only session, while creating opportunities for further work if it is requested by the client. What emerges is a collaborative,

direct, and transparent approach to providing services that puts the client in a very active role in determining the focus and length of the work.

As Young (2018; Chapter 6 this volume) has noted, Single Session Therapy/One-at-a-Time (SST/OAAT) is a service delivery approach that capitalizes on the natural help-seeking pattern of many clients. Thus, it is important to recognize that it was clients/patients—not therapists—who really "invented" Single Session Therapy! Subsequent investigations have endeavored to identify which clients find one session helpful and sufficient and what happens in sessions to enhance the likelihood of benefit—so that effective SST methods can be developed for more people. Schleider (Chapter 10) describes how the single session mindset has been usefully applied to digital client self-directed interventions.

Approaching each session one at a time (OAAT) is first of all a mindset and a service delivery. Indeed, from Talmon's (1990) original research and through the years to the present book, we see different ways to apply this kind of mindset: in clinical practice and for school, career, and human services counseling; by appointment and walk-in/drop-in; in person and online (even through digital services and software). Jay Haley's cover endorsement of Talmon's (1993) *Single Session Solutions: A Guide to Practical, Effective, and Affordable Therapy* seems more prophetic than ever: "We once assumed that long-term therapy was the base from which all therapy was to be judged. Now it appears that therapy of a single interview could become the standard for estimating how long and how successful therapy should be."

A Short History of SST

Occasional reports of successful one session therapies began with Sigmund Freud and are scattered through the psychotherapy literature (see Cannistrà & Piccirilli, 2021/2018; Hoyt, 2025). In the mid-1980s, Moshe Talmon, an Israeli psychologist then working at a large health maintenance organization (HMO: Kaiser Permanente) in Northern California, noticed that many patients came to the clinic and were seen only one time, regardless of the patient's diagnosis, the therapist's theoretical orientation (psychodynamic, cognitive-behavioral, family systems, etc.), or whether the patient was seen by the Adult Team, the Child & Family Team, or the Chemical Dependency Team. Although initially concerned that these cases were failures or "drop-outs," Talmon took the important step of contacting many patients to see what had actually happened and found that the great majority were satisfied with what they had accomplished in their one visit and didn't feel the need for more sessions. They had, in effect, achieved their therapy goal(s) and had "graduated" rather than "prematurely terminated" or "dropped out." Talmon then invited colleagues Robert Rosenbaum and Michael F.

Hoyt to collaborate on a prospective study of what might be accomplished in one deliberate visit. The books *Single Session Therapy* (Talmon, 1990) and *Single Session Solutions* (Talmon, 1993) were published, along with several chapters (Hoyt, 1994; Hoyt, Rosenbaum, & Talmon, 1992; Rosenbaum, 1990, 1993; Rosenbaum, Hoyt, & Talmon, 1990) and a training video (Talmon, Rosenbaum, Hoyt, & Short, 1990).

At approximately the same time, the Eastside Family Center (now called the Eastside Community Mental Health Service) in Calgary, Canada, began to offer no-appointment-needed walk-in therapy sessions—most of which were for a single session. They also reported considerable success in terms of client-reported outcomes and satisfaction (Slive, MacLaurin, Oaklander, & Amundson, 1995; Miller & Slive, 2004; Miller, 2008; Slive & Bobele, 2011; McElheran, 2021; Stewart et al., 2018; also see this volume, Bobele & Slive, Chapter 8, and McElheran, Chapter 14.

Since these early reports of the benefits of SST (by appointment or walk-in), numerous studies have been conducted and have consistently documented the value of SST—as will be seen in the References included with each chapter. Books in English, Italian, Swedish, Spanish, German, Japanese, and Dutch have appeared—including many by authors who contributed to this volume.[1]

There has been rapidly growing interest in SST, and there have been three previous international symposia, each resulting in a co-edited volume:

1. March 2012, on Phillip Island (near Melbourne, Australia)—see Hoyt and Talmon (2014)
2. September 2015, in Banff, Canada—see Hoyt, Bobele, Slive, Young, and Talmon (2018)
3. October 2019, again in Melbourne—see Hoyt et al. (2021)

The present volume, based on the international symposium held in Rome during November 2023, is the fourth.

What Is Mindset?

The term *mindset* refers to those beliefs, attitudes, and principles that underlie and guide one's perceptions, feelings, and actions. Concerning "The Vital Role of the Therapist's Mindset," Flavio Cannistrà (2021, p. 77) wrote:

> How we look—which is directed by our mindset—influences what we see, and what we see influences how we proceed. This [. . .] is about mindset, but also about epistemological and trans-theoretical matters. My meta-intention is that the reader becomes more aware of how our

mindset shapes clinical reasoning processes, the logic within how we listen and how we speak, the choice and clarification of the words we use, and thus, how we work with our clients—and how we may help them in a single session.

He notes that different theories predict (foretell in advance) different lengths of treatment, that different theories operate from different observations and opinions, and that "a choice must be made. Actually, a choice is always made. Here, I present my choices to be briefer in therapy" (p. 85) and then enumerates choices to be pragmatic, to be efficient, to avoid theory reification, and to adopt a multi-theoretical mindset. In a subsequent paper, "The Single Session Therapy Mindset: Fourteen Principles Gained through an Analysis of the Literature," Cannistrà (2022, p. 2) notes that it is essential to take mindset into account because "the organized series of ways in which we think and practice acts as a guide to a number of key points of the therapy itself."

Windy Dryden (2024, p. 3, emphases in original) distinguishes between three types of thinking that comprise the SST mindset:

SST 'orientation' thinking is the general thinking the SST therapist engages in when they are reflecting on the work and describes their orientation *to* the work. Such thinking is neither directly concerned with the active preparation the therapist makes before doing SST, nor is it concerned with how the therapist works with a particular client. On the other hand, SST 'pre-session thinking' is the thinking in which the therapist engages as they *actively prepare* to do the work and 'in-session' thinking is the thinking in which the SST therapist engages *in* during the session. It is more specific and directly concerned with how to help the client the therapist is working with.

The fundamental SST mindset is that each session—indeed, every chance to encounter a person—is approached (a) as though it may be the only one, a complete-unto-itself one-at-a-time (OAAT) event with a beginning, middle, and end; and (b) with the belief that the client is capable of making changes now. As will be seen in the chapters that follow, there are many variations of these SST/OAAT basic themes and how they can be put into practice in a wide range of contexts with an assortment of persons and problems.

The Book in Hand

The present volume explicates the continued exciting expansion of SST. In addition to some of the original investigators, a number of additional authors discuss new topics. The book is divided into five parts.

Part I. Opening. Editors' Introduction. This opening chapter welcomes readers, provides a brief overview of SST, its history and underlying mindset, and sets the stage for the chapters that follow.

Part II. What—Mindset, Theories, and Epistemologies Behind SST comprises six chapters in which various authors offer different perspectives on the essentials of single session thinking and practice. SST is not portrayed as a panacea, but the various authors emphasize how a flexible, here-and-now focus often yields positive outcomes.

Part III. Why, Where, and for Whom—Implementations, Applications, and Research offers ten chapters, with authors describing ways these ideas can be put into practice in various contexts with different populations and problems. Reports involving access systems, online SST and single session interventions (SSI), children and adolescents, adults, couples, and families come from the US, Canada, Italy, Australia, the UK, Holland, Japan, Israel, and Sweden. An update is also provided of recent supporting research.

Part IV: SST Techniques and Practices contains nine chapters describing additional specific SST techniques and methods drawn from different theoretical orientations. Reports come from around the globe. Goal setting, alliance building, and evoking client resources are emphasized; strategic, solution-focused, hypnotic, and narrative therapy methods are highlighted.

Part V. Closing . . . Until the Next Time—Editors' Conclusion: Themes, Lessons, and the Future garners key ideas and considers future possibilities.

References are gathered at the end of each chapter, and there is an overall Index at the end of the book.

One Size Does Not Fit All: Many Roads Lead to Rome

SST is not a particular psychotherapy theoretical orientation (such as psychodynamic, cognitive-behavioral, solution-focused). Much like the famous saying "All roads lead to Rome" ("*Tutte le strade portano a Roma*" in Italian), there are many ideas and methods that can inform SST. It was advantageous that when Talmon and his colleagues at Kaiser conducted their original study, they were of varying theoretical orientations. As Talmon (2014, p. 31) wrote:

> When we started our SST project, Rosenbaum had trained in brief psychodynamic therapy and was then fascinated with non-directive hypnosis à la Milton Erickson. Hoyt had done an internship with Carl Whitaker, trained in brief psychodynamic therapy, and was then taken by

the work of Goulding and Goulding (1979), which combined Trans-
actional Analysis (TA) and Gestalt into what they called Redecision
Therapy, a very directive form of treatment. I was primarily a systemic
therapist working with the Child and Family Team while Hoyt and
Rosenbaum worked with the Adult Team. When we started the project
I was quite intrigued by the simple elegance of solution-focused therapy
developed by de Shazer, Berg, et al. (de Shazer, 1985, 1988) in Milwau-
kee. I met them shortly before our project started and they were a main
force in spreading the word about our initial findings long before we
published anything.

Rather than narrowly conceiving of SST as a particular form of strategic, psychodynamic, solution-focused, or family systems therapy, this
multi-theoretical perspective helped promote the more capacious idea that
SST is essentially a delivery format ("OAAT") and that SST could be successfully conducted in various ways. One size doesn't fit all.

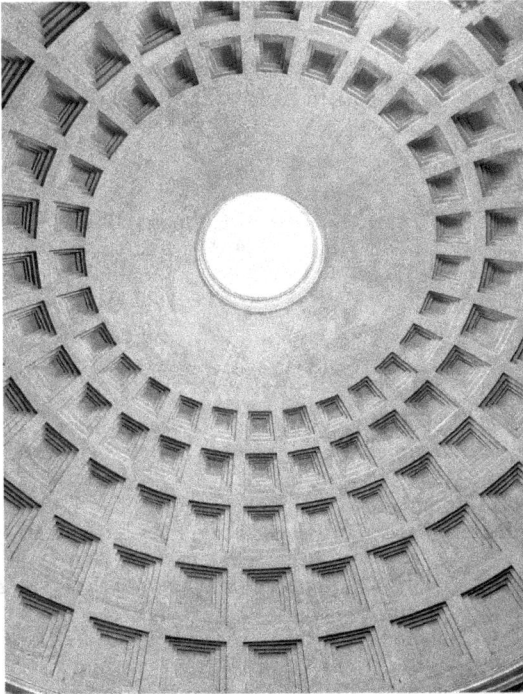

Figure 1.1 There are many ways to get to the light.

Source: (photo: Michael F. Hoyt © 2023. Used by agreement.)

Thus, as Cannistrà (2024, p. 105) recently commented:

When it comes to SST there is no one specific theoretical corpus to refer to. In our view, this illustrates one of the great strengths of SST, i.e., the fact that [it] is seen as a transtheoretical method, something that occurs and is located beyond the theoretical reference points of the practitioner. [. . .] The expression "Single Session Thinking" [. . .] highlights a way of thinking rather than a method of intervention: [. . .] it seeks to prioritize a mindset that accepts that a single session is possible (and from this, different ways of achieving it will then arise).

Perhaps it is fortuitous that Rome, the site of the 4th International SST Symposium, is also the home of one of the world's most revered ancient buildings, the Pantheon. The word *pantheon* comes from ancient Greek and means "all the gods." When one walks into the Pantheon and looks up, one sees (Figure 1.1) the Oculus surrounded by many coffers (panels).

In the chapters that follow, there are many ways that can lead to a successful SST. First we will consider some of the thinking and mindsets that inform SST; then we will look at a variety of implementation and practice contexts, examining closer some specific methods and techniques; and then will see what lessons can be learned and what likely trends can be predicted.

Note

1 See Cannistrà and Piccirilli (2018/2021), Cooper (2024), Dryden (2016, 2017, 2018, 2019a, 2019b, 2021), Hoyt (2024; Hoyt & Cannistrà, 2023), Schleider (2023), Slive and Bobele (2011; Bobele & Slive, in press), Söderquist (2023), and van Empel (2023).

References

Bloom, B.L. (1981). Focused single-session therapy: Initial development and evaluation. In S.H. Budman (Ed.), *Forms of Brief Therapy* (pp. 167–216). Guilford Press.

Bloom, B.L. (1992). Bloom's focused single-session therapy. In B.L. Bloom (Ed.), *Planned Short-Term Psychotherapy: A Clinical Handbook* (2nd ed., pp. 97–121). Allyn & Bacon.

Bobele, M., & Slive, A. (Eds.) (in press). *Implementing Single-Session Therapy in Open Access Services*. Routledge.

Budman, S.H., & Gurman, A.S. (1988). *Theory and Practice of Brief Therapy*. Guilford Press.

Cannistrà, F. (2021). The vital role of the therapist's mindset. In M.F. Hoyt, J. Young, & P. Rycroft (Eds.), *Single Session Thinking and Practice in Global, Cultural, and Familial Contexts* (pp. 77–88). Routledge.

Cannistrà, F. (2022). The single session therapy mindset: Fourteen principles gained through an analysis of the literature. *International Journal of Brief Therapy and Family Science*, 12(1), 1–26.

Cannistrà, F. (2024). How to maximize a single session? From a reflection on theoretical pluralism to the definition of five goals. *Journal of Systemic Therapies*, *43*(1), 104–117.

Cannistrà, F., & Piccirilli, F. (2021). *Single-Session Therapy: Principles and Practices*. Giunti. (Published in Italian as *Terapia a Seduta Singola: Principi e Pratiche* in 2018. An edition in Russian is in preparation.)

Cooper, S.J. (2024). *Brief Narrative Practice in Single-Session Therapy*. Routledge.

de Shazer, S. (1985). *Keys to Solution in Brief Therapy*. Norton.

de Shazer, S. (1988). *Clues: Investigating Solutions in Brief Therapy*. Norton.

Dryden, W. (2016). *When Time is at a Premium: Cognitive Behavioral Approaches to Single-Session Therapy and Very Brief Coaching*. Rationality Publications.

Dryden, W. (2017). *Single-Session Integrated CBT (SSI-CBT)*. Routledge.

Dryden, W. (2018). *Very Brief Therapeutic Conversations*. Routledge.

Dryden, W. (2019a). *Single-Session "One-at-a-Time" Therapy: A Rational-Emotive Behaviour Therapy Approach*. Routledge.

Dryden, W. (2019b). *Single-Session Therapy: 100 Key Points and Techniques*. Routledge.

Dryden, W. (2021). *Help Yourself with Single-Session Therapy*. Routledge.

Dryden, W. (2024). *How to Think and Intervene Like a Single-Session Therapist*. Routledge.

Goulding, M.M., & Goulding, R.L. (1979). *Changing Lives Through Redecision Therapy*. Brunner/Mazel.

Hoyt, M.F. (1994). Single session solutions. In M.F. Hoyt (Ed.), *Constructive Therapies* (pp. 140–159). Guilford Press.

Hoyt, M.F. (2025). *Single Session Therapy: A Clinical Introduction to Principles and Practices*. Routledge.

Hoyt, M.F., Bobele, M., Slive, A., Young, J., & Talmon, M. (Eds.). (2018). *Single-Session Therapy by Walk-In or Appointment: Administrative, Clinical, and Supervisory Aspects of One-at-a-Time Services*. Routledge. (Also available in Spanish and German.)

Hoyt, M.F., & Cannistrà, F. (2023). *Brief Therapy Conversations: Exploring Efficient Intervention in Psychotherapy*. Routledge. (Also published in Italian in 2023 as *Conversazioni de Terapia Breve: Esplorando Interventi Efficaci in Psicoterapia*. EPC Editore.)

Hoyt, M.F., Rosenbaum, R., & Talmon, M. (1992). Planned single-session psychotherapy. In S.H. Budman, M.F. Hoyt, & S. Friedman (Eds.), *The First Session in Brief Therapy* (pp. 59–86). Guilford Press.

Hoyt, M.F., & Talmon, M. (Eds.). (2014). *Capturing the Moment: Single Session Therapy and Walk-In Services*. Crown House Publishing. (Also available in Italian.)

Hoyt, M.F., Young, J., & Rycroft, P. (Eds.). (2021). *Single Session Thinking and Practice in Global, Cultural, and Familial Contexts: Expanding Applications*. Routledge. (Also available in German from Carl-Auer Verlag, Heidelberg.)

Hurn, R. (2005). Single-session therapy: Planned success or unplanned failure? *Counselling Psychology Review*, *20*(4), 33–40.

Hymmen, P., Stalker, C., & Cait, C.-A. (2013). The case for single-session therapy: Does the empirical evidence support the increased prevalence of this service delivery model? *Journal of Mental Health*, *22*(1), 60–71.

McElheran, N. (2021). The story of the Eastside Family Centre: 30 years of walk-in single session therapy. In M.F. Hoyt, J. Young, & P. Rycroft (Eds.), *Single Session Thinking and Practice in Global, Cultural, and Familial Contexts* (pp. 125–132). Routledge.

Miller, J.K. (2008). Walk-in single-session team therapy: A study of client satisfaction. *Journal of Systemic Therapies, 27*(3), 78–94.

Miller, J.K., & Slive, A. (2004). Breaking down the barriers to clinical service delivery: Walk-in family therapy. *Journal of Marital and Family Therapy, 30,* 95–105.

Rockwell, W.J.K., & Pinkerton, R.S. (1982). Single-session psychotherapy. *American Journal of Psychotherapy, 36,* 32–40.

Rosenbaum, R. (1990). Strategic therapy. In R.A. Wells & V.J. Giannetti (Eds.), *Handbook of the Brief Psychotherapies* (pp. 351–403). Plenum Press.

Rosenbaum, R. (1993). Heavy ideals: Strategic single-session hypnotherapy. In R.A. Wells & V.J. Giannetti (Eds.), *Casebook of the Brief Psychotherapies* (pp. 109–128). Plenum Press.

Rosenbaum, R., Hoyt, M.F., & Talmon, M. (1990). The challenge of single-session therapies: Creating pivotal moments. In R.A. Wells & V.J. Giannetti (Eds.), *Handbook of the Brief Psychotherapies* (pp. 165–189). Plenum. Reprinted in Hoyt, M.F. (1995). *Brief Therapy and Managed Care: Readings for Contemporary Practice* (pp. 105–139). Jossey-Bass.

Slive, A., & Bobele, M. (Eds.). (2011). *When One Hour is All You Have: Effective Therapy for Walk-In Clients.* Zeig, Tucker, & Theisen. (Published in Spanish in 2023 as *Cuando Solo Tienes Una Hora* by Paidós Editorial, Mexico City.)

Slive, A., MacLaurin, B., Oaklander, M., & Amundson, J. (1995). Walk-in single sessions: A new paradigm in clinical service delivery. *Journal of Systemic Therapies, 14,* 3–11.

Söderquist, M. (2023). *Single Session One-at-a-Time Counselling With Couples: Challenge and Possibility.* Routledge. (A version published in Swedish as *Ett Samtal I Taget* in 2020.)

Sproel, O.H. (1975). Single-session psychotherapy. *Diseases of the Nervous System, 36,* 283–285.

Steenbarger, B.N. (2002). Single-session therapy. In M. Hersen & W. Sledge (Eds.), *Encyclopedia of Psychotherapy* (Vol. 2, pp. 669–672). Academic Press.

Talmon, M. (1990). *Single Session Therapy: Maximizing the Effect of the First (and Often Only) Therapeutic Encounter.* Jossey-Bass. (Editions have appeared in many world languages.)

Talmon, M. (1993). *Single Session Solutions: A Guide to Practical, Effective, and Affordable Therapy.* Addison-Wesley.

Talmon, M. (2014). When less is more: Maximizing the effect of the first (and often only) therapeutic encounter. In M.F. Hoyt & M. Talmon (Eds.), *Capturing the Moment: Single Session Therapy and Walk-In Services* (pp. 27–40). Crown House Publishing.

Talmon, M., Rosenbaum, R., Hoyt, M.F., & Short, L. (1990). *Single Session Therapy.* Videotape. Golden Triad Films.

Van Empel, H. (2023). *Single Session Therapy: Help je Cliënt Korte en Krachtig Voorut.* Boom Publisher. [In Dutch: Translates as *Single Session Therapy: Help Your Client Move Forward Briefly and Powerfully.*]

Young, J. (2018). Single-session therapy: The misunderstood gift that keeps on giving. In M.F. Hoyt, M. Bobele, A. Slive, J. Young, & M. Talmon (Eds.), *Single-Session Therapy by Walk-In or Appointment: Administrative, Clinical, and Supervisory Aspects of One-at-a-Time Services* (pp. 40–58). Routledge.

Young, J., & Rycroft, P. (1997). Single session therapy: Capturing the moment. *Psychotherapy in Australia, 4*(10), 18–23.

Part II

What—Mindset, Theories, and Epistemologies Behind SST

Chapter 2

The Here and Now of Single Session Therapy

Questions That Need Answering

Flavio Cannistrà

What is Single Session Therapy (SST) for? The attempt to answer this question leads us to a multitude of further questions and possibilities. In this chapter we will look through the point of view of SST itself, discovering that the questions and possibilities raised can radically change our relationship with everything connected to our work as therapists.

A word of warning: there are many, many questions, but far fewer answers. The hope is that we can find them together.

Why Ask Ourselves What SST Is For?

When it comes to "therapy," we can't help but notice that we already have an enormous number of psychotherapies and intervention methods available (Norcross, 2005); it therefore seems reasonable to ask whether we really need another one. Indeed, adding to the list merely to satisfy a personal impulse to create something ("I want to invent my own way of doing therapy!") or to belong ("Nice to meet you, I'm a *Single Session Therapist*") makes no more sense than doing so in order to "fix" something that the other 500 approaches have inexplicably missed. However, it may be more helpful to take a different view. For example, we could begin with the observation that (1) albeit with some exceptions, there is widespread crisis in current mental health systems regarding service provision, cost-effectiveness, the usefulness of diagnoses, theoretical disputes, etc.[1], and (2) today's healthcare services are clearly not capable of solving this crisis. Are we asking the right questions?

At this point we should define the object in question ("What is a healthcare *system*?") and ask ourselves, "What does SST have to do with solving the crisis?" If we look at the definition of "system" in the Italian *Enciclopedia Treccani* we find that, in the scientific sphere, it is "any object of study that, although constituted by different *interconnected elements that interact* with each other and their environment, responds and evolves as a whole with its own general rules"[2] (*Sistema*, n.d.). In light of this definition,

DOI: 10.4324/9781032693828-4

I see SST as an element of healthcare systems that is capable of *influencing* the crisis: I highlight "influence" rather than "solve" because it would be erroneous to think that such a complex matter could be solved by a single method, activity, person, etc. Nevertheless, what SST does differently from other approaches or methods of therapy is actually to present itself as a paradigm[3] change on several levels.

So we can reformulate the question: *How, and at what levels, can SST have a positive influence on the crisis in healthcare systems?*

To answer this, allow me to cite the definition of another word, "crisis," from Latin and Greek roots meaning "*choice, decision*, critical phase of an illness," which in turn are derived from words meaning "*distinguish, judge*" (*Crisi*, n.d., italics added). We can therefore think of SST as an element of current healthcare systems that can influence its processes and activities of *evaluation, judgment, decision,* and *choice.*

But which evaluations, judgments, decisions, and choices can SST influence?

And here we can turn to another definition, that of "Single Session Therapy." In his 1990 book, Talmon wrote (p. xv): "Single-session therapy is defined here as one face-to-face meeting between a therapist and a patient with no previous or subsequent sessions within a year." Since then, there have been several definitions offered, and they have led to new terms (such as *single session intervention, single session work,* and *one-at-a-time*—for a comprehensive overview, see Hoyt, 2025; Hoyt, Young, & Rycroft, 2021a, 2018; Hoyt & Talmon, 2014). Here I would like to draw the reader's attention to three:

1. SST as a *mindset*—thus Hoyt, Young, & Rycroft (2021b, p. 3) wrote: "The essence of single session thinking is to approach the first session as if it will be the only session, while creating opportunities for further work if it is requested by the client."[4]
2. SST as an *approach to service delivery*—thus Young (2018, p. 44) wrote:

a fundamental definition of Single Session Therapy could be everything that derived attitudinally, clinically, and organizationally from accepting three findings [. . .] #1: that the most common number of service contacts that clients attend is one, followed by two, followed by three [. . .] irrespective of diagnosis, complexity, or the severity of their problem [. . .] #2: that the majority [. . .] of those people who attend only one session, across a range of therapies, report that the single session was adequate [. . .] #3: [. . .] that it seems impossible to accurately predict who will attend only one session and who will attend more, a proposition that had significant clinical and organizational ramifications.

3. SST as a *structured intervention method*—thus Cannistrà and Piccirilli (2021, p. 3) wrote:

> SST has progressively become a method for improving the utility of *every* session. Today especially, given the rapid changes to health and welfare which we are experiencing (whether we are public or private sector, health authorities or healthcare professionals), we must ask ourselves how we can make the therapeutic process more efficient (i.e., make every session prove useful and ideally, shorten the time needed for therapist and patient to achieve an agreed outcome) as well as more appropriate in terms of its response to people's needs and wants. [. . .] [T]he SST method is strongly resource-based, strength-oriented and person-centered.

These three definitions lead me to use the term "Single Session Therapy" and its variants with this meaning: *a series of heterogenous types of intervention with similar principles (mindset), which differ from other healthcare services primarily by their method of delivery and its implications.*

What I consider to have been the subject of the 4th International Symposium on Single Session Therapy, what emerges from this book, and the subject of reflection and discussion among all those involved in SST is *how to influence evaluations, judgments, decisions and choices made in the field of health and well-being in order to change the principles and practices of delivering healthcare services.* Or, to put it another way: by changing the principles and practices underlying the services we deliver, we seek to understand how we can influence the evaluations, judgments, decisions, and choices made in their inception and delivery.

In other words, what those working in SST are referring to is the *process* of change: change in psychotherapy, change in healthcare, change in how we think about change.

The Single Session Therapy Mindset (and Its Implications)

In actual fact, we're not only discussing these changes, we're already making them happen. For example, if we consider the fourteen principles of the single session mindset identified in "The Single Session Therapy Mindset: Fourteen Principles Gained Through an Analysis of the Literature" (Cannistrà, 2022), we find some interesting conclusions in our ways of conceiving therapy. Let's take a look at some of them.

- *Principle 1: A single session may be enough.*
- *Principle 6: Further sessions may be needed.*

Conclusion 1: Therapy, and change in general, might require one, a few, or many sessions, regardless of the diagnosis.

- *Principle 3: People have resources they can use to feel better.*
- *Principle 4: The client is the expert in their own life.*
  Conclusion 2: The outcome of therapy, and change in general, can start with something the person already has and may be able to use in order to feel better.

- *Principle 2: The therapist can play an active role.*
- *Principle 5: Different methods may be used.*
  Conclusion 3: To help people, we can draw on methods that are technically, theoretically, and epistemologically different from each other.

- *Principle 7: Single Session Therapy is suitable for different contexts and needs.*
- *Principle 8: It's fine to aim for small or simple goals and interventions.*
  Conclusion 4: Therapy should not be considered as a "cure," and neither should its end necessarily coincide with a "global" change in the person or the problem.

- *Principle 4: The client is the expert in their own life.*
- *Principle 11: Results are mainly achieved outside the session.*
  Conclusion 5: The power relation between the client and the therapist, the healthcare facility, the treatment process, and the approach to therapy is not one of subordination of the former to the latter.[5]

It does not follow that these conclusions are obvious and expected, particularly when it comes to their repercussions in clinical practice and, prior to that, in the organization of health services. But in any case, I believe they open the door to some questions that need answering.

A Few Questions and Reflections

(A) If therapy can require one, a few, or many sessions, regardless of the diagnosis (Conclusion 1), how do we decide the duration of therapy?

What is it that determines the length of a therapy? The diagnosis? The severity of the problem? Many studies do not appear to prove that these are the decisive factors. For example, in a review of the existing literature in the field, Cannistrà and Pietrabissa (2021) made an extensive list of studies—albeit not directly connected with SST practices—which demonstrates the effectiveness of the single session in tackling problems such as anorexia nervosa, self-harm, PTSD, alcohol and substance abuse, etc. This seems to be an undisputed fact, even in fields totally unrelated to SST. To quote one of many examples, in their article tellingly titled "Severe and Enduring Anorexia Nervosa? Illness Severity and Duration Are Unrelated to Outcomes from Enhanced Cognitive Behavior Therapy," Raykos, Erceg-Hurn, McEvoy, Fursland, and Waller (2018) measure the change in body mass index (BMI) over the first five sessions in patients diagnosed with low, moderate, and high levels of anorexia nervosa (AN), showing improvements indicating that "trajectories are almost perfectly parallel, demonstrating that the severity of problematic eating disorder attitudes and cognitions at pre-treatment has no impact on the amount of change in BMI during the early phase of treatment," and adding that there is "a small association between illness duration and the probability of completing treatment. [. . .] For example, a patient with illness duration of two years had the same likelihood of completing treatment (64%) as a patient with illness duration of 18 years" (p. 704), ultimately claiming that use

of the term "severe and enduring" has the potential to result in even greater stigma than is currently experienced by individuals with eating disorders. [. . .] It can be used as a justification for clinicians to avoid applying effective treatment, as demonstrated by the finding that individuals with enduring AN are more likely to be offered non-evidence-supported treatments.

(p. 706)

But why should we be concerned with Question A, i.e., what processes determine the duration of therapy? There may be a number of answers. Some insurance companies pay on the basis of duration, and some even ask mental health practitioners to sign an agreement with the client that specifies the length of treatment. As Jay Haley (1990, pp. 14–15) famously said: "The ideology and practice of therapy was largely determined when therapists chose to sit with a client and be paid for durations of time rather than by results." More generally, it is interesting to see how our mindset shifts when we see an insurance-reimbursable problem and not a person.

Added to this is the not at all obvious answer to what is meant by "diagnosis." As discussed in our book, *Brief Therapy Conversations* (Hoyt & Cannistrà, 2023), when we talk about *diagnosis* in the mental health sphere we almost take it for granted that we're referring to nosographic classifying diagnosis, a category-based system like the *DSM* or the *ICD*. But there are many ways to diagnose a problem attributable to a lack of well-being and mental health. To put it differently, there are many types of diagnosis, including systemic (Priest, 2023), operative

(Nardone & Watzlawick, 1990), hypnotic (Antonelli & Luchetti, 2011), psychodynamic (Lingiardi & McWilliams, 2017), and hierarchical taxonomic (Hopwood, Bagby, Gralnick, Ro, & Ruggero, 2019). And how do we respond to the success of therapies that do not feature diagnosis at all (e.g., Solution-Focused Brief Therapy—see Macdonald, 2007)?

(B) If the outcome of therapy, and change in general, can start with something the person already has and may be able to use in order to feel better (Conclusion 2), what is the role of the therapist?

In other words, what are the effective *whats* and *hows* of therapy? *What* should therapy do? What are its aims? What's the end result of successful therapy? The answers to these questions are not at all obvious. Let's consider a few examples, obtained by Googling "What's the aim of psychotherapy?":

- "to gain relief from symptoms, maintain or enhance daily functioning, and improve quality of life" (National Institute of Mental Health, NIMH, 2024)
- "not usually to give advice, but to provide a safe space to talk and to help you to find insight and understanding into your difficulties" (British Psychological Society, BPS, n.d.)
- psychotherapy "is considered the 'expert clinical response' to an illness. Over and above any possible definition, psychotherapy is an area of intervention for the purpose of curing" (Abbate, 2011, for the National Board of Italian Psychologists)
- "resolving problematic behaviours, beliefs, feelings and related physical symptoms. . . . Counselling is more likely to be on specific problems, changes in life adjustments and fostering the client's wellbeing. Psychotherapy is more concerned with the restructuring of the personality or self and the development of insight' (Psychotherapy and Counseling Federation of Australia, PACFA, n.d.)

Again, it's interesting to see how those definitions could lead to understandings of what are the aims of our therapeutic endeavors. Once we have established—if this is ever possible—the aims of psychotherapy and counseling, the next question is: *how* do we achieve them? Or rather, *how* do we achieve *what*? And even before that: what's the basis for our decisions about the *hows* and the *whats* of therapy? And once we've discovered that a single session may be all that's necessary, how will we alter our decisions? Might we even consider starting from this fact to decide the *whats* and the *hows*? Reflecting on the *what* and the *how* is anything but a mere exercise in style, considering the growing literature that shows us the importance of adopting pluralistic (Cooper & McLeod, 2010) or multi-theoretical (Cannistrà, 2024) perspectives. In short, this then brings us to a crucial question: *why* do we choose what we choose as our starting point for decisions about the aims (*whats*) of therapy and the methods (*hows*) we use to achieve them?[6]

> (C) *If to help people, we can (should?) draw on methods that are technically, theoretically, and epistemologically different from each other (Conclusion 3), what do we know about the* how?

In other words, what do we know about the more strictly methodological aspects and techniques of therapy?

In general, we know that one single way of doing things, however prevalent, is not always right for everyone, every problem, and every time. One size does not fit all. We also know that any way of doing things is determined by a way of seeing things. But if one way of doing things is not always appropriate, neither is one way of seeing things.[7]

What does this tell us? That each way of seeing things is not the map that describes the land: it's *one* of the possible maps. We can therefore expand on Korzybski's famous observation (1933, p. 58): not only is the map not the territory, the map is not *the* map.

And therefore, when we talk about the method we've chosen to use in order to help a person, do we know which map we're using? Further, do we know how we came to choose that map, that *how*, that method? And, in general, which map do we use to decide which map to use?

One of my favorite definitions of SST is that of Jeff Young (2018), who sees it as one of the possible services to deliver to our clients. How does our perception change, and also the perception of clients, healthcare systems, and approaches that produce psychological theories, when we assume we have access to a variety of services for delivery, all of them equally valid (as the Dodo Bird tells us[8]) and therefore to be chosen according to criteria other than effectiveness?

Conclusions

When I planned the three-day SST4 Symposium, I thought it was important to devote a whole day to reflection about the epistemology, mindsets, and theories surrounding Single Session Therapy.

- The idea that we can solve a lot of problems—even longstanding ones—in a day, an hour . . . what does that tell us about ourselves as human beings?

- What does it tell us about people's potential, their possibilities, what they're capable of?
- What does it tell us therapists about what we call "therapy"? About its aims, its methods, how it interacts with people?
- And, at this point, what is therapy? How is it different from what we think, decide, write and read it is? The words of Paul Watzlawick (1990, p. 55) come to mind, reminding us that therapy is what you say it is, "a name we give to something which, having been given a name, creates a reality of its own"; and also Ludwig Wittgenstein's advice (1922, §6.54) to ditch the ladder, the definition, the concept, once we've used it to get to where we want to go.[9]
- The idea that an hour may be enough, a single meaningful encounter—with the proviso of not trying too hard to make it so—what does that tell us, as therapists, about ourselves as therapists? Who are we? What is our role? How can we pursue it?
- These are the questions that need answering.

Notes

1 By way of example, we could point to the crises ongoing in Canada (Flood, Thomas, & McGibbon, 2023), France (Williamson, 2023), Germany (Bindewalt, 2023), Mexico (Miller, 2023), the U.K. (Landler, 2023), the U.S. (Glatter, Papadakos, & Shah, 2023), China (Kessel, 2019), Italy (Neri, 2019), and Japan (Suzuki, Nishida, Suzuki, & Kobayashi, 2008).
2 According to Google, the definition of *system* in the English-language *Oxford Dictionary* is essentially the same: "1. a set of things working together as parts of a mechanism or an *interconnecting* network. 2. a set of principles or procedures according to which something is done; an organized framework or method."
3 Wikipedia (retrieved February 28, 2024) tells us: "A *paradigm shift* is a fundamental change in the basic concepts and experimental practices of a scientific discipline. It is a concept in the philosophy of science that was introduced and brought into the common lexicon by the American physicist and philosopher Thomas Kuhn (1962). Even though Kuhn restricted the use of the term to the natural sciences, the concept of a paradigm shift has also been used in numerous non-scientific contexts to describe a profound change in a fundamental model or perception of events."
4 In "The Hope and Joy of Single Session Thinking and Practice" Hoyt (2021, p. 31) wrote: "Although different guiding models have been articulated, SST can be thought of more as an affirmative and optimistic mindset." In Hoyt and Cannistrà (2023, p. 52) he elaborated: "For me the *mindset* is how you set your mind, how you approach or what you believe—your orientation, your expectation, your hope, what you think is possible. *Mindset* refers to a set of beliefs that influence how you think, feel and behave in any given situation. And so the mindset with single session is, 'We could get something done today that would be good. And maybe one session is all the person needs.'"
5 To round out the list, the other principles:

- It's fine to have less prior knowledge.
- It's best to stick with process and the here and now.

- Results are mainly achieved outside the session.
- A structure is needed for the single session.
- A client-therapist relationship can be established rapidly.
- Nothing is taken for granted.

6 A good starting point might be the end point. This idea was inspired by Bertrand Russell, who maintains in *The Philosophical Importance of Mathematical Logic*: "The problem which we have to resolve, like every truly philosophical problem, is a problem of analysis; and in problems of analysis the best method is that which sets out from the results and arrives at the premises. [. . .] [I]t is the conclusions which have the greatest degree of certainty: the nearer we get to the ultimate premises the more uncertainty and difficulty do we find" (1913, p. 482). And the end point of any successful therapy, the outcome, is seen in two types of change in the person: changes in their way of signifying reality (e.g., beliefs, attitudes, perceptions) and changes in behaviors (simple and/or complex, such as interactions).

7 Obviously, even what I've just written is *one way* of seeing things, and this is a circle we can't escape.

8 See *Dodo Bird Verdict* (retrieved from Wikipedia February 28, 2024).

9 And so, in *The Name of the Rose*, Umberto Eco (1980/1983; quoted in Iveson, 1990, pp. 13-14) has the protagonist advise: "The order that our mind imagines is like a net, or like a ladder, built to attain something. But afterwards, you must throw the ladder away, because you discover that, even if it was useful, it was meaningless. . . . The only truths that are useful are instruments to be thrown away."

References

Abbate, L. (2011). *Parere pro-veritate sul confine tra attività psicologica e psicoterapeutica e i criteri che fondano la validità di una teoria scientifica della cura*. www.psy.it/documenti_utili/allegati/confine_psicologia_psicoterapia_CNOP_2011.pdf

Antonelli, C., & Luchetti, M. (2011). *Ipnosi Medica. Parola, Informazione, Esperienza*. Lulu.

Bindewalt, A. (2023). *Healthcare at the limit: How to cope with the crisis*. https://kpmg.com/de/en/home/insights/2023/06/health-care-at-the-limit-so-the-crisis-can- be-solved.html

BPS. (n.d.). *Counseling and psychotherapy*. https://explore.bps.org.uk/content/report-guideline/bpsrep.2014.rep101c/chapter/bpsrep.2014.rep101c.13

Cannistrà, F. (2022). The single session therapy mindset: Fourteen principles gained through an analysis of the literature. *International Journal of Brief Therapy and Family Science, 12*(1), 1–26.

Cannistrà, F. (2024). How to maximize a single session? From a reflection on theoretical pluralism to the definition of five goals. *Journal of Systemic Therapies, 43*(1), 105–120.

Cannistrà, F., & Piccirilli, F. (2021). *Single-Session Therapy: Principles and Practices*. Giunti. (Originally published in Italian in 2018.)

Cannistrà, F., & Pietrabissa, G. (2021). Single-session therapy: Data and effectiveness. In F. Cannistrà & F. Piccirilli (Eds.), *Single-Session Therapy: Principles and Practices* (pp. 33–50). Giunti.

Cooper, M., & McLeod, J. (2010). *Pluralistic Counseling and Psychotherapy*. Sage.

Crisi. (n.d.). In *Treccani*. https://www.treccani.it/vocabolario/crisi/

Eco, U. (1983). *The Name of the Rose*. Harcourt. (Work originally published in Italian as *Il nome della rosa* in 1980.)

Flood, C.M., Thomas, B., & McGibbon, E. (2023). Canada's primary care crisis: Federal government response. *Healthcare Management Forum, 36*(5), 327–332.

Glatter, R., Papadakos, P., & Shah, Y. (2023). The coming collapse of the U.S. health care system. *Time.* https://time.com/6246045/collapse-us-health-care-system/

Haley, J. (1990). Why not long-term therapy? In J.K. Zeig & S.G. Gilligan (Eds.), *Brief Therapy: Myths, Methods, and Metaphors* (pp. 3–17). Brunner/Mazel.

Hopwood, C.J., Bagby, R.M., Gralnick, T., Ro, E., Ruggero, C., Mullins-Sweatt, S., Kotov, R., Bach, B., Cicero, D.C., Krueger, R.F., Patrick, C.J., Chmielewski, M., DeYoung, C.G., Docherty, A.R., Eaton, N.R., Forbush, K.T., Ivanova, M.Y., Latzman, R.D., Pincus, A L., . . . Zimmermann, J. (2019). Integrating psychotherapy with the hierarchical taxonomy of psychopathology (HiTOP). *Journal of Psychotherapy Integration, 30*(4), 477–497.

Hoyt, M.F. (2025). *Single Session Therapy: A Clinical Introduction to Principles and Practices.* Routledge.

Hoyt, M.F., Bobele, M., Slive, A., Young, J., & Talmon, M. (Eds.). (2018). *Single-Session Therapy by Walk-In or Appointment: Administrative, Clinical, and Supervisory Aspects of One-at-a-Time Services.* Routledge.

Hoyt, M.F., & Cannistrà, F. (2023). *Brief Therapy Conversations: Exploring Efficient Intervention in Psychotherapy.* Routledge.

Hoyt, M.F., & Talmon, M. (Eds.). (2014). *Capturing the Moment: Single Session Therapy and Walk-In Services.* Crown House Publishing.

Hoyt, M.F., Young, J., & Rycroft, P. (Eds.). (2021a). *Single Session Thinking and Practice in Global, Cultural, and Familial Contexts: Expanding Applications.* Routledge.

Hoyt, M.F., Young, J., & Rycroft, P. (Eds.). (2021b). Single session thinking and practice going global one step at a time. In M.F. Hoyt, J. Young, & P. Rycroft (Eds.), *Single Session Thinking and Practice in Global, Cultural, and Familial Contexts: Expanding Applications* (pp. 3–26). Routledge.

Iveson, C. (1990). *Whose Life? Community Care of Older People and Their Families.* Brief Therapy Press.

Kessel, J.M. (2019). China's health care crisis. *The New York Times.* www.nytimes.com/2019/01/07/world/asia/chinas-health-care-crisis.html

Korzybski, A. (1933). *Science and Sanity: An Introduction to Non-Aristotelian Systems and General Semantics.* International Non-Aristotelian Library Publishing Company.

Kuhn, T.S. (1962). *The Structure of Scientific Revolutions* (2nd ed.). University of Chicago Press (rev. ed. 1970).

Landler, M. (2023). A national treasure, tarnished: Can Britain fix its health service? *The New York Times.* https://www.nytimes.com/2023/07/16/world/europe/uk-nhs-crisis.html

Lingiardi, V., & McWilliams, N. (2017). *Psychodynamic Diagnostic Manual* (2nd ed.). Guilford Press.

Macdonald, A.J. (2007). *Solution-Focused Therapy: Theory, Research and Practice.* Sage.

Miller, L. (2023). Mexico promised healthcare for all: Its failure to deliver made this smiling mascot famous. *Los Angeles Times.* www.latimes.com/world-nation/story/2023-03-01/la- fg-mexico-doctor-simi-mascot-healthcare-crisis

Nardone, G., & Watzlawick, P. (1990). *The Art of Change: Strategic Therapy and Hypnotherapy Without Trance.* Jossey-Bass.

Neri, S. (2019). The Italian National Health Service after the economic crisis: From decentralization to differentiated federalism. *E-cadernos CES, 31.*

NIMH. (2024). *Psychotherapies*. www.nimh.nih.gov/health/topics/psychotherapies

Norcross, J.C. (2005). A primer on psychotherapy integration. In J.C. Norcross & M.R. Goldfried (Eds.), *Handbook of Psychotherapy Integration* (pp. 3–23). Oxford University Press.

PACFA. (n.d.). *What is therapy?* https://pacfa.org.au/portal/Portal/Community/What-is- Therapy.aspx

Priest, J.B. (2023). *Systemic Diagnosis: The Application of Family Systems Theory*. Routledge.

Raykos, B.C., Erceg-Hurn, D.M., McEvoy, P.M., Fursland, A., & Waller, G. (2018). Severe and enduring anorexia nervosa? Illness severity and duration are unrelated to outcomes from enhanced cognitive behavior therapy. *Journal of Consulting and Clinical Psychology*, 86(8), 702–709.

Russell, B. (1913). The philosophical importance of mathematical logic. *The Monist*, 23(4), 481–493.

Sistema. (n.d.). In *Treccani*. https://www.treccani.it/vocabolario/sistema/

Suzuki, T., Nishida, M., Suzuki, Y., & Kobayashi, K. (2008). The imminent health-care and emergency care crisis in Japan. *The Western Journal of Emergency Medicine*, 9(2), 91–96.

Talmon, M. (1990). *Single-Session Therapy: Maximizing the Effect of the First (and Often Only) Therapeutic Encounter*. Jossey-Bass.

Watzlawick, P. (1990). Therapy is what you say it is. In J.K. Zeig & S.G. Gilligan (Eds.), *Brief Therapy: Myths, Methods, and Metaphors* (pp. 55–61). Brunner/Mazel.

Williamson, L. (2023). *France's health system under pressure of increasing demands*. https://www.bbc.com/news/world-europe-64216269

Wittgenstein, L. (1922). *Tractatus Logico-Philosophicus*. Routledge & Kegan Paul.

Young, J. (2018). Single-session therapy: The misunderstood gift that keeps on giving. In M.F. Hoyt, M. Bobele, A. Slive, J. Young, & M. Talmon (Eds.), *Single-Session Therapy by Walk-In or Appointment: Administrative, Clinical, and Supervisory Aspects of One-at-a-Time Services* (pp. 40–58). Routledge.

Chapter 3

The Golden Hour

SST as a Life-Long Event

Moshe Talmon

All kinds and all lengths of psychotherapy start with the first session. Often the first session, called an "intake," is just for psychodiagnostic purposes with no therapeutic goals. Many such first encounters are not even recorded or counted as the first session, for example, when it takes place outside the office or clinic. During the COVID-19 pandemic I was forced to conduct many first sessions using my phone and/or other digital applications like Zoom and WhatsApp, which were never recorded in my clinical or research data as a psychotherapy session.

In a wider and long-term view from both ancient times (with healers, witches and shamans conducting psycho-magical rituals) as well as modern times, starting from the early days of the "talking cure" with Sigmund Freud and hypnotherapy conducted by Milton Erickson, therapy often took place within one session—not only as a very common event but also as a highly effective one. Yet, as of today this highly and repeatedly evidence-based fact, indicating that SST is the most common length of therapy as well as the most cost-effective form of therapy, is still unknown to most psychologists during their academic and clinical training.

About our title: The "golden hour" is a term widely used in emergency medicine. Those of us who have faced extreme situations following a sudden life-threatening illness, accident, or even a combat situation might know that there is indeed a critical golden hour, which is the first hour after the event. The likelihood to help a person, often to even rescue a patient and to return him or her to their life, is taking place in the first hour.

Some Biographical Notes

Michael Hoyt, Robert Rosenbaum and I stumbled upon the SST phenomena with no prior scientific or clinical knowledge about it when we decided to launch an exploratory small study during the 1980s. At that time, we were already well trained and well experienced in conducting much longer terms of psychodiagnostic processes (using mental status exams,

DOI: 10.4324/9781032693828-5

psychological testing, and the *DSM* along 5 axes) and thereafter conducting an open-ended psychotherapy of various methods and lengths.

When we made our first 60 attempts to conduct planned and mutually agreed-upon SST we had a fairly humble assumption that it might be helpful only to the "worried well" and "first timers" who had never seen a psychologist and were not "psychologically minded."

Today, 38 years after our small exploratory study, I look now at any psychotherapy session as a golden hour, including those that are very complex and often involve life-threatening situations. From my present situation, as an old and medically quite sick person, after 48 years of practicing psychotherapy I view SST as a life-long event similar to what was named by the late Nicholas Cummings (Cummings & Sayama, 1995) as an "intermittent therapy throughout the life cycle." It is a lifelong event since I am practicing it for the last 30 years (with about half of my clients) while being available to see them for as long as I am alive and practicing in my solo private practice. I'm glad to have their trust in me whenever they select to work with me for as long as it is helpful and cost-effective in their resources and judgment. I now have in my practice many clients I have seen only once as well as very long-term clients who I have seen for a series of SSTs. Practicing in a small country (Israel) within a highly inter-connected community I can keep in touch and follow up with most of them along many years.

Today, Hoyt, Rosenbaum and myself are seen as founders and leading advocates of SST. The fact is that we did not invent Single Session Therapy. We simply didn't know anything about SST until we stumbled upon it.

I joined the Child & Family Team at the Kaiser Permanente Medical Center in Hayward, California, in 1985 following a long and intensive training in three main models of psychotherapy: analytical, contextual, and medical. When I joined Kaiser, I already had 10 years of experience in conducting individual and family therapy, including two in-depth, long-term Jungian analyses for myself as a training analyst. Both in my role as a clinical director of a child and family clinic serving the Kibbutz movement in Israel as well as in my private practice I worked mostly with highly motivated, highly psychological-minded and articulate clients. I was very proud to have long waiting lists as signs of good and needed service. In such settings nobody dropped out of treatment after the 1st session or in the 10th session or in the 20th session.

I never noticed the option for SST.

When I joined Kaiser, Hoyt and Rosenbaum were already part of the Adult Team. All three of us were educated and well trained to be clinical and medical psychologists, mostly under psychoanalytical and medical models. We assumed that therapy takes a few years and psychodiagnostic processes take a few sessions.

When I arrived to work in the Child & Family Team at Kaiser Permanente I was asked by the head of our team, Paul Opsvig, how many families I could see every week. I replied: "Well, since I don't have any clients at
the moment, I would start with two new cases every day till my schedule is
filled." Dr. Opsvig was very grateful because we had a long waiting list and
were short-staffed. After a while I realized that I continued to see two new
cases every day and my calendar never got filled. It took me a little while
to realize that many of them simply didn't show up to the second appointment. I was bewildered. I had never encountered such a phenomenon. After
a few months of trying to overcome my fears and sense of sure rejection
I went to study those who dropped out after one intake session. I began to
study the practice of other people in the team during the 10 years prior to
my arrival. That was my first time to realize it's extremely common and a
lot of wasted time and money for the medical group, which employed us
and paid our salaries, for so many no-shows. I understand why others did
not notice it: (1) it gave you a free paid hour during the working day, and
(2) nobody wants to notice such a high percentage of immediate rejection.

I first launched by myself an informal study following my own
no-shows (later labeled as "un-planned SSTs"). I collected the data from
200 no-shows after the first intake. I presented the outcome to the entire
staff at the Department of Psychiatry: 78% of the "un-planned SSTs" indicated that they were improved, satisfied, and did not seek further therapy
elsewhere. These "no shows" counted for one-third of all clients served in
our department as well as in my own caseload. Such findings seemed to all
of us as "much too good to be true." How one can be improved from a single intake session? In trying to understand these unexpected outcomes, a
few staff members suggested that it might be the result of me seeing mostly
children who may improve faster than adults, while others hypothesized
that since I often saw the "IP" (identified patient) together with his or her
family it could be possible that one member (or more) from the family
served as a "co-therapist" to support the child following the one session.

I decided to ask two of my colleagues (and by that time already friends)
from the Adult Team, Michael and Bob, to join me. We reviewed the psychotherapy literature and found a few scattered reports of unplanned
one-session therapies. We launched a formal exploratory study with random new clients in a course of one year. Michael was at that time the head
of the Adult Team, had a Ph.D. from Yale, and was the senior member
among us. We gladly agreed that he would be our principal investigator
(PI) in seeking a research grant from the Garfield Foundation of Kaiser's
research department. The grant was for one year. In 1986, we did an
exploratory study, 60 random new intakes. When given the clients' consent, we recorded the session and/or watched one another via the one-way
mirror.

None of us knew how to conduct SST and had no supervision about it. We agreed on several ground rules:

1. No one-size-fits-all. No attempt for a unified protocol. No attempt for a unified theory of practice.
2. At the beginning of the session we would inform the clients about the option of one session.
3. At the end of the first session, we would be clear that they are all most welcome to continue on a weekly basis with us. They all had 20 sessions a year available as part of their medical coverage (pre-paid by their employer to the HMO).
4. We would be flexible with the 50-minute-hour to meet last-minute issues clients often raise.

At times, we added a suggestive induction that together with the clients we will do the best we can in that one session, while we will be available and ready for more sessions as needed. At the conclusion of the session we made it explicit to leave an open door to more sessions, offering an option for either ongoing weekly sessions or leaving the door open for more sessions as needed.

When a client elected to continue to the second session, we scheduled the appointment and re-affirmed the mutual responsibility to keep the next appointment in order to reduce the level of no-shows.

During 1987, we continued the follow-up research with planned SST clients (58% of the sample) as compared with the ongoing therapy clients (42% of the cases). We found (Talmon, 1990, p. 16):

> Of all the SST patients contacted, 88 percent reported either "much improvement" or "improvement" since the session [. . .] 79 percent thought that the SST had been sufficient [. . .] and 65 percent reported having other positive changes. [. . .] The SST patients showed slightly more improvement and more satisfaction than the patients who were seen for more therapy, but the differences were not significant. Three patients reported no improvement or felt that SST had not been sufficient, and they received further therapy.

A year later we were able to get a small grant to complete the follow-ups, and we started to develop a training tape based on some of the cases (Talmon, Rosenbaum, Hoyt, & Short, 1990) and an outline for SST training. Soon after, we started to teach SST all around the world and published books (Talmon, 1990, 1993) and several articles (Hoyt, 1994a; Hoyt, Rosenbaum, & Talmon, 1992; Rosenbaum, 1990, 1993; Rosenbaum, Hoyt, & Talmon, 1990).

The Post-Kaiser Years: 1992–2024

Unfortunately, due to a crisis in my own family, I had to leave and go back to Israel after 5 and a half years at Kaiser, while Bob and Michael continued to work at Kaiser until retirement. In retrospect, clearly those were the best years of my long practice. We were able to enjoy our friendship, do some research together, some teaching, while taking good care of clients. I now know that public settings like HMOs as well as public walk-in clinics, call-in centers, and other primary and emergency care systems are best suited to notice and utilize SST. In walk-in situations without long intake processes SST may be 80% of the practice (see Slive & Bobele, 2011; Bobele & Slive, in press).

When I arrived in Israel in 1992, I elected to make most of my living from a private practice. I was hoping not to need to attend too much to SST. In private practice you don't look for single session clients. Like in most other professional services in our Western consumer societies we are paid for our time and not for our results or effectiveness. You basically wish to get good-paying clients and keep them for as long as you can, mostly for the purpose of income safety. In psychodynamic terms (which is the most common approach in Israel) you offer a client "the safety of the set and the setting" in order to allow the development of the transference and counter-transference as the main tools for your psychotherapy work.

The two books (Talmon, 1990, 1993) I wrote for American publishers about SST were translated to Hebrew. Once published in Hebrew I was invited to give a few interviews to the Israeli media. Soon after a lot of people came requesting Single Session Therapy. I was also invited to teach SST in Israel, but unlike my worldwide teaching, most of the invitations in Israel came from oncology departments in hospitals, from suicide hotlines, services for homeless youngsters who live on the streets, and centers treating sexually and physically abused women. They all treated very difficult and highly pathological cases. When I got such calls, I explained to them that I have no research or clinical data or experience to support SST in such severe situations. All the agencies repeatedly claimed they had a lot of single sessions anyhow and that they needed some training in how to do it. We agreed to try and learn together, and in most cases I was the student and the staff were my teachers. In most places I volunteered my time and when they insisted on paying I charged a symbolic fee.

I would like to describe a little bit of my own summary of these challenging 32 years (1992–2024) where I am trying to offer "the golden hour" to people who are faced with very severe problems. The reason I was asked a lot of times to teach SST with very difficult cases was the repeated claim of the staff that very often they have only one session, regardless of the severity of the problem. It forced me to learn how to treat each and every session knowing that my aim was not anymore to cure the client from illness or life problems. All we need is to be respectful to our clients' choices, including their decision about when to start and when to end the course of therapy—at any point along their life span and for as long as they allow me to be of help to them.

Only when my professional judgment strongly convinced me that the client was in a much worse condition without ongoing therapy, might I go the extra mile to convince him or her to give ongoing therapy a second chance.

The length of therapy is at times not the client's choice. For example, the Israeli public mental health system has very limited resources and is short staffed. A lot of therapists can't plan SSTs nor can they treat people for as long as they wish. As I write this chapter (April 2024), there is an ongoing long and difficult conflict along all of our borders, and mental health needs are overwhelming, yet the staff and budget for mental health services is very limited and can't meet the needs.

The Three Foundations

The three foundations of our professional practice as psychotherapists are (1) science, (2) craft and (3) creativity. Each one is a necessary building block of our professionalism, but none of them is good enough by itself.

Psychology as a science uses quantitative, qualitative and theoretical methods. The main goal of science is to discover reliable and validated data that can be replicated by other studies. Our very small study at Kaiser with a relatively small N was fortunately replicated by many others in many states and countries.[1]

Just as illustration I will mention here two large-scale statistics. The first one is the measure of the frequency of SST as done by our Australian partners in the State of Victoria, Australia, during the years 2002–2005. As reported by Jeff Young, Shane Weir, and Pam Rycroft (2012, 2014; Young, 2018, pp. 47–48; also see Chapter 6 this volume, including Figure 6.1), the vast majority of clients chose to attend 1–3 sessions, and 42% of clients chose to attend for only 1 session even though Australia has a relatively generous mental health service and more sessions were readily available. What you cannot see in the Australian diagram of attendance percentages is one kind of therapy that is even higher in frequency than SST and that is "Zero Session Therapy"—many people manage their mental health (for better or worse) without professional assistance.

A second large-scale study: The World Health Organization (WHO, 2009) looked worldwide and reported that:

1. The vast number of patients in mental health services cost much less for their care, whereas there is a much smaller number of patients for whom the cost of their long-term and intensive treatments in inpatient

and outpatient settings is much higher. The largest number of patients are under self or informal community care.

2. Much more important than the economics of health care is the well-established (yet often ignored) fact that most people, during most of their lives, deal with psycho-physical problems and challenges by themselves and with the help of family, friends and the community. For large part, these "informal services" require few mental health providers simply due to the fact that in most cases clients' psycho-immune systems and human resources are effective and successful in dealing with many of the psycho-physical challenges people face daily.

My conclusion is that the essence of any good psychotherapy at any length is *to help people help themselves*. Dependency and co-dependency between patient and therapist are rarely therapeutic nor are they necessary for the mental health patient. The well-known assumption among many psychodynamic theories that the slow and deep development of the transference and counter-transference relationship is the master key for effective psychotherapy is clearly false. (See Frank, 1990, regarding the "go slow" and "gradual" mindset that underlies such approaches). At difficult and stressful times people may experience severe demoralization about their ongoing ability to take care of themselves or trust the help from others (Frank & Frank, 1991); at such times accessible and immediate professional services are necessary. However, research (see Bohart & Tallman, 1999) also repeatedly indicates that most of the positive changes that take place in formal/professional psychotherapy services are done with the active involvement and great help of the client. Within primary care there are now large numbers of walk-in/drop-in, hotline, and call-in services. In all those primary and first-line services SST, as well as very brief therapy (of 1–3 sessions), is both common and effective.

Going back to the scientific base in clinical psychology, we need to consider also qualitative research, which is not based on the nomothetic law of large numbers of statistics but more on the idiographic narrative of one or a few cases. In our original study we looked at the recordings of our sessions and analyzed what clients told us during the session as well as in the follow-up. Some questions were quantitative; others were more qualitative and non-directive in nature. Asking, for example, "On a scale of 1 to 7 how much is the problem the same or changed?" yields a different quality of understanding then asking, "What do you remember from the session?" and "How did you help that to happen?" Both can have value.

I will share with you my own personal experience. I have seen many clients as a clinical and medical psychologist for many years starting at age 26, including those faced with very difficult and life-threatening situations, such as AIDS in the early helpless days of the epidemic in the San Francisco Bay Area in the 1980s, many stage-4 kinds of cancers, highly suicidal youngsters, psychotic patients with paranoia, and others. Being fairly healthy myself at that time my clients were my main teachers both for understanding great human suffering along with unbelievable human abilities in facing very severe conditions I had never encountered in my lifetime. I felt truly lucky and grateful being their psychologist. They were my heroes, and I was their student. In the last few years, as part of getting older I got sick myself. In the last few years, I was faced twice with an immediate danger to my life through two severe medical conditions. I was hospitalized, I was operated on and later I found myself for the first time in my life in the ICU (intensive care unit) connected to a lot of tubes and pipes and unable to control most of my basic functions.

The only thing I had in mind from the first day I woke up after a major surgery was how soon can I get out of the hospital and go back home? From my years of working in hospitals I kept thinking about the many ways a hospital is the last place you want to be when you are really sick. It took a lot of effort on my part to convince the hospital staff and my family members that going back home as soon as possible is the best choice for me. And indeed, after a few days (much shorter than planned), they allowed me to go back home. Even—or especially when—in a very severe psycho-physical condition and even in life-threatening cases, some of us prefer to go back to self-care and family care as soon as possible. In any case it was a very strong reminder of how critical listening to your clients is when the provider is forming the diagnosis, the treatment plan and the prognosis.

Constructive Minimalism

The theoretical basis of our view of SST was only briefly mentioned in my first book. It was primarily developed and elaborated after the conclusion of our SST Kaiser studies and is well reflected in the later books written and edited by Hoyt (1994b, 1996, 1998, 2000, 2017, 2025) focusing on the constructive mind's views and theories, as well as the Zen view as written by Rosenbaum (1999, 2013, 2014, 2021, 2022). Clearly, like any theoretical approach, the outstanding books by Hoyt and Rosenbaum are addressing much wider, deeper, and bigger issues than SST per se.

I tend to define my mind's view as a *constructive minimalism approach* (Talmon, 2014, 2018). A lot has already been written about helpful mindsets for the single session therapist (see Cannistrà, 2021, 2022; Porter et al., Chapter 7 this volume). I will mention here just two very old, basic and seemingly the simplest ones:

1. First, do no harm (*Primum non nocere* in Latin).
2. Help people to help themselves.

The Professional Base (Craft/Tools)

The second base is professional craftmanship, namely, the tools and techniques we may employ when conducting psychotherapy in general and SST in particular.

The first challenge for Hoyt, Rosenbaum and myself operating as clinical psychologists in a large medical center and hospital:

- How do you convert regular first intake sessions where you are only gathering information for *DSM* diagnostic purposes into a therapeutic one as well, if indeed it may be the last session?
- How do you form questions, inquiries and feedback that are both diagnostic and therapeutic at once?

Let me describe how the therapist's mindset is translated into his or her action during the therapy when you attempt to capture the moment and be fully present with your client.

a. **Presence:** Proactive
b. **Present:** Pro-here and now
c. **Exchanging Presents (gifts):** Pro-client, Pro-solutions, Pro-hope, Pro-resources (internal and external) and so on

It's derived from the three meanings of the word **Present:**

1. *Presence.* The power of *presence* is well described by Proverbs 18:21: "Death and life are in the power of the tongue," as well as in the saying, "When two people meet everything may happen." It is your ability to be fully present in the session by proactively conversing with your client. It is done by your attempts to get closer and affiliate with your client's narrative, needs, character and values. (For example: "What do you see as my role in our session today?" or "How I can be of help to you in helping yourself?")
2. The second one is the present as *time*, to be pro- the here and now. For example: "What are your best hopes for our meeting today?"
3. The third one is present as a *gift*. You may look at therapy as an exchange of presence/presents/gifts where the client opens up to you in order to share his or her authentic story and you reply expressing your empathic and compassionate understanding of his or her pain while offering new re-framing and re-affirmation that may offer a reliable hope. Rosenbaum calls it a "pivot chord" (Rosenbaum et al., 1990). Some elements in the therapist gifts are:

   1. being pro-client/cheerleader of the client
   2. being pro-solution

3. being pro-hope
4. being pro-resources (internal and external ones)

Being pro-resources is often done with our feedback to what the client told us. For example:

- "What you just said is very important. Can you repeat it for me so I fully understand your point?"
- "I am quite moved by the way you coped with such a difficult situation like ____."
- "What you did when _____ impressed me deeply since I never imagined I could _____ as you did."
- "I see here several options you have right now. I will mention them based on what you told me today. I don't know which one you will choose but I fully trust you will do it in the right timing and the right way for you."

Clearly, each therapist adopts his or her own craft and use of his or her own tools. Here are a few tools I have used sometimes: hypnotherapy, EMDR, mindfulness, cognitive and contextual reframing, visual imagery, enactment, joining, dream interpretations. The tools may give us the sense of mastering professionalism, and it is nice to know we have tools we can use. It is important but never enough simply because each client responds differently to our tools. Sometimes clients don't recall dreams at all or don't enter a stage of trance to your hypnotic suggestion or simply "Yes, but . . ." all of your reframing or suggestions and so on.

Creativity

That bring us to the creative basis, which in Single Session Therapy, in my experience, is the most important one and most fun for the therapist. Regarding creativity I want to acknowledge a great researcher and a psychologist who passed away a few years ago, Mihaly Csikszentmihalyi, whose books include *The Evolving Self: A Psychology for the Third Millennium* (1994), *Creativity: Flow and the Psychology of Discovery and Invention* (1997), and *Flow: The Psychology of Optimal Experience* (2008). Most Americans could not pronounce his Hungarian name, so they called him "Mike." He was a leading qualitative researcher at the University of Chicago for many years and after retirement moved to Claremont College in California. In studying in-depth 91 highly creative people via long interviews, Csikszentmihalyi found an interesting common characteristic among all of them: Creative people are able to hold opposing characteristics of themselves without internal conflict or rejecting one side of the poles. For example, they can be lazy as well as hard-working, they can be childlike and adult-like, they can think quickly and intuitively and they can think thoroughly and slowly. They can be very organized and very chaotic, and so on. No side of the poles is labeled as "good" or "bad."

In "The Eternal Now" (Talmon, 2018, p. 153), I wrote:

> Treating each session as the *first* session (for the rest of therapy), while knowing it could be also the *last* one (accepting that one day it will be also true), has been the most creative force in my work as a therapist. Holding these two poles (beginning and endings) together and working with both at once—a fresh beginning and possible ending—has proved for me to be very critical for the creative force clients and therapists bring into each therapeutic session. I have found that OAAT therapy is the best force for my creativity in psychotherapy. Such creativity often takes place when I walk in curious and open-minded and allow patients to surprise me and teach me something new in each session.

Here are a few of my guidelines for staying creative in conducting psychotherapy:

- The beginner's mind ("walk in and stay curious")
- Holding and using opposing poles (e.g., hope for the best while being ready for the worst)
- Stay tuned: attunement for the intersubjectivity in the meeting of the minds and trying to synchronize the exact therapeutic alliance with every new client. Utilizing both the common and unique therapeutic factors. The common factors are mostly based on the fact that we are all humans and share similar genetic codes. Thus, things that are helpful to us might be helpful to others, yet each new client is also a unique person with his or her own fingerprints and a unique narrative that each client brings to the room, including their own belief system, their culture and personality.
- Psychological flexibility. Always be ready to be surprised. Be aware of your mistakes and errors as your best teacher. ("Life is what happens when we make all kinds of plans and mistakes.") In psychotherapy sessions it is often us saying something that is "right," "smart" or logical in our mind, and as you watch for the client response you may realize you may be right but not helpful to the person in front of you.
- Encourage mindful, kind and compassionate encounters of beginnings and ends (hello and goodbye) in each session as a whole and each life as a whole. (We are all humans. We are all born and die.)
- The client is your best teacher. The spiral of life from birth to death: Our life is composed with beginnings and ends, hellos and goodbyes.

The Creative Spiral of Intermittent SSTs Throughout the Life Cycle

Being a creative therapist is not only an individualistic professional ability. It is also intersubjective creativity between at least two people. At times the interaction is "symmetrical" when we agree with one another, share similar personal qualities or similar values and points of view. That is clearly fun and easier when we identify as "lovable" and have a clear sense of affinity and familiarity with new clients. Other times, the mind's views I presented here are "complementary" (Watzlawick, Beavin, & Jackson, 1967, p. 67) with those of the client.

For those clients I will share here my spiral model. As an example, I present here one such spiral. On the left-hand side my mind's views as described earlier: positive, common, present, psycho-health, solution talk, active, non-directive and empathic. I may consider it as the "correct" side. As psychotherapists, when we meet clients they might not be on the same pole as we are. In such cases they invite me to use an intersubjective creative spiral. Such poles may present themselves as we move through our life from birth to death, from the positive pole to the negative one, from the common to the uncommon, from the present backward to the past or from the present to looking ahead to our future. For example, I may address the present by asking, "What brings you here today?" and the client may dive right into a long history talk of the painful past. I may address the client's strengths, resources and abilities and he or she in return addresses

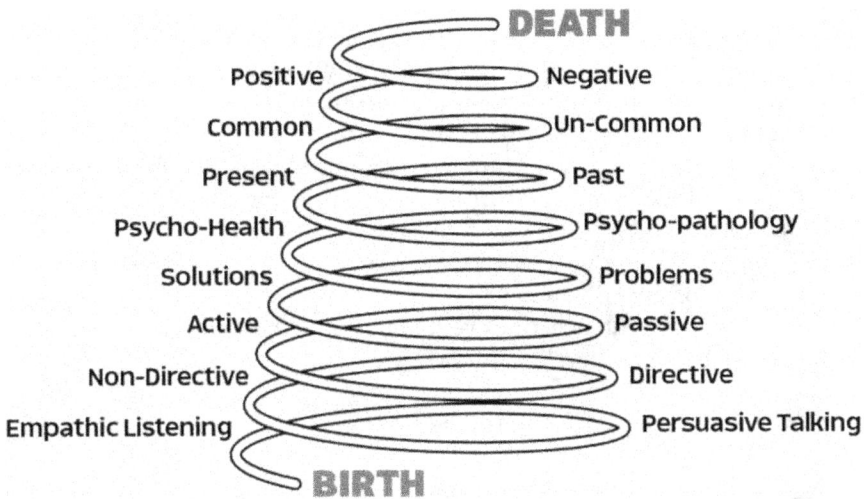

Figure 3.1 The creative spiral of intermittent SSTs throughout the life cycle.
Source: (©M. Talmon, 2013. Used by agreement.)

his or her weaknesses and disabilities. You may prefer to host a solution talk and the client may insist on a problem talk. I may tend to be proactive from the first session, while some clients require that I shut up and listen silently. Such encounters call for both your internal creativity and your intersubjective creativity. You want in such cases to allow things to come together and hopefully meet somewhere in the middle or in a better balance or better non-judgmental communication between seemingly opposing poles. This is where I search and re-search for the golden path. For sure it doesn't always happen. Our job in such cases is to keep looking and listening and use our creative flexibility while deeply respecting our client being as they are.

Clients come to us often to talk about their psycho-physical suffering, pains, and traumas. Our job is to work with both poles, where in one hand we express our deepest empathy, compassion and attunement to their pain, while on the other hand offering a sense of relief, hope and potential and accessible solutions. If we offer only one end of the pole (the empathy) we may induce in them only the sense of victimhood, blame on others (parents, boss, spouse) and/or self. If we hold only the "positive" pole of being overly optimistic we might leave the client with the sense of us minimizing or even ignoring their suffering. That might lead to an inappropriate early drop-out from therapy. That creative balance and creative communication between seemingly opposing poles is so important to our work.

Finally, after conducting intermittent Single Session Therapy throughout the life cycle for many years with many clients, I have also had the opportunity and the pleasure to follow up with the lives of many of my clients. As I learned back in the 1980s as part of our research, at times when I ask my clients if they remember anything from our SST, sometimes many years later, often they remember only one sentence from our one-hour conversation, at times it was only one word. Yet that one thing was remembered as an anchor, a pivot chord (Rosenbaum et al., 1990) that led to big changes in their life and sometimes in the lives of other people.

Once and for all/All you need is one:
One word, one sentence, one event and timing that may change the lives of one and or many.

That might be the essence of constructive minimalism.

Note

1 *Editors' note*: For a summary of recent findings, see Chapter 13 (Pietrabissa) in this volume.

References

Bobele, M., & Slive, A. (Eds.) (in press). *Implementing Single-Session Therapy in Open Access Services.* Routledge.

Bohart, A.C., & Tallman, K. (1999). *How Clients Make Therapy Work: The Process of Active Self-Healing.* APA Books.

Cannistrà, F. (2021). The vital role of the therapist's mindset. In M.F. Hoyt, J. Young, & P. Rycroft (Eds.), *Single Session Thinking and Practice in Global, Cultural, and Familial Contexts: Expanding Applications* (pp. 77–88). Routledge.

Cannistrà, F. (2022). The single session therapy mindset: Fourteen principles gained through an analysis of the literature. *International Journal of Brief Therapy and Family Science, 12*(1), 1–26.

Csikszentmihalyi, M. (1994). *The Evolving Self: A Psychology for the Third Millennium.* Harper Perennial.

Csikszentmihalyi, M. (1997). *Creativity: Flow and the Psychology of Discovery and Invention.* Harper Perennial.

Csikszentmihalyi, M. (2008). *Flow: The Psychology of Optimal Experience.* Harper Perennial.

Cummings, N.A., & Sayama, M. (1995). *Focused Psychotherapy: A Casebook of Brief, Intermittent Psychotherapy Through the Life Cycle.* Brunner/Mazel.

Frank, J.D. (1990). Foreword. In M. Talmon (Ed.), *Single-Session Therapy: Maximizing the Effects of the First (and Often Only) Therapeutic Encounter* (pp. xi–xiii). Jossey-Bass.

Frank, J.D., & Frank, J.B. (1991). *Persuasion and Healing: A Comparative Study of Psychotherapy* (3rd ed.). Johns Hopkins University Press.

Hoyt, M.F. (1994a). Single-session solutions. In M.F. Hoyt (Ed.), *Constructive Therapies* (pp. 140–159). Guilford Press. Reprinted in Hoyt, M.F. (1995). *Brief Therapy and Managed Care* (pp. 141–162). Jossey-Bass.

Hoyt, M.F. (Ed.). (1994b). *Constructive Therapies.* Guilford Press.

Hoyt, M.F. (Ed.). (1996). *Constructive Therapies* (Vol. 2). Guilford Press.

Hoyt, M.F. (Ed.). (1998). *The Handbook of Constructive Therapies.* Jossey-Bass.

Hoyt, M.F. (2000). *Some Stories Are Better Than Others: Doing What Works in Brief Therapy and Managed Care.* Brunner/Mazel.

Hoyt, M.F. (2017). *Brief Therapy and Beyond: Stories, Language, Love, Hope, and Time.* Routledge.

Hoyt, M.F. (2025). *Single Session Therapy: A Clinical Introduction to Principles and Practices.* Routledge.

Hoyt, M.F., Rosenbaum, R., & Talmon, M. (1992). Planned single-session psychotherapy. In S.H. Budman, M.F. Hoyt, & S. Friedman (Eds.), *The First Session in Brief Therapy* (pp. 59–86). Guilford Press.

Rosenbaum, R. (1990). Strategic therapy. In R.A. Wells & V.J. Giannetti (Eds.), *Handbook of the Brief Psychotherapies* (pp. 351–403). Plenum Press.

Rosenbaum, R. (1993). Heavy ideals: Strategic single-session hypnotherapy. In R.A. Wells & V.J. Giannetti (Eds.), *Casebook of the Brief Psychotherapies* (pp. 109–128). Plenum Press.

Rosenbaum, R. (1999). *Zen and the Heart of Psychotherapy.* Brunner-Routledge.

Rosenbaum, R. (2013). *Walking the Way: 81 Zen Encounters With the Tao Te Ching.* Wisdom Publications.

Rosenbaum, R. (2014). The time of your life. In M.F. Hoyt & M. Talmon (Eds.), *Capturing the Moment: Single Session Therapy and Walk-In Services* (pp. 41–52). Crown House Publishing.

Rosenbaum, R. (2021). Gradually and suddenly: What Zen teaches us about change in SST. In M.F. Hoyt, J. Young, & P. Rycroft (Eds.), *Single Session Thinking and Practice in Global, Cultural, and Familial Contexts: Expanding Applications* (pp. 89–97). Routledge.

Rosenbaum, R. (2022). *That is Not Your Mind! Zen Reflections on the Surangama Sutra.* Shambhala Publications.

Rosenbaum, R., Hoyt, M.F., & Talmon, M. (1990). The challenge of single-session therapies: Creating pivotal moments. In R.A. Wells & V.J. Giannetti (Eds.), *Handbook of the Brief Psychotherapies* (pp. 165–189). Plenum Press. Reprinted in Hoyt, M.F. (1995). *Brief Therapy and Managed Care* (pp. 105–139). Jossey-Bass.

Slive, A., & Bobele, M. (Eds.). (2011). *When One Hour is All You Have: Effective Therapy for Walk-In Clients.* Zeig, Tucker, & Theisen.

Talmon, M. (1990). *Single-Session Therapy: Maximizing the Effect of the First (and Often Only) Therapeutic Encounter.* Jossey-Bass.

Talmon, M. (1993). *Single Session Solutions: A Guide to Practical, Effective, and Affordable therapy.* Addison-Wesley.

Talmon, M. (2014). When less is more: Maximizing the effect of the first (and often only) therapeutic encounter. In M.F. Hoyt & M. Talmon (Eds.), *Capturing the Moment: Single Session Therapy and Walk-In Services* (pp. 27–40). Crown House Publishing.

Talmon, M. (2018). The eternal now: On becoming and being a single-session therapist. In M.F. Hoyt, M. Bobele, A. Slive, J. Young, & M. Talmon (Eds.), *Single-Session Therapy by Walk-In or Appointment: Administrative, Clinical, and Supervisory Aspects of One-at-a-Time Services* (pp. 149–154). Routledge.

Talmon, M., Rosenbaum, R., Hoyt, M.F., & Short, L. (1990). *Single Session Therapy.* Videotape. Golden Triad Films.

Watzlawick, P., Beavin, J.H., & Jackson, D.D. (1967). Pragmatics of Human Communication: A Study of Interactional Patterns, Pathologies, and Paradoxes. Norton.

World Health Organization (WHO). (2009). *Improving Health Systems and Services for Mental Health Self-Care.* World Health Organization.

Young, J. (2018). Single-session therapy: The misunderstood gift that keeps on giving. In M.F. Hoyt, M. Bobele, A. Slive, J. Young, & M. Talmon (Eds.), *Single-Session Therapy by Walk-In or Appointment: Administrative, Clinical, and Supervisory Aspects of One-at-a-Time Services* (pp. 40–58). Routledge.

Young, J., Weir, S., & Rycroft, P. (2012). Implementing single session therapy. *Australian and New Zealand Journal of Family Therapy, 33*(1), 84–97.

Young, J., Weir, S., & Rycroft, P. (2014). Implementing SST: Practical wisdoms from down under. In M.F. Hoyt & M. Talmon (Eds.), *Capturing the Moment: Single-Session Therapy and Walk-In Services* (pp. 121–140). Crown House Publishing.

Chapter 4

Single Sessions

Beyond "Is" and "Is Not"

Robert Rosenbaum

The seeds of the development of Single Session Therapy (SST) sprouted from an act of courage. Moshe Talmon (1990; see Chapter 3 this volume) looked at some clinic data about client visits and noticed the modal number was one. This was true, without exception, for every therapist in our clinic. Moshe thought if so many clients were coming in once and not returning, we must be doing something wrong. Then he did something brave: he called his clients who had only come in for a single visit and asked them why.

Moshe braced himself to hear about our clinic's—and his personal—failures. He was surprised to hear most of them say "I felt that was enough, I got what I needed."

Moshe invited Michael Hoyt and myself to join him in a research project on planned SST. There were times during the project when each of us felt we'd been particularly skillful at how we met a client and devised some clever therapeutic intervention. We were initially a bit disheartened, looking at the follow-up data, to discover our feelings of how well we'd done in a session had little bearing on the client's report of how good an outcome they'd experienced.

We shouldn't have been so surprised. The research literature is clear: the most important factor in psychotherapy outcome—accounting for somewhere between 40% and 87% of the variance—is the client (Bohart & Tallman, 1999). Relationship factors account for about 30%, techniques account for at most 15%, possibly much less (Cooper, 2010).

I love to quote how Moshe phrases this finding to psychotherapists: "Remember, psychotherapy is not about *you*." This provides all us do-gooders with a sense of relief, but also with a narcissistic injury. Hey, if psychotherapy is not about us, what are we in the therapy process? Is it possible that what we say doesn't really matter? Most of us have had a client say, "I took what you said to heart," but then we don't recognize their

DOI: 10.4324/9781032693828-6

version of what they say we said. (I've sometimes not only thought "I don't think I said that" but even "I don't think I *would* say that.")

I think what we say, and how we interact with a client, is important—*and* not at all important. The better we are able to be important, not important, both important and not important, as well as neither important nor not-important, the better we can fully engage with our clients and ourselves.

I got a clue about how to dance with these swirling currents from Michael Hoyt. While studying Redecision Therapy with Mary and Robert Goulding (1979), Michael had been impressed with the power of committing to a course of action compared to what we (and our clients) more commonly say to a suggestion to do something different: "I'll give it a try." During one conversation with Michael, he said to me: "Too often saying 'I'll try . . .' is something kids say to satisfy parents, but they don't really mean it. When adults say 'I'll try' to a therapist, they usually mean 'I'll go through the motions to get you off my back but my heart's not really in it and I don't expect anything to come of it.'"

So I stopped *trying* to help clients decide on a course of action. I acknowledged I usually don't know what (if anything) they should do. I became less interested in what they'd decide to do and more interested in *how* they'd come up with some new choices. I wanted to enjoy the process, so before each session I asked myself: "How can I enjoy myself in this session?"

When I began doing this, I sometimes felt anxious that I might fail. I sometimes felt guilty: weren't therapist and client supposed to be working hard, and didn't that mean we shouldn't be having fun? Very often, before seeing a difficult client, I "knew" they were impossible and I was "justified" to feel put-upon. I gradually discovered I had to learn a different way to enjoy each client, each time—and that it was possible.

Whenever I found a way to enjoy being with a client, they seemed to like it. Most clients come to therapy feeling bad about themselves; to have someone enjoy being with them eases some of their negative thoughts and feelings. It makes it easier for clients to connect with themselves, the therapist, and the therapy. My clients and I became collaborators, and we could have a good time sparking each other to a process of mutual discovery. Instead of worrying about what we might achieve or fail to achieve, we could explore, roam freely, and create a space for the familiar and the unexpected to unfold intriguing horizons. Therapy became less like work and more like play.

In the context of developing ways to enjoy ourselves while enjoying our clients, I found I could take The Bouverie Centre's excellent map for single sessions[1] and adapt it as the steps to hosting a good party:

Bouverie	Steps to a Good Party	Party Processes
Connect, Set Context, Contract Find a Focus, Establish Priorities	Invite	Meet & Greet—Let's Do This! Validate—Empathize, Accept the Client's Perceptions Collaborate—Hear the Music, Partner in the Dance
Gather Information, Avoid Dead Ends, Raise Possibilities Avoid Therapeutic Drift Intervene	Entertain Host & Guest	Explore—Prepare to Be Surprised Cut to the Chase—How Is the Problem a Problem? Expand—You're Bigger Than Your Problem Pivot—Turn the Wheel, Oil the Hinge
End Well	Adieu	Integrate—Client Meanings, Values, Identity Revisit to Fare Well

Work and play, partying and trudging don't contradict each other. They *complete* each other. Our challenge—both as therapists and in everyday life—is to find a way to embrace (or at least acknowledge and appreciate) all the myriad facets of whatever we're facing without getting stuck in one isolated aspect of it. Sometimes, when we anticipate a session, we may experience dread or weariness, anxiety or annoyance. When I'm experiencing these uncomfortable feelings, I look for a way to enjoy my discomfort. I remember I was initially put off by the bitterness of IPA beer and the spiciness of Indian food—both of which I now enjoy. I call to mind a Zen saying:

Health and sickness subsume each other.
The whole world is medicine.
What is your true self?

This may seem overly philosophical. But therapy is, like any activity, an existential paradox:

As everyone is who they are and everything is as it is, there are
problems and solutions, therapists and clients, misery and delight.
As everyone and everything is continuously in flux and ungraspable,
there are no problems and no solutions, no therapists and clients, no
misery or delight.
Moments are meetings, so there are problems, solutions, therapists,
clients, misery, and delight.

Yet when people hold on tight, flowers wither, and when people push away, weeds spread.

I've just paraphrased the opening lines of an essay by 13th-century Zen teacher Eihei Dogen (Dogen, 1233/2010). The title of the essay is *Genjo Koan*, which means something like "actualizing the fundamental point." When we get right down to it, what is the fundamental point of Single Session Therapy?

(A confession: I don't think SST is a big deal. Forty years ago, when Moshe, Michael, and I first learned many clients improve in a single therapy session, I had trouble believing it. I found it remarkable and exciting. These days, I see it as simply being in line with the way everything works: every moment something happens, life and death continuously flowing.)

Every therapy session is an event—actually, a series of events—expressing our lives completely for that place and time. We and the world are constantly realizing ourselves together with all beings. Usually we don't notice it, but that doesn't mean it's not happening. When we are fully present to each expression of arising and vanishing, why should we be surprised that sometimes a single meeting is enough?

But there's a paradox. A little later on in the same essay by Dogen, he says—I'm paraphrasing here—"When you first catch on to the marvel of each moment, you feel it's enough. But when each moment fills your body and soul, you realize something is always missing." My Zen teacher's teacher, Shunryu Suzuki (see 1970), expressed it in a way I think therapists should adopt as a guide for forming relationships with their clients: approach each person with the attitude "You are perfect just as you are . . . *and* you could use a little improvement."

Perfect, Flawed, Both, Neither: The *Tetra Lemma*

When we completely accept people as who they are while acknowledging we are all, always, works in progress, we create the conditions for wholesomeness. "I love you, you're perfect, now change" is not hypocritical. It's an acknowledgment of our basic existential condition. Neither we nor our clients can begin to cope with people or situations until we accept each as it is: "this is what I need to deal with!" As soon as we accept whatever's going on as it is—dropping our pre-conceived ideas of what they're supposed to be while removing our filters of how we want them to be—our experience of the situation has already changed, and we've changed along with it.

One obstacle to doing this is our tendency to confuse acceptance with resignation. We think if we accept something or someone, it means we resign ourselves to its being that way. Actually it's the opposite. We can only accept something when we know that it can't stay that way—that it will inevitably change.

Gregory Bateson (1980) liked to point out that all stability is maintained by change, and all change depends on stability. The two don't contradict each other; they complete each other. We have a tendency, though, to see things as either-or. This goes back thousands of years, to the development of Western logic based on the rule of the excluded middle, which basically says something cannot be A and not-A at the same time.

Around 200 C.E., the Indian Buddhist philosopher Nagarjuna proposed a different logic: the *tetra lemma*. In this schema all phenomena are approached from four perspectives: A ("is"), not-A ("is not"), *both A and not-A* ("both *is* and *is not*"), and *neither A nor not-A* ("neither *is* nor *is not*"). All four perspectives apply equally at all times to all phenomena. Translating this to the language of therapy: every presenting problem is a problem, is not a problem, both is and is not a problem, and neither is nor is not a problem.

There's an old Jewish joke about a husband and wife who have an intense argument they cannot resolve, so they bring their dispute to their rabbi. The rabbi listens to the wife's side of the story and, after she's finished, says: "You're right!" Then the husband says, "but Rabbi . . ." and tells him his side of the argument. At the end, the rabbi says to the husband: "You're right!" At that point the rabbi's student, who's been listening in, turns to the rabbi and objects: "Rabbi, they can't both be right." The rabbi turns to his student and says, "You're also right!" To complete the tetra lemma, all we need do is add that none of them are right—*Oy Vey!*

On a profound level, this joke contains a truth not just about arguments but also about people and personalities. We say to ourselves "I'm *me*"— but we also sometimes say "I'm not myself today." When we realize that I can be both at the same time (both me and not myself) as well as neither myself nor not-myself, our horizons expand exponentially.

If this seems confusing, it's because we're accustomed to "is or isn't" mindsets. This may seem obvious: a person is either alive or dead, healthy or ill. Actually, each moment we are a conglomeration of some cells that are fully alive, some cells that are inert and being sloughed off, not to mention all the cells in our microbiome that don't even have human DNA. When we cannot breathe without the aid of an artificial lung, perhaps we feel we're neither alive nor dead—while remaining very much alive!

To clarify this, consider the Kanizsa triangle (see Figure 4.1), an optical illusion first described by the Italian psychologist Gaetano Kanizsa in 1955 (Gregory, 1997). Do you see the white triangle? Is the white triangle "really" there, or is it not there? Is it both there and not-there? Is it neither

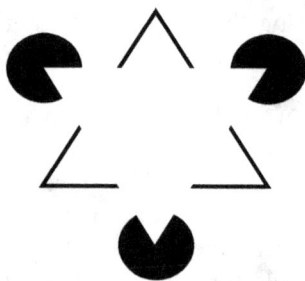

Figure 4.1 Kanizsa triangle.

there nor not-there? Each of these statements evokes one aspect of how we experience the white triangle.

We easily dismiss this as an illusion arising from how our neurology shapes our perception. It's a bit shocking, but ultimately liberating, to realize: *everything* we experience is a "perceptual illusion," shaped by the limitations of our bodies and brains, our minds and the environments in which they're embedded. All the seeming "facts" of our physical sensations and impulses are perceptions, as are all our ideas and feelings, along with everything we encounter in the world "out there" and the world "in me." Mystics and neuroscientists might call them illusions, but they are the means by which we live: very real, yet unreal; both real *and* unreal, neither real *nor* unreal.

We joke that a person cannot be half-pregnant. We create wider possibilities for ourselves when we understand that everybody—men and women alike—is continuously pregnant, not pregnant, as well as both and neither. Children are pregnant with possibilities; men can be mid-term in the gestation of an idea or going through the labor pains of a rebirth of wonder. When a woman's ovum has been inseminated but has not yet attached to the uterine wall, we might say she is both pregnant and non-pregnant; later on, if her body is at risk of miscarriage and she experiences some spotting, she may feel neither pregnant nor not-pregnant.

Saying a person cannot be half-pregnant isn't true, but it does intuitively acknowledge that finding a halfway point between two extremes often is not satisfying. If we exist on a two-dimensional continuum of being either mentally healthy or mentally unwell, being "kind of OK" will be as unsatisfying as being "kind of" pregnant. When we assume a person cannot be both pregnant and non-pregnant, cannot be both alive and dead and both and neither, we set the stage for fights over when life begins and ends. Then we have political and legal battles over abortions, and conflicts over withdrawal of life support in terminal illness.

It's healthier—and truer to reality—to treat life and death as a process. The same holds for psychotherapy. If we see people as either having a problem or problem-free, we can get into battles over when therapy starts and stops, how many sessions a client needs, and whether they're better or worse.

We can't always know whether we're better or worse off, because we, and everything around us, keeps changing. We're all married to ourselves, for better *and* worse, in sickness and health, in life and in death. All of us have had experiences that first seemed to be disastrous but turned out to lead to new growth, and getting what we wished for is often a mixed blessing and curse. The same holds true for the changes clients experience in psychotherapy: they're usually a mixed bag.

The *Tetra Lemma* and Psychotherapy

Reality shimmers. This may seem counter-intuitive, overly abstract, or irrelevant to our psychotherapy work, but when you think about it (or, better yet, meditate on it), you may appreciate how the tetra lemma accords with therapeutic experience much better than either-or approaches. There are more degrees of freedom in a four-dimensional therapeutic space than in a two-dimensional one.

All our concepts about therapy are just that: concepts, not therapy itself. As my friend Art Bohart (see Rosenbaum & Bohart, 2007) likes to emphasize, therapy is not a thing: it's a process people act out with other people, with their world, and with themselves. Even our concepts, according to recent developments in perceptual psychology, philosophy, and neuroscience, are processes we enact and embody. Research (see Carney, 2020) based on the "4E" model highlights how we live in a four-dimensional world: all our thoughts, feelings, and sensations are

- Embedded in a context
- Embodied physically
- Enacted behaviorally, and
- Extend beyond their seeming boundaries.

Let's take emotions as an example. A lot of people think that therapy is a process of finding your "true feelings." I think we can agree emotion plays some role in psychotherapy, but if we imagine there is such a thing as a "true feeling" we'll fall into a trap. It's the same trap that holds out the illusion that the "real me" exists as some graspable, unchanging thing, the same trap that holds there is a cure that will heal all my hurts and take care of all my problems once and for all.

Psychotherapy stumbles when we treat feelings as if events "out there" trigger a primitive part of the brain "in me," which then generates chemical secretions and electrical impulses along unchanging, hard-wired paths. When we use this model to treat depression—whether pharmacologically or with psychotherapy—we have at best modest success.

Systemic, humanistic, and interpersonal approaches point out that "depression" is a dormitive principle: it groups together a diverse set of experiences (interrupted sleep and excessive sleep, agitation and lethargy, sadness and irritability), assigns a name to them, and confuses the name with the lived experience. The 4E research goes further by emphasizing *every occurrence of emotion is unique.*

Each time we feel something it is the first and only time, because our nervous system is engaged in a continuous process of interoception, taking stock each moment of multiple psycho-physical parameters, interpreting them, anticipating needs, and allocating our mind's and body's resources. Each instant depends on a unique confluence of multiple factors that are never repeated exactly.

If you're a passenger in a small car at night careening around curves at high speed, your heart will beat faster, your eyes will dilate, and your breathing will change. If the car is on a narrow country road being driven by a frenzied companion, you're likely to fearfully yell "Whoa!"—but if the car is on the track of an amusement park roller coaster you may shriek with glee. Each scenario involves a similar body experience, but the body goes beyond the skin to include the type of car and track it's on. The context in which it's embedded—amusement park or country road, daylight or dark—alters how we interpret the experience. Our interpretation changes the way we act out a feeling (shouting "Whee!" rather than "Whoa!")—which in turn changes how we feel. Are we scared or not (or both or neither)?

Our feelings are always in flux; diagnostic labels deaden them into supposedly stable underlying entities. This makes them easy targets for medical treatment, at the expense of making them harder to treat. Saying a client is "depressed" or "anxious" seems to explain what we're feeling, but emotions are never the "why" of our experience. They are the weather, arising from confluences of conditions—the clouds and clearings of our being. The tetra lemma and the 4E framework remind us that all our forecasts are subject to uncertainty.

This is good news for SST practitioners seeking the proverbial Brazilian butterfly whose wings will influence whether there are tornadoes in Kansas. We learn that when it's raining, we need not despair at our inability to stop the downpour. We can seek shelter; we can substitute an indoor get together for the ruined picnic; we can go singing in the rain even without a Gore-Tex jacket, dancing with an umbrella, and enjoy making a splash.

Case Examples

A forty-year-old woman came to therapy because she worried she was becoming anorexic. She was concerned she'd suffer a relapse of problems she'd suffered earlier in her life. During her adolescence and early twenties she trained to be a professional dancer in a company that assigned the best roles to women who had long, lean legs (as my client did) and were thin to the point of wispiness: narrow hips, little or no fat deposits, small breasts and delicate arms. As a result, aspiring dancers often starved themselves intentionally. For many of them—my client amongst them—this turned into intractable anorexia. My client almost died. Over several years of treatment she recovered, quit ballet, found a different life path. She married, had two children, and became a full-time housewife.

Now her children had grown old enough so that she had some free time for herself. She'd always loved classical ballet, so she enrolled in a local dance studio to return to the art of dance. Most of the women in her class, though, were twenty years younger. They were thinner than she, and she found herself comparing herself to them. She went on a diet. She noticed she was becoming self-conscious about her weight and came to me worried that she was spiraling into anorexia again.

During the session I learned she was happy in her marriage, enjoyed being a mother (even while dealing with the usual ups and downs of daughters in early adolescence), had a good social network, and was in good health. At the ballet studio, though, she felt she couldn't measure up to the younger women. "How could I?" she protested. "I'm forty years old, I've had children, my body has changed, I'm a grown woman in a grown woman's body."

I asked her to repeat what she just said. She was a little puzzled, but dutifully recited again, in a perfunctory fashion. I asked her to say it again and notice how she felt as she said it. "I'm a grown woman in a grown woman's body," she said, more slowly this time. Then, unasked, she said it again, more forcefully, with an exclamation point! "Hey, *I'm a grown woman in a grown woman's body*! There's *no way* I could be like a twenty-year-old anymore. And I don't have any desire to be a twenty-year-old. I'm much happier now! And my weight is fine! There's no way I'm going to starve myself again. I'm going to just dance the way I like and enjoy it as I am!" From the 4E perspective, this successful single session offered a different context to embed the experience of her current body, extending it to include her daughters' births, enacting it by speaking her truth out loud in the presence of a listener who'd confirm her current manifestation of herself. To put this in terms of the tetra lemma: my client was a dancer, even though she could no longer be a dancer. As a forty-year-old, when she capered at a disco with her husband, she was both a dancer and not a dancer. As a mother, wife, a competent and happy grown woman, she was neither a dancer nor not a dancer.

Another, perhaps more dramatic, single session case involved a referral from the Neurology clinic.

A thirty-year-old man was suffering multiple complex partial seizures every day. These kinds of seizures often involve psychiatric symptoms.

In this man's case the seizures were accompanied by agitation, obsessive rumination, and intrusive thoughts of harming himself. These were only present during the seizures and stopped as soon as the seizure activity ended, usually within five to ten minutes. The thoughts of self-harm were dramatic (slashing his wrists, taking a kitchen knife and cutting his throat), but they were ego-dystonic; he'd never acted on the impulses. He was not otherwise depressed, though of course he was concerned and unhappy at how the seizures were interfering with his life.

Since the neurologist had not been able to bring the seizures under control with medication, he referred the client to me. At our first—and what turned out to be the only—appointment I met with the client and his wife. It soon became clear that the wife was caught in a state of continuous anxiety—more even than her husband, whose anxiety at least calmed down when he was in between seizures. His wife, however, hovered non-stop over her husband, scanning vigilantly for early warning signs of seizure onset so she could be ready to prevent him from cutting his wrists or acting on his impulses.

It's a well-established fact that anxiety lowers seizure thresholds. For people with epilepsy, the more anxious they are, the more likely they are to have seizures. A common behavioral treatment for seizures is to teach patients relaxation techniques. In this case, however, the client's wife held more anxiety than the client.

When I pointed out to the couple how her anxiety exacerbated his seizures and his seizures exacerbated her anxiety, they readily agreed. Each acknowledged their role in the vicious cycle. They knew relaxation methods but had found they couldn't use them effectively. How could he relax when she was hovering? He'd asked her to give him more space. His wife felt badly about her hovering, but how could she back off while she feared he'd lose control during a seizure and harm himself?

I empathized and validated their experience. I acknowledged it wouldn't work for either of them to just tell themselves to relax. I suggested instead they both needed to help the other person by giving their partner relaxation challenges.

Specifically, I suggested they arrange for the husband to go into a separate room several times a day to practice his relaxation . . . and for the wife to interrupt him unexpectedly, so he could learn how to stay calm even while she intruded. Meanwhile, I suggested that in addition to whatever seizures occurred naturally, three times a day the husband should *pretend* to have seizures. That would give the wife a chance to practice relaxation by pausing, taking a few breaths, and asking herself whether she was facing a seizure or pseudo-seizure: did she really need to act immediately to protect him? Could she take a little more time and a few more breaths to calm herself down?

As soon as they started doing this, the seizure frequency decreased to one seizure every few days. At this point, the neurologist was able to institute an effective medication regimen.

This is a good illustration of how the 4Es play out in concrete clinical phenomena. The man's seizures were certainly embodied, and so was the wife's anxiety. These body experiences, though, extended beyond their individual bodies into and through each other; they were embedded in the context of their loving relationship of mutual concern and enacted in the ways they treated each other. As an aside, I'd like to mention I do not view the intervention as "paradoxical reverse psychology." There's an unfortunate tendency in our field to view paradox as a technique you apply to a case. The tetra lemma reminds us that paradox is the shimmering reality of being who we are intertwined with who we are not.

In both these cases, the therapy process avoided getting caught in "is" or "is not." If we'd focused on whether the worried mother was or was not in danger of developing anorexia, narrowing our attention might have missed an opportunity for her to realize her self as she is, was, and will be. In the case involving seizure disorders, research has shown people with pseudo-seizures are also prone to "real" seizures, and epileptics with documented seizures are also prone to pseudo-seizures: focusing on "accurately" assessing the husband's seizure risk might have missed addressing the risk of their marriage imploding.

Are Single Session Therapies "Really" Single Sessions?

We are not who we think we "really" are, and our therapies are not what we think they "really" are. Single session therapies are not "really" defined according to whether they are, or are not, confined to one session.

I'm reminded of a client who was struggling to break free from self-disgust after a childhood trauma of sexual abuse unexpectedly resurfaced. After a few sessions, she experienced a transformative "Aha!" moment and exclaimed: "I'm *me*. I'm not what *happened* to me!" This is an important realization. Of course, it's also true we *are* what happened to us—we're affected by our conditioning. Still, on a fundamental level, we are not who we were, nor who we will be. As for who we are—best to get accustomed to being surprised.

In this case, I'd met with the client numerous times before the pivotal session, and I met with her several times thereafter to help her consolidate her experience. It was that one session, though, that was the turning point within a treatment course that ran about fourteen sessions. So I include this case when I'm teaching therapists SST.

Pivotal moments (Rosenbaum, Hoyt, & Talmon, 1990) can occur in therapies short or long, because time is not a tick. An important foundation for SST is understanding that we can't do *now* later.

The tetra lemma's "is, isn't, both is-isn't, neither is-isn't" applies to time as it does to all phenomena. Physicists debate whether time and space are illusions, or if they have inherent existence. Physicists generally agree, though, that time and space are not fixed absolutes. For a hundred years we've known time and space are relative, but we still have a tendency to think of clock time as some inexorable tyrant, as if it's something separate from us. We ignore how the mind arises in a moment, *and* a moment arises in the mind. Zen teacher Dogen says, "this is the understanding that the self is time." I like to say (Rosenbaum, 2014, 2021): we cannot "have" the time of our life, because we *are* the times of our lives.

Moments are not very short ticks of time: moments are meetings. Our subjective experience of time is every bit as valid—perhaps more so—than what mechanical chronographs proclaim. We've all had the experience of time seeming to move fast or slow. We have multiple internal biological clocks, working at different rhythms. Realizing "I'm *me*, I'm not what *happened* to me" is another way of understanding that we are a process, not an object. We are not one thing which then turns into another. A little girl is not a half-grown woman; an eighty-year-old person is not a decayed adult. Every person is complete every moment: every therapy session is complete every moment.

> The evening becomes night. Yet the night is not a conclusion drawn from the evening, as death is not a conclusion drawn from a life. Neither is the night the fruition of the evening, as death is not the fruition of life. There is evening, and there is night, each of them eternal in its own right and mode.
> —Erazim Kohak (1984), *The Embers and the Stars*

Meeting the Moment: Pivot Chords in Psychotherapy

During one formal Zen question-answer ceremony I was doubting whether my practice would lead to fruition and was questioning my commitment. When it was my turn to get up and ask a question, I walked over to the open doorway and stood on the threshold with one foot in the Zendo and the other foot outside.

> Standing there, I asked my teacher: "Am I in or out?"
> He replied, "turn around."
> I made a 360 degree turn and wound up back where I'd started.
> My teacher said, "keep turning."

We're continuously turning and being turned: moment to moment, non-stop flow. In therapy, we look for turning points. These are like pivot chords in music, where a theme is simultaneously in two keys at once. When we can find an aspect of a presenting issue that's in two "musical keys," it facilitates change. We can find pivot chords whenever we discern problems contain seeds of their dissolution. Seemingly irrelevant aspects of a situation often are the key to unlocking change.

In one of our first published cases of SST (Rosenbaum, 1993), a 27-year-old woman came in asking for hypnosis for weight control. I was the therapist, and I was initially flummoxed. Although I do hypnotherapy, I'm skeptical about its long-term efficacy for weight loss.

During the course of our conversation it turned out the client was living with her parents and her mother was harping on her to lose weight. When I asked if her mother nagged her other siblings in the same way, the client responded: "I have always had the weight of being the ideal child." Here was a possible pivot point: finding an intervention to ease the burden of being an ideal child offered an avenue for losing weight.

I agreed to do hypnosis. First, though, I suggested that if the client lost weight to please her mother rather than herself, it wouldn't work. She readily agreed. I suggested that, since she couldn't avoid her mother trying to monitor the ups and downs of her weight loss program, she should post a chart on their family refrigerator. On the chart, she would post her weight for that day—but rather than putting down what the scale said, she should make up whatever number she felt like.

"You mean, *lie?*" she said. Then she broke out into a big smile—the first of the session.

We then did some hypnosis, during which the client went to a clothing store, entered a changing room, then put on and took off clothing until she felt she'd found what was just right for her. On follow-up the client had lost weight and kept it off; she'd moved out of her parents' home and was pursuing her passion for singing. Perhaps the hypnosis played some role, but I think it was mostly a matter of morphing a weight loss program away from being a grim battle into a fun game that was also a path to autonomy.

Another way of finding pivot chords is by helping clients apply their skills in an overlooked, seemingly irrelevant area of their life to their problem. For example, I was seeing a client who still loved her alcoholic husband but was angry at his abusive outbursts; she felt caught between her religious beliefs that forbade divorce and her fears for her safety, as well as her family's urging her to leave him. Her favorite hobby was spending time in the kitchen, creating new meals of fusion cuisine. She found a way of applying her cooking skills to her conjugal problems and developed a recipe for deciding her next steps.

This kind of pivot chord is a core component of solution-oriented therapy. Solution-oriented approaches are helpful, very much in the spirit of "both/and." However, I think this is sometimes still a bit two-dimensional. The tetra lemma expands the field beyond "both/and" to liminal spaces spanning is, isn't, both, and neither. Here's a clinical example:

> I was seeing a woman in therapy who'd survived a truly horrific childhood but had not emerged unscathed. She'd needed lifelong treatment for severe episodes of major depressive disorder. By the time I saw her for supportive therapy she'd succeeded in building a life for herself with friendships, a good job, and a spiritual practice. She often felt satisfied, but she still had some intense downs.
>
> One session she told me she'd been sleeping poorly; she had trouble getting out of bed, couldn't concentrate, moved slowly; she got no pleasure from her usual activities but forced herself to keep going. She had no intention of killing herself but did have to brush away intrusive suicidal thoughts.
>
> Her affect was a bit flatter than usual, but she didn't present as obtunded or swaddled in sadness. Rather, she seemed down-to-earth and pragmatic. I said I was impressed at how she could describe her difficulties so matter-of-factly. She was a little surprised. "Why should you be impressed?" she said, then added: "Just because I'm depressed—why should I be miserable?"

Would that all our clients could find a way of being in distress *and* not being in distress, *both* and *neither*. She had found freedom from pigeonhole-ing herself into diagnostic categories.

Being free from "is" and "is not" helps us break free from dichotomies of problems and solutions, of psychopathology and mental health. In Buddhism, we say that if you want to experience enlightenment and nirvana, you can only find it in samsara and delusion. Healthy wholeness does not preclude feeling something is missing, and a sense of incompleteness does not get in the way of being undividedly yourself.

Let me conclude with a Zen koan that calls this forth:

> Zen teacher Dongshan was unwell.
> A student said to him, "You've been sick. Is there anyone who doesn't get ill?"
>
> *Dongshan replied:* "There is."
>
> [Note: this contradicts not only our everyday experience, but a fundamental Buddhist teaching].

The student was surprised. Could it be that if he practiced Zen faithfully he could become enlightened and wouldn't get sick?! So he asked Dongshan, maybe a little hopefully:

Student: Does the one who doesn't get ill take care of you?

Dongshan replied: *"I have the opportunity to take care of him."*

The student was confused. He said, "I don't understand! You're sick, and *you're* taking care of the one who doesn't get sick? What happens when you take care of the one who doesn't get ill?"

Dongshan replied: "Then I don't see any illness."

If you want to be a good therapist, stop being a therapist, but continue to engage with your clients in psychotherapy. Then you can meet them, and meet yourself meeting them, and not worry about it. Just enjoy the people you meet. Enjoy your life.

Don't look for problems, and don't seek for solutions. Put the fundamental point of your life, together with your client's life, in play.

Note

1 Editors' note: see Figure 20.1 in Chapter 20 (Rycroft) of this volume.

References

Bateson, G. (1980). *Mind and Nature: A Necessary Unity*. Dutton.

Bohart, A.C., & Tallman, K. (1999). *How Clients Make Therapy Work: The Process of Active Self-Healing*. APA Books.

Carney, J. (2020). Thinking avant la lettre: A review of 4E cognition. *Evolutionary Studies of Imaginative Culture*, 4(1), 77–90. https://doi.org/10.26613/esic/4.1.172

Cooper, M. (2010). *Essential Research Findings in Counselling and Psychotherapy: The Facts are Friendly*. Sage.

Dogen, E. (2010). Actualizing the fundamental point. In K. Tanahashi (Ed.), *Treasury of the True Dharma Eye: Zen Master Dogen's Shobogenzo* (pp. 29–33). Shambhala Publications. (original work published 1233)

Goulding, M.M., & Goulding, R.L. (1979). *Changing Lives Through Redecision Therapy*. Brunner/Mazel.

Gregory, R. (1997). *Eye and Brain*. Princeton University Press.

Kohak, E. (1984). *The Embers and the Stars: A Philosophical Inquiry into the Moral Sense of Nature*. University of Chicago Press.

Rosenbaum, R. (1993). Heavy ideals: Strategic single-session hypnotherapy. In R.A. Wells & V.J. Giannetti (Eds.), *Casebook of the Brief Psychotherapies* (pp. 109–128). Plenum Press.

Rosenbaum, R. (2014). The time of your life. In M.F. Hoyt & M. Talmon (Eds.), *Capturing the Moment: Single Session Therapy and Walk-In Services* (pp. 41–52). Crown House Publishing.

Rosenbaum, R. (2021). Gradually and suddenly: What Zen teaches us about change in SST. In M.F. Hoyt, J. Young, & P. Rycroft (Eds.), *Single Session Thinking and Practice in Global, Cultural, and Familial Contexts: Expanding Applications* (pp. 89–97). Routledge.

Rosenbaum, R., & Bohart, A.C. (2007). Psychotherapy: The art of experience. In S. Krippner, M. Bova, & L. Gray (Eds.), *Healing Stories: The Use of Narrative in Counseling and Psychotherapy* (pp. 295–324). Puente Press.

Rosenbaum, R., Hoyt, M.F., & Talmon, M. (1990). The challenge of single-session therapies: Creating pivotal moments. In R.A. Wells & V.J. Giannetti (Eds.), *Handbook of the Brief Psychotherapies* (pp. 165–189). Plenum Press.

Suzuki, S. (1970). *Zen Mind, Beginner's Mind: Informal Talks on Zen Meditation and Practice*. Weatherhill.

Talmon, M. (1990). *Single Session Therapy: Maximizing the Effect of the First (and Often Only) Therapeutic Encounter*. Jossey-Bass.

Chapter 5

The SST/OAAT Mindset and Using Single Session Thinking to Teach an SST Workshop

Michael F. Hoyt

The 1990 publication of Talmon's *Single Session Therapy: Maximizing the Effect of the First (and Often Only) Therapeutic Encounter* was a watershed event. As Jerome Frank (1990, pp. xi–xiii) noted in his Foreword to the book, rather than focusing on the "go slow" ethos of long-term therapy:

> In *Single-Session Therapy*, Moshe Talmon, by refreshing contrast, has seized upon and developed the implications of improvement after a single session, and he has succeeded in specifying at least some of the features of a single therapeutic contact that contributes to this outcome. His central assumption is that most outpatients, by virtue of the fact that they are functioning in the community, have considerable powers of spontaneous recuperation, as well as ability to resolve their problems. The therapist can mobilize these latent potentials in single-session therapy, empowering the patient by showing understanding of his or her problems and symptoms and offering alternative solutions and encouragement. [. . .] Talmon's presentation of single-session therapy is convincing. His style is exceptionally clear and refreshingly free of jargon. He makes no exaggerated claims, and his points are amply illustrated by clinical examples and supported by systematic empirical findings from his own experience and the relevant literature.[1]

Jay Haley (1993) also said, in his backcover endorsement of Talmon's (1993) follow-up book, *Single Session Solutions*:

> We once assumed that long-term therapy was the base from which all therapy was to be judged. Now it appears that therapy of a single interview could become the standard for estimating how long and how successful therapy should be.

DOI: 10.4324/9781032693828-7

Single Session Therapy heralded a significant shift. As Moshe (Talmon, 1993, p. 73) wrote:

> These concepts represent an alternative to the traditional model in psychiatry and psychotherapy: psychohealth replacing psychopathology, solutions replacing problems, and partnership replacing patronization, domination, and hierarchy.

The SST Mindset

Mindset refers to the guiding attitudes and beliefs that shape how we approach and make sense of the world—including how we think about psychotherapy (Hoyt & Cannistrà, 2023). As Talmon (1990, p. 116) wrote:

> Since much evidence suggests that a single session is likely to be the most common treatment duration during most professional careers, the development of more positive and productive attitudes toward SST is of crucial importance.

While an assortment of theoretical orientations (SFBT, strategic, narrative, CBT, psychodynamic, etc.) have all been shown to be useful, to my mind underlying SST are four fundamental mindset ideas:

1. Change is possible NOW.
2. Approach each single session one-at-a-time (OAAT), each visit a one-and-done event or episode complete unto itself—although more sessions might occur in the future, with the recognition that "one-at-a-time" doesn't necessarily mean "only one time."
3. The session is largely driven by the client's goals and skills—although, as Dryden (2020) and others (see Moccia, 2023) have noted, the therapist may also contribute skills and resources as well as help identify those of the client.
   and
4. Constructive minimalism, that is, focusing therapeutically on what will help the client now rather than on diagnostic assessment (Talmon, 1990, 2018). *CURE* is a very problematic concept. I used to have a supervisor who had a sign on the wall in his office that said "Bacon can be cured. People grow and change."[2]

For some, this "meta perspective," as Martin Söderquist (2023, p. 46) has called it in his excellent book on SST/OAAT with couples, can be new and maybe a bit overwhelming. The basic ideas involve making fundamental mindset shifts:

1. From the conventional idea that therapy must take a long time and that we should proceed slowly to the idea that there is no time but the present and that change can occur NOW. "Moments are Forever" (Talmon & Hoyt, 2014); *this* is "The Eternal Now" (Talmon, 2018). As Bob Rosenbaum has neatly put it (2014, 2021, p. 95): "Psychotherapy ceases to be short or long, gradual or sudden. [. . .] We exist not *in*, but *as* the time of our lives." Indeed, there is really no time but NOW—as Dante Alighieri (c. 1265–1321) said in *The Divine Comedy*: "Everywhere is here and every when is now."[3]
   and
2. From the conventional idea that it is the expert therapist who determines what is wrong and how to fix it, to the idea that the client is competent and capable. Our therapeutic job may be more to bring forth the client's solution rather than to "fix" or "cure" the patient.

Different therapy models can inform SST, but in the moment creativity involves "a genuine *process* of undetermined becoming: it cannot be the mere unfolding of an already completely determined sequence of steps to a ready-made conclusion" (Morson, 1994, p. 24). I like the way Nobel Prize laureate Bob Dylan (2022, p. 128) said it:

One of the ways creativity works is the brain tries to fill in holes and gaps. We fill in missing bits of pictures, snatches of dialogue, we finish rhymes and invent stories to explain things we do not know.

How and where you look determines what you see, and what you see influences what you do, around and 'round. Our mindset—our basic guiding beliefs—shapes the lenses through which we see the world and ourselves. Gray (2020, p. 54) notes that the term *theory* comes from the Greek *theorein*, meaning "to look at." As Einstein said, it is our theories—our mindset—that determine what we can see. Alas, much traditional psychotherapy training inculcates beliefs that clients are not capable (that's why they're called "patients"—see Hoyt, 1979/2017) and that the therapist is The Expert on what is required and that we should proceed slowly and gradually. Economics that reward us for long-term therapy reinforce this mindset. And these mindset beliefs are not only held by therapists. We've all seen cartoon images of therapy that depict a patient laying on a couch or television programs in which the patient is endlessly "in treatment." They teach the public long-term therapy prophecies. That's why the term *Single* Session Therapy is so powerful—as Jeff Young (2018) has written, it is "in your face" and disruptive of the usual "go slow" mindset.

Applying SST Principles When Teaching an SST Workshop

My intention here and now is to highlight some ways I organize and teach SST workshops using the mindset of single session thinking so that process mirrors content, form follows function, and the medium becomes the message. These parallels or isomorphisms can help reinforce learning and application of an SST/OAAT mindset.[4]

1. General Philosophy for Teaching a Workshop

I believe that a good workshop, like a good therapy session, should be always engaging, usually educational, and occasionally inspirational (Hoyt, 2017, p. 227). Wouldn't it be grand to take a workshop that was "continuing inspiration" as well as "continuing education"? My primary intent is to get SST workshop participants to be excited to recognize and use their own existing knowledge and skills optimally, plus learn some new ones. The same is true with SST clients: excitement, opening the door, evoking possibility, asking, "What are your best hopes for today's session?"

SST works better when the therapist has the mindset that *change is possible NOW*. At the 2nd International SST Symposium, held in 2016 in Banff, Canada, I asked (Hoyt, 2017, p. 306) *"Where is the magic?"* and answered, *"THE MAGIC IS WITHIN, BETWEEN, and AROUND."*

I think therapy takes place within a "Context of Competence" (Hoyt, 2014; see Figure 5.1). Effective therapy occurs when the client's GOALS are identified and their RESOURCES brought to bear via the THERAPEUTIC ALLIANCE.

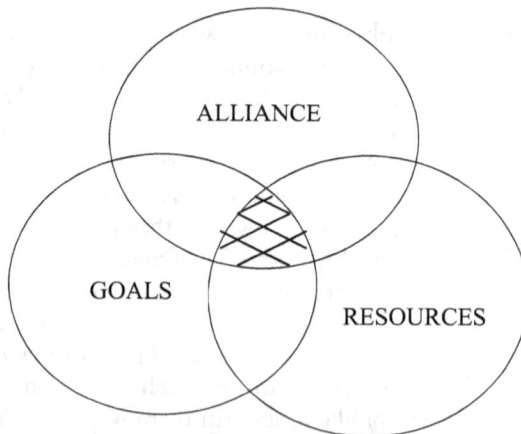

Figure 5.1 Context of competence.

Source: (from Michael F. Hoyt 2014. © Michael F. Hoyt 2014. Used by agreement)

Therapy takes place where the three intersect. If you have GOALS and an ALLIANCE but don't access RESOURCES, nothing happens. If you have RESOURCES and an ALLIANCE, but don't have GOALS, there's nothing to do, no direction. If the client could match up their GOALS and RESOURCES on their own, they wouldn't need the therapist. Hence, all three are needed: the *Context of Competence* is where GOALS and RESOURCES come together through the ALLIANCE. The work is collaborative. Effective therapy involves all three (Hoyt, 2017, p. 300).

This can sometimes be achieved in one session—especially if therapist and client believe it can be so. Insistence produces resistance, imposition produces opposition, push produces pushback—so I think it is important to offer and invite, but not demand, one visit (Hoyt, 2017, p. 296). Asking "Why now?" and highlighting the benefits of changing and the consequences of not changing may be helpful.

2. SST Workshop Goals

A basic SST workshop purpose is to help attendees understand and embrace a single session/one-at-a-time (SST/OAAT) mindset, which requires a shift from the usual "We'll just keep meeting until we're done" approach to an appreciation of what Talmon (Chapter 3 this volume) called "The Golden Hour." When teaching, I like to point out, quoting my colleagues Monte Bobele and Arnie Slive (2014), that rather than thinking "We *only* have one hour" we could instead think "We have a WHOLE hour"—noting that lots can be covered in a single session. ONE is *de facto* the most frequent number of sessions attended. (The most frequent length of therapy is actually ZERO sessions; people think of going to therapy but never do.) Amongst those who do attend, 1 session is most frequent, followed by 2, followed by 3; and since it was clients (not therapists) who invented SST, and since SST is often helpful with a wide variety of problems, I think we are being respectful and ethical to appreciate and work with clients' natural help-seeking patterns.

Sometimes it is beneficial to note that it was Sigmund Freud—often thought of as the father of long-term therapy—who was the first single session therapist. I may quote Jay Haley, who would sometimes ask, "IF I told you that we were only going to meet once, what would you want to focus on today?" and/or Mary and Bob Goulding (1979), who would ask their basic redecision therapy contract question, "What are you willing to change today?" In her new book, Jessica L. Schleider (2023) speaks of "meaningful moments." We can cite the abundant empirical evidence (see Hoyt, 2025; Pietrabissa, Chapter 13 this volume) for frequency and effectiveness of SST with a wide variety of problems.

Our mindset and psychotherapy theories direct us toward different time orientations, toward focusing on the past, the present, or the future.

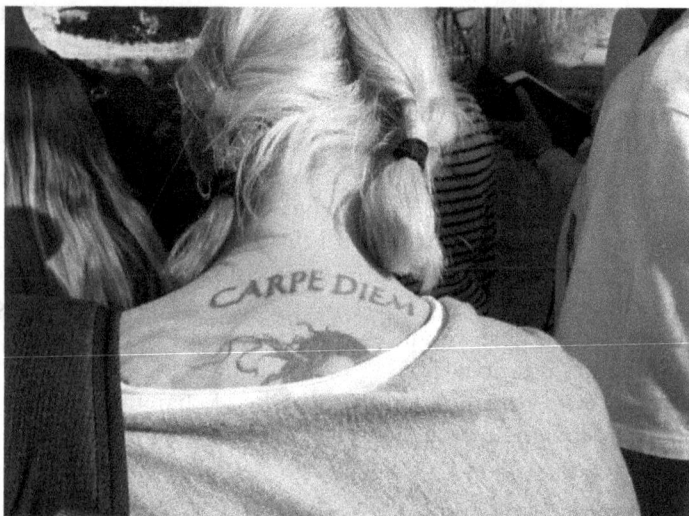

Figure 5.2 Thank you, Horace!
Source: (© 2017 Michael F. Hoyt. Used by agreement)

All may be useful, but as Milton Erickson (1954, p. 127) reminded us, "Emphasis should be placed more upon what the patient does in the present and will do in the future than upon a mere understanding of why some long-past event occurred." Indeed, the Roman philosopher Horace in 20 BCE said (quoted in Scott Samuelson, *Rome as a Guide to the Good Life*, 2023, p. 242): "Dare to be wise: do it. If you don't strike off now for the good life, you're like the bumpkin waiting to cross the river until it flows by. It keeps flowing. It just keeps flowing."

When I was walking around the Roman Forum a few years ago, I saw this woman in front of me:[5]

When the famous American baseball player Yogi Berra was asked "What time is it?" he answered, "Do you mean NOW?" Dr. Martin Luther King Jr. spoke of "the fierce urgency of now." Leo Tolstoy (1885) said: "Remember then: there is only one time that is important—Now! It is the most important time, because it is the only time when we have any power." It is good to "capture the moment" (Young & Rycroft, 1997; Hoyt & Talmon, 2014) and motivate people by asking, "Why now did you decide to call?" and by perhaps noting that "If you don't change directions, you're going to wind up where you're heading." As Giorgio Nardone and Paul Watzlawick (1990, 2005; see Chapter 18 this volume) and others have noted, we need to address how IN THE PRESENT the client is staying "stuck."

We should pay attention to what we pay attention to. Therapists don't need to give up useful things we have learned, but it should be mindset, not *mind-set-in-concrete* (Hoyt & Cannistrà, 2023; also see Cannistrà, 2021). As Erickson said (Erickson, Rossi, & Rossi, 1976, p. 213), "There is nothing wrong with having rigid sets. But if you want to alter yourself in some way, you must be unashamedly aware that you do have sets and it's better to have a greater variety of sets."

We can see the limiting role of certain mindset belief systems when, teaching and practicing SST, we encounter "therapist resistances to brief and single session therapy" (Hoyt, 1985/1995) such as the belief that "more is better," belief in the myth of the "pure gold of analysis," the belief in the inappropriateness of greater therapist activity, and the confusion of clients' interests (usually efficient problem solving) with what may interest therapists (often comprehensive exploration of psychosocial issues).

The response "Hmmm, that's interesting" (*or* "That's a really good question") often signals that someone has bumped up again their underlying mindset and that a second-order change, an alteration in the rules that govern their attitudes and beliefs, may be in the air. Sometimes eyes roll up and search to the side when this happens (Ziegler & Hoyt, 2023)—a sign of what Neurolinguistic Programming (retrieved from Wikipedia on August 22, 2023) would call a *transderivational search*.

Just as clients who want help NOW may elect to have a single session by calling a counseling center that specializes in SST or by responding to an option for SST on a website or by walking into (or online, clicking into) a clinic that offers OAAT without appointment, by signing up for an SST symposium or workshop therapist-trainees wanting to help NOW have selected for themselves the goal of learning about single session thinking and practice. I think that would include those of us who are here today.

Paralleling the identification of specific therapy goals with clients, I have found that early in a workshop it is good to ask attendees, "What do you want to make sure we address today?" I write their responses on a whiteboard or large flip-pad and ask, "How will you know if we've achieved that goal?" As in SST, a variant of the Miracle Question (de Shazer, 1988) can be used: "Suppose this turns out to be a great workshop. What will be different, how will you know?" I might also comment, using a golf metaphor to highlight the importance of clear goals, that "It's a long day on the course if you don't know where the hole is" (Hoyt, 1996/2017, p. 33). Near the end of an SST workshop, we take time to review the list to make sure attendees' concerns have been attended to. I might also ask another version of the Miracle Question: "Suppose tomorrow, when you wake up in your office, you're an even more effective single session therapist than you were before! What will you be doing differently now that you've taken this workshop?"

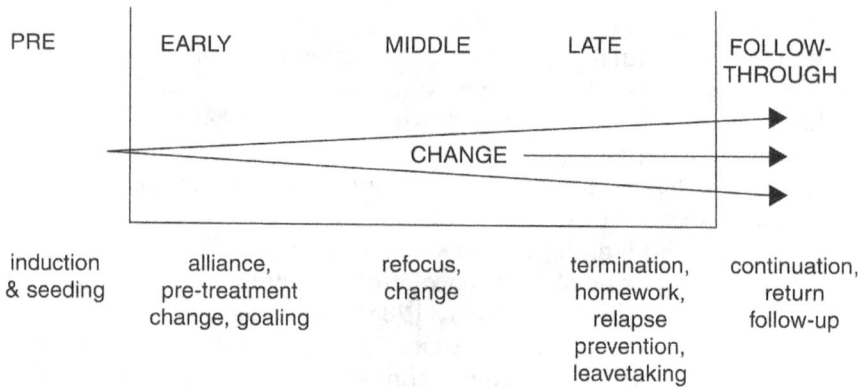

Figure 5.3 The structure of Single Session Therapy: tasks and skills associated with different phases of a session.

Source: (from Michael F. Hoyt 1995; ©Michael F. Hoyt 1995. Used by agreement.)

3.   SST Thinking and the Structure of a Typical One-Day Workshop

There is often a temporal structure to SST (see Figure 5.3), with early phases of a session focused on induction, alliance, and goal setting; the middle phase focused on making changes; and the later phases focused on termination and follow-through.

Aspects of the client-therapist relationship may be repeated in the therapist-supervisor relationship (Ekstein & Wallerstein, 1972; Frances & Clarkin, 1981; Hoyt, 1991/1995), including, as Pam Rycroft (2018) has noted, in both therapeutic and supervisory single sessions. Indeed, a parallel time structure may be used in organizing an SST workshop: early workshop stages involve building alliance,[6] changing mindset, and identifying workshop goals with the audience; the middle phase involves focusing on learning and practicing skills; and the latter stages involve discussion of how trainees will follow through, applying single session thinking and practice, and continuing to develop their SST skills.

4.   Favorite SST Workshop Exercises/Processes

When a goal is improvement of skills, not just acquisition of theoretical information, learning is usually much enhanced by experiential practice activities in addition to reading or attending a lecture. Quoting Erickson (in Zeig, 1980, p. 72) again, "I believe that patients and students should do things. They learn better, remember better." Along related lines, Carl Whitaker (1983, p. 40) commented: "Explanation leads to recognition. Experience leads to change."

Here are four workshop activities I have found useful:

1. To help participants see the potential value of a single session, early on I will often ask workshop attendees to think of a time when, through a single meeting or even a single interaction, they made a significant change in their life. To give some encouragement, range, and flavor, I might cite some single session experiences from my own life. I also note that every single session need not have "zingers" (Ritterman, 2019) nor produce dramatic changes—that most times just some support and incremental gain (or avoidance of worsening) is what clients want and will be a good SST result. I watch for nodding heads and may ask a few folks to share their thoughts.

2. A second process involves providing attendees with handouts containing lots of questions useful in an SST—and having the attendees break into small groups and experiment with asking and answering the questions. Numerous examples of these typical SST questions—which can be divided into pre-treatment, early, middle, late, and follow-through (again, see Figure 5.2)—can be found in various publications, including extensive lists in my recent book, *Single Session Therapy: A Clinical Introduction to Principles and Practices* (Hoyt, 2025).[7] Here are just a few such questions, informed by an SST/OAAT mindset:

Pretreatment

Change begins even before we have contact with the client. He or she or they have decided there is a problem and would like assistance to resolve the difficulty. Some questions to ask while making an initial appointment (online or phone call):

- What's the problem—why have you called now?
- How have you tried to solve the problem so far—how did it work?
- When the problem isn't present (or isn't bad), what is going on differently?

Early in the Session

As we begin a session, we attend carefully to forming a good alliance, inquiring about possible changes since our last contact, and establishing goals for the session. Some useful questions might include:

- Since we last spoke (*or*, Since you decided to call), what have you noticed that may be a bit better or different? How did that happen? What did you do?

- If we were only going to meet once or a few times, what problem would you want to focus on solving first? How would you prefer the future to be?
- What needs to happen here today so that when you leave you can feel this visit was worthwhile?
- What decided you to call now? What will happen if you don't change?

In the Middle of the Session

We keep track of the client's goal(s) and whether we have a good working alliance and are going in the right direction or if some course "corrections" need to be made. Possible refocusing is directed by the client's response to questions such as these:

- How did that work?
- Is this being helpful? What can I do to be more helpful to you now?

Late in the Session and Follow-Through

Termination—extracting the therapist from the successful equation (Gustafson, 1986, p. 279; also see Hoyt & Rosenbaum, 2018)—becomes central:

- When we finish meeting today, what do you want to be taking with you?
- Which of the helpful things you've been doing do you think you should continue to do? How can you do this?
- Who can be helpful to you in doing _____? What might interfere, and how can you prepare to deal with those challenges?
- Who will be glad to hear about your progress? Who in your present or past (family, friends, colleagues) would support your efforts?

3. A third process involves describing episodes (and sometime showing brief video clips) from different SST therapy sessions, demonstrating examples of clients practicing solutions, of identifying and prioritizing a therapeutic focus when the client presents multiple issues, and of the use of an imagined other as a helper or ally—and then asking attendees to consider and describe in detail, perhaps role-playing, how they might adapt the methods to their own clients.

4. A fourth process, which I call "What Can We Learn from Our Internalized Clients?" was developed with my colleague David Nylund (Hoyt & Nylund, 2000/1997; see Hoyt, 2025, Chapter 7). In workshops, I want participants to recognize that they already have SST skills.[8] This to me is consistent with (or parallel to) the idea of helping clients to better utilize their own skills to solve their problems.

Instructions are printed on a handout. The practice of *internalized other questioning* is explained, the idea that the "self" is made up of a person's internalized community of significant others and that one can "step into" the experience of the other by being addressed by the name of the other person and imagining that person as best you can—the way they talked, what they said, their intonation, how they sat, how they looked, and so forth. Workshop participants are invited to think of a specific person (client) they worked with in an SST or other effective brief therapy. A list of guideline questions is provided, and they are then interviewed *as that person* to see what our internalized clients can offer to nurture and inform us.

We then have the subject step out of her or his client's experience and return to being interviewed as herself or himself and have somebody ask a variety of questions.

We then have the participants switch roles: the interviewer becomes the interviewee and vice versa. Again, they work through the internalized other questions for 10–15 minutes, then interview as self. Interesting discoveries and greater appreciations often occur. I'll ask interviewers and interviewees to share what they learned.

A NOTE ABOUT DEMONSTRATION INTERVIEWS

A live demonstration interview at a conference or in a workshop can be an exciting in-the-moment single session learning experience. Indeed, Joseph Barber (1990, p. 437) in his paper "Miracle Cures? Therapeutic Consequences of Clinical Demonstrations" cited one of the first SST presentations (Talmon, Hoyt, & Rosenbaum, 1988) by Moshe, Bob, and myself ("When the First Session May Be the Last"), given at the 1988 Brief Therapy Conference, and highlighted several of our key mindset points:

- Expect change.
- View each encounter as a whole, complete unto itself.
- Don't rush or try to be brilliant.
- Emphasize abilities and strengths, rather than pathology.
- Life, not therapy, is the great teacher.

I caution, however, that when possible it is good to screen the client beforehand, even if only for a moment ("What problem do you want help with?") lest you find yourself in front of an audience with someone very unlikely to get benefit and be able to stop with a single session. It is important that the therapist manage the demonstration session in a way that leaves the client in a safe place and lets the audience see the positive potential of one session.

A NOTE ABOUT THE NEED FOR CULTURAL ADJUSTMENTS

When attempting SST (or any therapy) it is wise to appreciate cultural contexts. Therapy can be much more effective and efficient if you work within someone's cultural context, and especially if you don't work against their culture (Hoyt, Young, & Rycroft, 2021, pp. 336–337). Or, as Flavio and I (Hoyt & Cannistrà, 2021/2023) put it in our ironic tongue-in-cheek paper "Common Errors in Single Session Therapy," if you want to *avoid* single session success, rub the client's culture the wrong way.

The same is true in teaching SST. I'm American, and I've learned when teaching in places such as Japan and Mexico that it is important to consider ways personal, familial, regional, and national cultures may influence my and the audience's mindsets and create expectations about goals and roles and about topics and pace that can either promote or interfere with successful SST. I imagine the same to be true in Italy (where this chapter was first presented)—for example, how to connect, what can be talked about and when, how is feedback given and received?

Conclusion

Effective Single Session Therapy helps people organize and catalyze, integrate and motivate so that they can better access their own resources. [. . .] Our primary therapeutic effort and expertise should be directed toward encouraging, eliciting, evoking, exploring, and elaborating whatever the client brings that can be helpful to get them to where they want to go (Hoyt, 2014/2017, p. 285).

To me (Hoyt, 2025), the basics of SST are working in a collaborative and culturally appropriate way:

1. Plan for one visit ("one-at-a-time").
2. Identify the client's goal for the session (which may involve hearing their "problem" or "complaint" and helping them recognize that something different needs to be done to get a different result).
3. Look for client strengths and abilities that can be used to make a desired change ("empowerment").
4. Encourage application in problematic situation.
5. Leave the door open for possible follow-up. (Remember: "OAAT" does not mean necessarily "only one time.")

As my colleagues Moshe and Bob and I (Hoyt, Rosenbaum, & Talmon, 1992, p. 63) wrote:

The therapist needs to be versatile, innovative, and pragmatic, asking: "What would help this [client] today?" [. . .] Nothing works all the time, but what might work this time?

And, as my colleagues Jeff, Pam, and I (Hoyt et al., 2021, p. 3) wrote:

> The essence of single session thinking is to approach the first session as if it will be the only session, while creating opportunities for further work if it is requested by the client. What emerges is a collaborative, direct, and transparent approach to providing services that puts the client in a very active role in determining the focus and length of the work.

I hope these remarks about mindset and using single session thinking when doing therapy—and when teaching and attending SST workshops—will provide a few keys and clues for seeing, as our symposium title says, how and why SST is effective, efficient, and excellent.

Notes

1 Frank (1990, p. xiii) also commented: "Readers should not overlook the author's explicit recognition that, while perhaps as many as four-fifths of psychiatric outpatients receiving single-session therapy respond favorably, the remaining one-fifth, as well as most inpatients, require considerably more treatment."
2 In English the terms *heal, whole, health, hale,* and *holy* all derive from the same old Middle English and Anglo-Saxon words (*hole, hale*; Hoyt, 2017, p. 133). People who are happy seem complete in the present, "integral in the moment rather than distended across time by regret or anxiety" (Grudin, 1982, p. 188). Treatment is something that comes from the outside, but as Milton Erickson (quoted in Short, Erickson, & Klein, 2005, p. 19) and others have emphasized, healing occurs within the person.
3 Aristotle (quoted by Gleick, 2016, p. 251): "To start, then: the following considerations would make one suspect that [time] either does not exist at all or barely, and in an obscure way. One part of it has been and is not, while the other is going to be and is not yet." Luigi Boscolo and Paolo Bertrando (1993, p. 34) in their book *The Times of Time,* quote St. Augustine (354–430 C.E.) making a similar observation in his *Confessions*: "What is by now evident and clear is that neither future nor past exists, and it is inexact language to speak of three times—past, present, and future. Perhaps it would be exact to say: there are three times, a present of things past, a present of things present, a present of things to come. In the soul there are these three aspects of time, and I do not see them anywhere else. The present considering the past is the memory; the present considering the future is expectation." T.S. Eliot (1943) asked, "How do we live in time to conquer time?" Jorge Luis Borges (1947/1964, p. 234) wrote: "Time is the substance I am made of. Time is a river which sweeps me along, but I am the river; it is a tiger which destroys me, but I am the tiger; it is a fire which consumes me, but I am the fire." Octavio Paz (1963, pp. 124–125) wrote: "Yesterday is today, tomorrow is today, today everything is today." Nikos Kazantzakis (1957/1965, p. 478) also said: "No other moment exists: before and behind this moment is Nothing." Poet Mary Dorcey (1995, p. 19) cautioned that tomorrow will come suddenly and slip into yesterday and take the good times. Meditation teacher Ram Dass (1971) advised, "Be here now," Eckhart Tolle (1999) spoke of "The Power of Now," and American singer-songwriter Billy Joe Shaver (2009)

exhorted us to "Live Forever Now." For more, see Hoyt (1990/2017, especially "On Time in Brief Therapy").

4 A Google search for "How to be an effective presenter" will yield many resources on the general topic of successful presentations, all emphasizing knowing your material, organizing and rehearsing, being enthusiastic and connecting with the audience, using humor, checking your AV equipment, etc. Here I will focus on specific uses of single session thinking when teaching SST workshops. Others (e.g., Young, Rycroft, & Weir, 2014; Young, 2021; Dryden, 2021; Cannistrà & Piccirilli, 2021/2011; Miller, Xing, Yaorui, & Yilin, 2021) have also described methods for teaching SST workshops; and Hoyt (1995) and Rycroft (2018) have explicated how an SST framework can be used in one-on-one supervision sessions.

5 Samuelson (2023, p. 101) notes that while "seize the day" is the most common translation of Horace's *carpe diem*, "the verb [*carpe*] is closer to 'pluck,' like picking a daisy or an apple. I've gone with 'reap' to keep in mind that the time is ripe."

6 How one responds to the first audience question or two can help set the tone. *Alliance*: it is especially important to be welcoming. The authors (Bowles et al., 2022, p. 170) of *How to Tell a Story* report: "Takeoffs and landings are considered the most dangerous parts of a flight. And so it goes with stories." The same can be said about therapy and workshop teaching. Arrivals and departures, beginnings and endings, primacy and recency effects (Hoyt, 2025, pp. 51–55) are often crucial.

7 See Cannistrà and Piccirilli (2020); Connie and Froerer (2023); Dryden (2016, 2019); Hoyt (1990, 1995, 2000, 2009, 2017, 2025); Hoyt and Talmon (2014); Hoyt and Rosenbaum (2018); Ratner, George, and Iveson (2012); Rycroft and Young (2021); Slive and Bobele (2011); K. Young, (2018).

8 I agreed when I read Brett Steenbarger (2012, p. 123, emphasis in original): "My goal [. . .] is not to enable you to conduct brief therapy in the manner of recognized practitioners. I also do not intend to encourage you to do therapy my way. Instead, I wish you to *consider becoming more of the effective helper that you already are when you are at your best*. Identify what you are already doing when you are an efficient, effective facilitator of change, and then do those things more consistently and intentionally."

References

Barber, J. (1990). Miracle cures? Therapeutic consequences of clinical demonstrations. In J.K. Zeig & S.G. Gilligan (Eds.), *Brief Therapy: Myths, Methods, and Metaphors* (pp. 437–442). Brunner/Mazel.

Bobele, M., & Slive, A. (2014). One session at a time: When you have a whole hour. In M.F. Hoyt & M. Talmon (Eds.), *Capturing the Moment: Single Session Therapy and Walk-In Services* (pp. 95–119). Crown House Publishing.

Borges, J.L. (1964). A new refutation of time. In *Labyrinths: Selected Stories & Other Writing* (pp. 217–234). New Directions. (Work originally published in Spanish in 1947)

Boscolo, L., & Bertrando, P. (1993). *The Times of Time: A New Perspective in Systemic Therapy and Consultation*. Norton. (Work originally also published in Italian in 1993)

Bowles, M., Burns, C., Hixson, J., Jenness, S.A., & Tellers, K. (2022). *How to Tell a Story: The Essential Guide to Memorable Storytelling from the Moth*. Crown.

Cannistrà, F. (2021). The vital role of the therapist's mindset. In M.F. Hoyt, J. Young, & P. Rycroft (Eds.), *Single Session Thinking and Practice in Global, Cultural, and Familial Contexts* (pp. 77–88). Routledge.

Cannistrà, F., & Piccirilli, F. (Eds.). (2021). *Single Session Therapy: Principles and Practices*. Giunti. (Work originally published 2012 in Italian.)

Connie, E.E., & Froerer, A.S. (2023). *The Solution Focused Brief Therapy Diamond: A New Approach to SFBT That Will Empower Both Practitioner and Client to Achieve the Best Outcomes*. Hay House.

Dass, R. (1971). *Be Here Now*. Lama Foundation/Crown Publishing.

de Shazer, S. (1988). *Clues: Investigating Solutions in Brief Therapy*. Norton.

Dorcey, M. (1995). The good times. In *The River That Carries Me* (p. 19). Salmon Publishing.

Dryden, W. (2016). *Single Session Integrated Cognitive Behavior Therapy (SSI-CBT): Distinctive Features*. Routledge.

Dryden, W. (2019). *Single-Session Therapy: 100 Key Points and Techniques*. Routledge.

Dryden, W. (2020). Single-session one-at-a-time therapy: A personal approach. *Australian and New Zealand Journal of Family Therapy*, 41(3), 283–301.

Dryden, W. (2021). Sign up, meet up, speak out: Single sessions in the context of meet-up groups. In M.F. Hoyt, J. Young, & P. Rycroft (Eds.), *Single Session Thinking and Practice in Global, Cultural, and Familial Contexts* (pp. 153–162). Routledge.

Dylan, B. (2022). *The Philosophy of Modern Song*. Simon & Schuster.

Ekstein, R., & Wallerstein, R.S. (1972). *The Teaching and Learning of Psychotherapy* (2nd ed.). International Universities Press.

Eliot, T.S. (1943). Burnt Norton. In *Four Quartets* (pp. 3–8). Harcourt, Brace, & World.

Erickson, M.H. (1954). Special techniques in brief hypnotherapy. *Journal of Clinical and Experimental Hypnosis*, 2, 109–129.

Erickson, M.H., Rossi, E.L., & Rossi, S.I. (1976). *Hypnotic Realities: The Induction of Clinical Hypnosis and Forms of Indirect Suggestion*. Irvington.

Frances, A., & Clarkin, J.F. (1981). Parallel techniques in supervision and treatment. *Psychiatric Quarterly*, 53, 242–248.

Frank, J.D. (1990). Foreword. In M. Talmon (Ed.), *Single Session Therapy* (pp. xi–xiii). Jossey-Bass.

Gleick, J. (2016). *Time Travel*. Pantheon Books.

Goulding, M.M., & Goulding, R.L. (1979). *Changing Lives Through Redecision Therapy*. Brunner/Mazel.

Gray, J. (2020). *Feline Philosophy: Cats and the Meaning of Life*. Picador.

Grudin, R. (1982). *Time and the Art of Living*. Ticknor & Fields.

Gustafson, J.P. (1986). *The Complex Secret of Brief Psychotherapy*. Norton.

Hoyt, M.F. (1979). "Patient" or "client": What's in a name? *Psychotherapy: Theory, Research, and Practice*, 16(1), 46–47. Reprinted in Hoyt, M.F. (2017). *Brief Therapy and Beyond* (pp. 1–2). Routledge.

Hoyt, M.F. (1985). Therapist resistances to short-term dynamic psychotherapy. *Journal of the American Academy of Psychoanalysis*, 13, 93–112. Reprinted in Hoyt, M.F. (1995). *Brief Therapy and Managed Care* (pp. 219–236). Jossey-Bass.

Hoyt, M.F. (1990). On time in brief therapy. In R.A. Wells & V.J. Giannetti (Eds.), *Handbook of the Brief Psychotherapies* (pp. 115–143). Plenum. [An expanded version appears in Hoyt, M.F. (2017). *Brief Therapy and Beyond* (pp. 6–32). Routledge.]

Hoyt, M.F. (1991). Teaching and learning short-term psychotherapy within an HMO. In C.S. Austad & W.H. Berman (Eds.), *Psychotherapy in Managed Health Care: The Optimal Use of Time and Resources* (pp. 98–108). American Psychological Association. Reprinted in Hoyt, M.F. (1995). *Brief Therapy and Managed Care: Reading for Contemporary Practice* (pp. 63–68). Jossey-Bass.

Hoyt, M.F. (1996). A golfer's guide to brief therapy (with footnotes for baseball fans). In M.F. Hoyt (Ed.), *Constructive Therapies* (Vol. 2, pp. 306–318). Guilford Press. Reprinted in Hoyt, M.F. (2017). *Brief Therapy and Beyond* (pp. 33–43). Routledge.

Hoyt, M.F. (2000). *Some Stories Are Better Than Others*. Brunner/Mazel.

Hoyt, M.F. (2009). *Brief Psychotherapies: Principles and Practices*. Zeig, Tucker, & Theisen.

Hoyt, M.F. (2014). Psychology and my gallbladder: An insider's account of a single session therapy. In M.F. Hoyt & M. Talmon (Eds.), *Capturing the Moment: Single Session Therapy and Walk-In Services* (pp. 53–72). Crown House Publishing. Reprinted in Hoyt, M.F. (2017). *Brief Therapy and Beyond* (pp. 272–286). Routledge.

Hoyt, M.F. (2017). *Brief Therapy and Beyond: Stories, Language, Love, Hope, and Time*. Routledge.

Hoyt, M.F. (2025). *Single Session Therapy: A Clinical Introduction to Principles and Practices*. Routledge.

Hoyt, M.F., & Cannistrà, F. (2021). Common errors in single session therapy. *Journal of Systemic Therapies*, 40(3), 29–41. [Reprinted in Hoyt, M.F., & Cannistrà, F. (2023). *Brief Therapy Conversations* (pp. 157–169). Routledge.]

Hoyt, M.F., & Cannistrà, F. (2023). *Brief Therapy Conversations: Exploring Efficient Intervention in Psychotherapy*. Routledge.

Hoyt, M.F., & Nylund, D. (2000). The joy of narrative: An exercise for learning from our internalized clients. In M.F. Hoyt (Ed.), *Some Stories Are Better Than Others* (pp. 201–206). Brunner/Mazel. [An earlier version appeared in *Journal of Systemic Therapies*, 1997, 16(4), 361–366.]

Hoyt, M.F., & Rosenbaum, R. (2018). Some ways to end an SST. In M.F. Hoyt, M. Bobele, A. Slive, J. Young, & M. Talmon (Eds.), *Single-Session Therapy by Walk-In or Appointment* (pp. 318–323). Routledge.

Hoyt, M.F., Rosenbaum, R., & Talmon, M. (1992). Planned single-session psychotherapy. In S.H. Budman, M.F. Hoyt, & S. Friedman (Eds.), *The First Session in Brief Therapy* (pp. 59–86). Guilford Press.

Hoyt, M.F., & Talmon, M. (Eds.). (2014). *Capturing the Moment: Single Session Therapy and Walk-In Services*. Crown House Publishing.

Hoyt, M.F., Young, J., & Rycroft, P. (Eds.). (2021). *Single Session Thinking and Practice in Global, Cultural, and Familial Context: Expanding Applications*. Routledge.

Kazantzakis, N. (1965). *Report to Greco*. Simon & Schuster. (Work originally published in 1957 in Greek.)

Miller, J.K., Xing, D., Yaorui, H., & Yilin, X. (2021). Single session team family therapy (SSTFT) in China: A seven-step protocol for adapting Western methods in Eastern contexts. In M.F. Hoyt, J. Young, & P. Rycroft (Eds.), *Single Session Thinking and Practice in Global, Cultural, and Familial Contexts* (pp. 245–254). Routledge.

Moccia, F. (Mod.) (2023, November 10). *Is it possible to practice it with any theoretical approach?* SST Conversation Panel with M. Bobele, W. Dryden, A.

Slive, and H. van Empel at 4th International Symposium on Single Session Therapy, Rome.

Morson, G.S. (1994). *Narrative and Freedom: The Shadows of Time*. Yale University Press.

Nardone, G., & Watzlawick, P. (1990). *The Art of Change: Strategic Therapy and Hypnotherapy Without Trance*. Jossey-Bass.

Nardone, G., & Watzlawick, P. (2005). *Brief Strategic Therapy: Philosophy, Techniques, and Research*. Jason Aronson Publishers.

Paz, O. (1963). The endless instant/*No hay salida?* In D. Levertov (Trans.), *Early Poems 1935–1955* (pp. 124–125). New Directions.

Ratner, H., George, E., & Iveson, C. (2012). *Solution Focused Brief Therapy: 100 Key Points & Techniques*. Routledge.

Ritterman, M. (2019). The single stroke: What makes "zingers" zing? In M.F. Hoyt & M. Bobele (Eds.), *Creative Therapy in Challenging Situations: Unusual Interventions to Help Clients* (pp. 163–171). Routledge.

Rosenbaum, R. (2014). The time of your life. In M.F. Hoyt & M. Talmon (Eds.), *Capturing the Moment: Single Session Therapy and Walk-In Services* (pp. 41–52). Crown House Publishing.

Rosenbaum, R. (2021). Gradually and suddenly: What Zen teaches us about change in SST. In M.F. Hoyt, J. Young, & P. Rycroft (Eds.), *Single Session Thinking and Practice in Global, Cultural, and Familial Contexts: Expanding Applications* (pp. 89–97). Routledge.

Rycroft, P. (2018). Capturing the moment in supervision. In M.F. Hoyt, M. Bobele, A. Slive, J. Young, & M. Talmon (Eds.), *Single-Session Therapy by Walk-In or Appointment* (pp. 347–366). Routledge.

Rycroft, P., & Young, J. (2021). Translating single session thinking into practice. In M.F. Hoyt, J. Young, & P. Rycroft (Eds.), *Single Session Thinking and Practice in Global, Cultural, and Familial Contexts* (pp. 42–53). Routledge.

Samuelson, S. (2023). *Rome as a Guide to the Good Life: A Philosophical Grand Tour*. University of Chicago Press.

Schleider, J. (2023). *Little Treatments, Big Effects: How to Build Meaningful Moments That Can Transform Your Mental Health*. Robinson.

Shaver, B.J. (2009). *I'm Gonna Live Forever*. Luck Films.

Short, D., Erickson, B.A., & Klein, R.E. (2005). *Hope and Resiliency: Understanding the Psychotherapeutic Strategies of Milton H. Erickson, M.D.* Crown House Publishing.

Slive, A., & Bobele, M. (Eds.). (2011). *When One Hour is All You Have: Effective Therapy for Walk-In Clients*. Zeig, Tucker, & Theisen.

Söderquist, M. (2023). *Single Session One at a Time Counseling for Couples*. Routledge. [Work originally published in 2020 in Swedish.]

Steenbarger, B.N. (2012). Solution-focused brief therapy: Doing what works. In M.J. Dewan, B.N. Steenbarger, & R.P. Greenberg (Eds.), *The Art and Science of Brief Psychotherapies: An Illustrated Guide* (2nd ed., pp. 121–155). American Psychiatric Publishing.

Talmon, M. (1990). *Single Session Therapy: Maximizing the Effect of the First (and Often Only) Therapeutic Encounter*. Jossey-Bass.

Talmon, M. (1993). *Single Session Solutions: A Guide to Practical, Effective, and Affordable Therapy*. Addison-Wesley.

Talmon, M. (2018). The eternal now: On becoming and being a single-session therapist. In M.F. Hoyt, M. Bobele, A. Slive, J. Young, & M. Talmon (Eds.), *Single-Session Therapy by Walk-In or Appointment* (pp. 149–154). Routledge.

Talmon, M., & Hoyt, M.F. (2014). Moments are forever: SST and walk-in services now and in the future. In M.F. Hoyt & M. Talmon (Eds.), *Capturing the Moment: Single-Session Therapy and Walk-In Services* (pp. 463–485). Crown House Publishing.

Talmon, M., Hoyt, M.F., & Rosenbaum, R. (1988, December). *When the First Session is the Last: A Map for Rapid Therapeutic Change.* Short course at 1st Brief Therapy Conference, sponsored by the Milton H. Erickson Foundation. San Francisco, CA.

Tolle, E. (1999). *The Power of Now: A Guide to Spiritual Enlightenment.* New World Library.

Tolstoy, L. (1885). *What Men Live By, and Other Tales.* [Work originally published in Russian; English version available from Wildside Press, 2005.]

Whitaker, C.A. (1983). Comment. *Voices, 19,* 40.

Young, J. (2018). Single-session therapy: The misunderstood gift that keeps on giving. In M.F. Hoyt, M. Bobele, A. Slive, J. Young, & M. Talmon (Eds.), *Single-Session Therapy by Walk- In or Appointment* (pp. 40–58). Routledge.

Young, J. (2021). Single-session therapy in practice: Concepts, training, and implementation. In F. Cannistrà & F. Piccirilli (Eds.), *Single Session Therapy: Principles and Practices* (pp. 169–184). Giunti.

Young, J., & Rycroft, P. (1997). Single session therapy: Capturing the moment. *Psychotherapy in Australia, 4*(10), 18–23.

Young, J., Rycroft, P., & Weir, S. (2014). Implementing SST: Practical wisdoms from down under. In M.F. Hoyt & M. Talmon (Eds.), *Capturing the Moment: Single-Session Therapy and Walk-In Services* (pp. 121–140). Crown House Publishing.

Young, K. (2018). Change in the winds: The growth of walk-in therapy clinics in Ontario, Canada. In M.F. Hoyt, M. Bobele, A. Slive, J. Young, & M. Talmon (Eds.), *Single-Session Therapy by Walk-In or Appointment* (pp. 59–71). Routledge.

Zeig, J.K. (Ed.) (1980). *A Teaching Seminar with Milton H. Erickson, M.D.* Brunner/Mazel.

Ziegler, P.B., & Hoyt, M.F. (2023, September). Effective goal-constructing conversation in single-session/brief therapy. *The Science of Psychotherapy, 11*(9), 20–29 (online).

Chapter 6

How Single Session Thinking Could Revolutionize Mental Health Care Delivery

Jeff Young

The concept of Single Session Therapy (SST) is surprisingly disruptive, that's why it evokes such strong reactions in professional therapists and other helpers. Interestingly, it is more readily accepted by clients. Inflamed by an outrageous name, SST is disruptive to how we think about therapeutic change, how we conduct therapy, and importantly—given the state of mental health systems worldwide—how we provide services. The impact of SST has been so profound that the essential ideas derived from thinking about therapy differently have begun to influence an ever-widening range of professional and personal activities, which has given rise to a broader concept, *single session thinking,*[1] a concept that goes beyond SST and extends the emerging ideas around the single session mindset. Single session thinking can be thought of as *making the most of any encounter or event, conscious of the time available*—in work, love, and play, not just in therapy.

Overwhelming demand for mental health services across the world is creating a major crisis. An already emerging trend of increased demand for mental health services has been exacerbated by COVID. In Australia, for example, mental health distress and demand for mental health services rose significantly, as measured by the use of Medicare Benefits Schedule (MBS) subsidized mental health–related services, Pharmaceutical Benefits Scheme (PBS) mental health–related prescriptions, government-funded crisis counseling services, and emerging research (Shelly, Lodge, Heyman, Summers, & Young, 2021). Meanwhile, the pre-existing underlying structural impact of an aging population has led to fewer people in the workforce, translating to less public funding and human resources available to simply expand mental health services to keep up with demand. Many countries are stuck with unacceptably long wait times for people to access services. In the UK, for example, wait time for adolescent mental health services commonly stretches to years, not months or weeks.[2] At the same time as wait times are expanding, we also have an increasingly informed community expecting immediate access to high-quality services, including

DOI: 10.4324/9781032693828-8

mental health services, when and where they want them. Put simply, the inability of current services to respond to demand in line with consumer expectations is creating increasing pressure to review the ways we provide mental health care (Young, Rycroft, & Hoyt, 2020). This growing crisis in service delivery provides incentive to draw on single session thinking to redesign service delivery in ways that reduce wait lists and the pressure on professional resources, and at the same time improves the overall client experience and access to services.

In what follows, I will expand on four common misunderstandings I raised in Young (2018) that if left unchallenged are likely to restrict the expansion of SST and reduce its relevance to the redesign of services. I'll provide a broad definition of SST to facilitate a wider application of the approach and float *single session thinking* as an overarching concept. The chapter raises a neglected area in the thinking about single session mindset and provides a brief account of an innovative walk-in online family therapy service and how it fits into a planned comprehensive service delivery system, inspired by single session thinking. I conclude with situations in which SST doesn't work and what to do instead.

Four Common Misunderstandings About SST

Misunderstanding #1—SST Is a Brief Therapy Model Rather Than Responding to Clients' Natural Help-Seeking Behavior

The view that SST is a brief therapy model, rather than simply responding to the natural help-seeking behavior of clients, is likely to restrict the spread of SST internationally. Whilst brief therapy models have gained popularity, seeing SST as an approach to therapy that mirrors the community's natural help-seeking behavior rather than as a brief model of therapy will help SST appeal to more practitioners, irrespective of their therapeutic orientation.

A consultation that my colleague Colin Riess, the director of Bouverie at the time, and I were asked to conduct with Community Health Counselling Services across Victoria, Australia, led to us to a powerful data set that entrenched my thinking about client help-seeking behavior. Colin and I were asked to provide advice on how to improve the quality of care—which equated with how to get clients attending more sessions—because we were told that about 50% of Community Health Counselling clients only attended one or two sessions. Familiar with the SST research, we advised that this client contact data was consistent with most services across the world and that it would be a waste of time trying to change natural human help-seeking behavior. Instead, we advised that Community Health Counselling services could give those clients who only attend once (or twice) a more effective and satisfying service experience.

It should be noted that Community Health Services are based on a social model of health and hence are very pro-counseling. Counseling services are also charged relative to income. Hence, the common constraints to accessing services do not exist. There were no restrictions on the number of sessions clients could access at the time this data was collected, yet the mode of sessions that Community Health Counselling clients attended was one.

Figure 6.1 shows the number of counseling sessions 115,206 clients attended in community health centers across the state of Victoria, Australia, from 2003 to 2005, prior to the introduction of SST.

The graph shows 42% of the 115,206 clients attended once—whilst clinicians no doubt were trying to offer ongoing sessions. Of the 115,206 clients attending counseling over the three years, 18% attended two sessions and 10% attended three sessions. Whilst the pattern of these figures is in keeping with SST research more generally, the percentages of clients attending 1–3 sessions is still confronting. At the same time, it is also important to emphasize that 30%, nearly 35,000 clients, attended four or more sessions and some attended 20+ sessions. I will return to this point—but single session thinking needs to appreciate that a comprehensive service delivery model must cater for the need some clients have for longer-term work if it is to significantly influence mental health service delivery.

Whilst approaching therapy from a single session perspective is likely to make therapy briefer, I would argue that this is not the main purpose. The main purpose is to align the therapeutic work with client help-seeking behavior and what the client wants—which incidentally typically makes it more efficient and hence briefer. Emphasizing that single session therapeutic approaches are a direct response to the help-seeking behavior of clients also creates the groundwork for public information programs pointing out that most therapies only last one, two, or three sessions, potentially demystifying therapy for the broader community and potentially encouraging

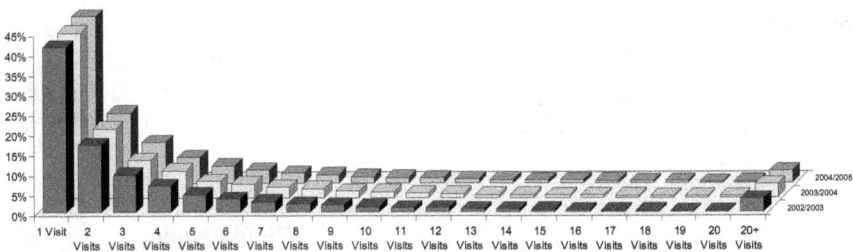

Figure 6.1 Number of sessions clients attended at Community Health Counselling in Victoria, Australia, between 2003 and 2005.

Source: (Used by agreement with The Bouverie Centre.)

people to seek help earlier. Long-term representations of therapy typically portrayed in the media may be a constraint to members of the general community seeking therapeutic support.[3] On the other hand, defining SST as a brief model may put off some clinicians and clients. It is also likely to imply that SST is a particular model of brief therapy, thus dividing clinician support for the approach, which brings us to the second misunderstanding.

Misunderstanding #2—SST Is a Specific Therapeutic Model Rather Than a Model of Service Delivery

SST is in fact often seen as a specific model of brief therapy, typically solution-oriented therapy, but its greatest strength is that clinicians trained in different therapeutic models can all provide services in a single session way—thus avoiding the somewhat fruitless ongoing battles over which model of therapy is most effective and allowing a unifying model of care, potentially across an entire organization. Seeing SST as a service delivery model, rather than as a specific therapeutic model, will allow single session thinking to be more relevant to the current crisis of overwhelming demand in mental health services.

Defining SST as a service-delivery model, rather than a specific therapeutic model, also has significant advantages when attempting to implement the approach in an organization. When Bouverie won the tender to implement SST into Victorian Community Health Counselling Services following Colin's and my initial consultation, branding it as a service delivery model meant that clinicians were not required to give up their preferred model of therapy, a model they had often spent many years and many dollars perfecting. They were confident using their preferred approach and would have been very resistant to giving it up to adopt a new model of therapy. Rather than throwing out their model of therapy, they simply had to adapt it and deliver it differently. As a result, along with other factors outlined in Young, Weir, and Rycroft (2012), our three-year project led to 84% of the 57 services who responded to a post-implementation survey reporting that they had implemented SST in some way, 58% at an organizational level and 42% up to the discretion of individual clinicians. Given that the success of most implementation projects at the time was less than 10% (Greenhalgh, Robert, Macfarlane, Bate, & Kyriakidou, 2004), this result was unusually successful.

Misunderstanding #3—SST Is Not Suitable for Clients Facing Serious or Complicated Problems

No research that I am aware of has clearly defined which clients find one session sufficient and which clients decide they need further sessions. Our experience of over three decades of offering single session family therapy suggests that trying to determine who will attend once and who will attend further sessions is a rather pointless activity. We, and many of the leading SST practitioners, have accepted that it is not possible to accurately predict attendance clinically. Rather than being a constraint to good work, the impossibility of predicting attendance can lead to an open-mindedness about how change will occur. Accepting that it is a waste of time trying to predict who will attend one session and who will attend further sessions informs the definition of Single Session Therapy provided later in this chapter and is an important consideration when designing single session–inspired service delivery systems.

When we started training practitioners in SST in the 1990s, slow adopters often held the view that SST might lead to superficial change but not to "deep" change and that SST was possibly suitable for simple, clearly defined, minor presenting problems. Frustrated that our experience that it was difficult to predict the outcomes of an initial single session on client families, whether they faced serious or less serious problems, led me and my colleague Pam Rycroft to design and conduct an exercise exploring what led to major changes in therapists' personal lives at the 28th Annual Australian and New Zealand Family Therapy Conference in Hobart, Tasmania, in 2009. We found that roughly half of the professional audience reported one-off experiences such as watching a film, reading a book, or witnessing an event had led to major changes in their lives, and roughly half attributed major changes to longer experiences such as academic courses, mentorship, etc. Interestingly, when we asked about their professional theory of change there was not a strong alignment with their personal accounts of change. Extensive experience with SST practice gives the impression that clients find SST approaches helpful irrespective of the degree of complexity they are facing. We have found that complexity of the presenting problem is not a good predictor of length of therapy. In fact, many clients facing major complex problems often don't have the time, finances, or motivation to engage in ongoing long-term work.

Anyone who has established an SST service soon realizes that, if anything, SST is more appealing to clients with more complex problems. Also, in many low-income countries around the world, clients are not able to afford travel costs or time off work to attend long-term therapy. When I presented SST in 2015 at a national psychiatric conference in Sri Lanka the audience found SST more relevant to their context than complex and longer-term approaches; similar preferences have been found in a variety of cross-cultural/non-Western contexts, including Mexico, Haiti, Aotearoa New Zealand, China, Indigenous Australia, Cambodia, First Nations Canada, and elsewhere (see Hoyt, Bobele, Slive, Young, & Talmon, 2018; Hoyt, Young, & Rycroft, 2021). However, the paradox that offering easy access to ongoing work can lead to shorter-term work brings us to the fourth misunderstanding.

Misunderstanding #4—SST Is One Session Therapy Rather Than the Number of Sessions Clients Decide They Need

Returning to the fact that 30% of Community Health clients decided to attend more than three sessions, a comprehensive single session service delivery model needs to provide options for easy access to further help. Paradoxically, providing clear and easy options for additional assistance is likely to create greater confidence for clients to treat the first session as potentially sufficient and therefore increase the number of complete one-off encounters. Offering ongoing services without any impediments to accessing them is key to making the most of SST efficiency and hence, reducing wait lists.

The first piece of research we conducted at The Bouverie Centre (Boyhan, 1996, 2014, 2021) evaluated the first 50 families attending our newly established single session family therapy service and found that after one year, roughly:

- 50%[4] of families had decided they were content with one session
- 25% of families decided they wanted a second single session
- 25% decided they wanted ongoing work.

The statistics were perfect to create a no-failure context for families who wanted further work. We used to say to clients that surprisingly half of the families we see find one session enough but half require more sessions. We emphasized that either was fine.

In a more recent attempt to reduce a growing waitlist (von Doussa, Tsorlinis, Cordukes, Beauchamp, & McIntosh, 2021), a one-off session was offered to clients waiting for an ongoing service. If clients wanted further sessions, they had to return to the waitlist until their turn came up for ongoing work—we didn't offer them ongoing work at the time of the one-off session. Our effort to reduce the waitlist and the pressure on our service didn't work. Only one of the 25 families we followed up with (4%) decided that the one-off session was sufficient. The other 24 families (96%) elected to stay on the waitlist.

How could this be so different than our initial SST outcomes—same organization, similar staff, similar clientele, similar context? However, when the client families who elected to go back on the waitlist were finally offered ongoing family work, four families (16%) reported that they didn't need further help and 13 families (52%) only needed a second session (one further session)—see Table 6.1.

Although these numbers are very small statistically, they suggest that when you don't offer further service options, clients will hold on to the service, especially to a waitlist. Interestingly, when we combined

Table 6.1 Percentage of families electing one, two, or three-plus session(s)

Percentage of families electing:	Study 1 (1996)	Study 2 (2021)
One session only	50%	4%
Two sessions	25%	68%
Three-plus sessions	25%	27%

Table 6.2 Percentage of families electing one to two sessions and three-plus sessions

Combining percentage of families electing one or two sessions:	Study 1 (1996)	Study 2 (2021)
One to two sessions	75%	72%
Three-plus sessions	25%	27%

the numbers for one to two sessions and ongoing work, the figures were very similar to our original foundational research in 1996—see Table 6.2.

Put simply, it is possible that the goal of providing effective help in the shortest amount of time, which may not be all SST practitioners' goal, but is in keeping with reducing the world's wait times for mental health services, relies on providing easy access to ongoing services.

In my clinical experience, providing options for ongoing work, not at the end of the first session, but in a follow-up phone call sometime later, creates a supportive context after the session and prior to the follow-up phone call for clients to take responsibility for change. Clients have new information and possibly practical strategies to try out because of the initial session, have the support of expecting a follow-up phone call, and in our service, the open and ongoing invitation to contact us at any time. This support, combined with the message that the client is expected to put the ideas generated in the session into practice, creates a fertile context for change to occur.

More recently, The Bouverie Centre has developed a one-off online family therapy service called Walk-in Together (WIT) that has no waitlist (Hartley, Moore, Knuckey, von Doussa, & Painter, 2023). In two years of operation, 82% of client families have found one session sufficient. At first glance, this seems contradictory to the argument given earlier. But this service is clearly advertised as a one-off session from the get-go, and client families can return for a second or third one-off session or elect to go on a waitlist for ongoing family therapy. Hence, the key principle may be about expectations and options for further work. The WIT program is described in greater detail as part of a comprehensive single session–inspired service delivery model later in this chapter. But first, let me reintroduce a definition of SST that makes the approach sympathetic to a wide range of services.

A Broad Definition of SST

In a 2018 chapter called "SST: The Gift That Keeps on Giving," I suggested that a pragmatic definition of SST is everything that results clinically and organizationally from accepting three findings. The first two findings are supported by research and the third by clinical experience. They are:

1. That the mode of sessions clients choose to attend is one
2. Most of these clients who choose to attend once find this one session sufficient, even when offered more
3. As mentioned earlier, it is not possible to predict who will attend once and who will attend further sessions.

Accepting these three findings has significant ramifications for how to conduct your first session and how to provide those services organizationally. Over the years I have used these three research findings to explain SST succinctly. I articulate these findings as part of my "lift speech"—what I would say to a clinician, middle manager, senior executive, policymaker, or funder if I found myself in a lift with them and only had seconds to explain what SST is and how it could impact their service. These findings essentially inform:

SST as a Clinical Approach (for further details see Rycroft & Young, 2021)

- Approaching the first session as if it could be the last; irrespective of diagnosis, complexity, or severity
- Exploring what each client would want to walk away with at the end of the session at hand (rather than the usual question of what the client wants from a course of therapy)
- Prioritizing what to focus on—negotiated between client and clinician
- Checking in at various points throughout the session to ensure the work is on track
- Sharing directly, albeit in a tentative way, feedback, advice, strategies, commendations, and information that the clinician feels is helpful, driven by the idea "What would I want to share with the client if I knew they would not return?"
- Providing resources and clarifying next steps.

SST as Service Design (for further information see Young et al., 2012)

- Embedding SST services within the organization so that clients have follow-up support if they need and want it whilst supporting the possibility that one session may be sufficient, irrespective of diagnosis, severity, or complexity
- Creating processes that accept that clients may or may not seek further help and establishing a no-failure context that supports clients to choose to attend one or multiple sessions.

Moving forward, I think we should also begin to include in the definition the impact that SST ideas have on our thinking about broader work practices and our personal lives outside of the therapy room.

The Client's Mindset: A Missing Element in the SST Literature

Preparing for a session, we tend to focus on the *therapist*'s mindset, which Flavio Cannistrà and Michael Hoyt have done a wonderful job exploring (Cannistrà, 2021; Hoyt & Cannistrà, 2023). In preparing my plenary talk for the 4th International Single Session Therapy and Walk-in Services symposium, I reflected on the absence of the client's voice from our symposia. Pam Rycroft and I thought about how to include the client's voice in the 2019 SST symposium in Melbourne but failed in practice. I do think it is something we should rectify in future symposia—and in the literature.

In his second book, *Single Session Solutions*, Moshe Talmon (1993) argued it is important to help the client get into the SST mindset—so they can get into therapy quickly and out of it quickly. Interestingly, *Single Session Solutions* didn't take off like his first book did —maybe because it didn't have a provocative title like *Single Session Therapy* (Talmon, 1990), and maybe because it focused on empowering clients to get the best out of us therapists.

The therapist adopting an SST mindset is not sufficient to get the most out of a therapeutic encounter. Getting the most out of a therapeutic encounter requires the therapist and client to be in sync. In a single session approach this requires the client to also embrace making the most of every encounter, embracing the limited time available, and appreciating that each session might be the last. When Katy Stephenson and I presented an SST workshop to Exeter University recently (Young & Stephenson, 2023) one of the participants reminded us of a concept articulated by John Burnham (2018) called relational reflexivity. Burnham talks about "warming" the therapeutic context for change and, like my colleague Pam Rycroft (personal communication), encourages us to talk about the talking. For example, asking clients:

- As we begin/continue to talk about this issue would you prefer to focus on the past, the present, or the future?
- Are you someone who would like to start making changes straight away or get to know me first and start to address change down the track?

We all know the excitement when client and therapist engage each other to work on an agreed problem, in an agreed way, at an agreed pace, for an agreed purpose. Sharing ideas and thoughts as they emerge, co-creating hypotheses and solutions takes the pressure off the therapist, engages the resources of the client, and hence makes therapy more collaborative, efficient, and often briefer. The goal of getting people into therapy quickly and out of it just as quickly is key to addressing the current overwhelming demand for mental health services.

Comprehensive Service Delivery Systems Informed by Single Session Thinking: An Early Pilot Program

As mentioned earlier, one of the constraints to SST and walk-in services having a greater influence on the design of our mental health services internationally is that they are seldom presented as part of an integrated comprehensive SST-inspired service system.

The Bouverie Centre is currently exploring how to provide a comprehensive SST-inspired tiered service delivery model, inspired by Peter Cornish's Step Care 2.0 work (Cornish, 2020). Clients will be able to access 24/7 self-help support online[5] to address relationship issues. Jessica L. Schleider and her colleagues have found that making "little interventions" available online to a broad audience can have a significant impact on mental health issues, especially in younger people (Schleider & Weisz, 2017; also see Chapter 10 this volume). If client families need professional support, they can seek a one-off online family therapy session called the Walk-in Together service[6] (maybe it should be called the Click-in Together project—but in the future it may also be delivered face-to-face). Having learned from our waitlist research, client families can return to the walk-in service for further one-off sessions or elect to have ongoing single session–oriented family therapy sessions, either face-to-face or online.

Exploring what a comprehensive single session–inspired service delivery model might look like raised a further area for exploration: How can single session thinking make our ongoing family therapy work more efficient?

This is an important question if single session thinking is going to help design models of service delivery to satisfy current demand. Ideas may include reviews done collaboratively with the client every three sessions; inviting a colleague to consult on the change process every so often, where the consultant approaches the review as a single session; designating a particular session within the ongoing work as a single session, etc. Whilst much of the comprehensive SST-inspired service delivery project is yet to be completed, The Bouverie Centre's early Walk-in Together (WIT) pilot is showing promise as a key part of the strategy.

Early Evaluation of the Walk-in Together Pilot

In the first 14 months of operation, the WIT service only operated on a Monday afternoon, and during this time 147 families were seen. Several family members shed tears of relief when told they could be seen immediately (waitlists were six months or longer elsewhere, and our own waitlist for ongoing family therapy work was not much better). Reassured that they could walk back in for another one-off session or go on the waitlist for ongoing family therapy, 88% of families decided they only needed one session, 12% decided two sessions were sufficient, and one family elected to return for a third single session. No families elected to go on the waitlist for ongoing family therapy (Moore, Knuckey, Barrington, Tsorlinis, & George, in press).

Evaluation of the first 22 families at three time intervals (T1, prior to WIT session; T2, at the conclusion of the WIT session; and T3, six weeks following the WIT session) found client families were positive about the WIT service (Hartley et al., 2023). At T3 69% ($n = 11$) of families reported that the session had helped resolve the problem they had come with, and 94% of adults ($n = 15$) reported that they would recommend the WIT program to others. Although only 69% of families felt the session had solved the problem they presented with, 88% ($n = 14$) of family members reported that they knew what to do next and 81% ($n = 13$) reported having followed through with the decisions made during the session.

Although only in the pilot and planning stages, the results to date suggest that immediate access to one-off sessions, embedded in a service delivery model where options for ongoing work are clearly available with the minimum of fuss may help address demand for services and reduce waitlists. The nuanced balance of creating a service delivery context where the possibility that one session will be enough whilst making it easy for further work, seems to create safety for clients to potentially let go of therapy after one session and to take charge of their own recovery.

Single Session Thinking: Expanding SST Outside of the Therapy Room

Single session thinking, which at its simplest is to make the most of every encounter, can inform any model of therapy but also models of care that don't define themselves as therapy, such as case management, mental health support services in general, and possibly even non-health services such as legal, housing, and homecare support services.

I have found single session thinking increasingly informs my professional work in general, such as how to conduct staff meetings or an executive meeting (for example, asking "What is the most important thing we need to discuss this meeting?"). I have drawn on single session thinking when planning presentations and talks, asking myself, "What is the most important thing I want to convey to the audience given the time I have been allocated?" and when running out of time during a presentation, asking, "What is the most important thing I want to get across given how much time is left?" rather than naively ploughing on or alienating the audience by talking faster and leaving out key bits.

The broader concept of single session thinking has allowed our center to negotiate a large contract to help a rural mental health service of 360 staff with 17 different services to introduce the approach across their entire organization. SST would not work for some of the 17 services.

Single session thinking has started to influence aspects of my personal life. For example, I teach martial arts, and when I ask students to perform their forms *as if* it is the last time they will ever be able to perform it, they tend to have a smile on their face, don't spend nearly as much time rebuking themselves for mistakes, perform in the moment, and often do a better "last" effort.

When SST Doesn't Work and What to Do About It

The argument that if we take an SST mindset into each session, embed each clinical single session into our service system so there are no impediments to further work, create a context for clients to also have an SST mindset and balance the possibility that one session may be enough whilst making further work easily available, and not a failure—then theoretically SST works as a service delivery model in all situations, for all models of therapy, and for all clients. But arguing that such a simple phenomenon always works, as I have been guilty of, is neither accurate nor a good sell. Hence, I have reflected on times when a single session approach has not been practically effective.

Reflecting on my own clinical work there are four areas in which SST has not practically worked.

Client Does Not Embrace the SST Rationale

In my experience, SST doesn't work practically when the client is not convinced of the SST rationale; essentially, they cannot adopt or be persuaded to adopt an SST mindset. It doesn't happen very often, especially if further work is clearly and accessibly made available, but it does happen. The solution for me is to simply offer ongoing work, inspired by SST.

Overwhelming Documentation

SST has not worked very well when I've had to digest copious legal documents relevant to the therapy. It is simply overwhelming to absorb the information in a single session. The simple solution is to allocate additional time to read the documentation, prior to or during the session, and emphasizing that further sessions are available if needed.

Safety Concerns

The suitability of SST approaches when there are ongoing safety concerns has been raised in the broader therapeutic literature. My response to this concern is to respond to risk as you would in traditional work—a safety plan, an emergency hospitalization or safe house. Conceptualizing and articulating how to deal with risk, especially in single session approaches without follow-up contact, such as walk-in services, is essential. Whilst Bobele and Slive (2021) have written about risk in their walk-in service, it remains an important area for further exploration, including the articulation of clinical guidelines in the literature, if SST is to become a powerful force in redesigning services.

Involuntary Clients

What is not so simple is when clients attend therapy under pressure from an external source. For example, when clients are mandated, involuntary, or not quite voluntary. This might include clients who are "partner mandated" ("get some help or I'm out of here"), pressured to attend therapy by parents or other family members, pressured by other helping professionals or institutions to seek further help, or legally mandated by the courts or parole officer to address their problems. The solution is to take a very different approach to the work. An approach I have developed called *No Bullshit Therapy (NBT)*, is briefly described here (for a comprehensive understanding of NBT please refer to Young, 2024).

No Bullshit Therapy

I love therapy. I decided to make it my career. It took me decades to realize that not everyone in the community shared my love of therapy. There is a continuum from people who love therapy to those who hate it. Most models of therapy have been designed by professionals who love therapy for clients who love therapy or are at least open to it. People who hate therapy are often pathologized, typically seen as uncooperative and resistant to change. I use the terms *therapy lovers* and *therapy haters* as provocative terms to encourage us to have the debate I think we need to have—that therapy should be designed to fit people, not the other way around—and that most of our current models of therapy are not designed for therapy haters.

The lovely SST-inspired questions that work for therapy lovers do not work for therapy haters, who if they could respond honestly, would respond something like that outlined in Table 6.3.

Inspired by the cutting to the chase core element of SST (Rycroft & Young, 2021), No Bullshit Therapy consists of four clinical guidelines, all designed to create a context for mutual honesty and directness between therapist and therapy hater:

1. Get a mandate on how to work, what to work on, or whether to work at all
2. Marry honesty and directness with warmth and care
3. Make a feature of constraints
4. Avoid jargon

These NBT clinical guidelines, which are outlined separately here but in practice are interconnected, are particularly helpful to engage people who don't want to work with you.

Table 6.3 The imagined honest responses of therapy haters to common SST questions

Common SST questions	Honest response of a therapy hater
How would you like to work together today?	I expect you'll tell me—yah wanker!
What would you like to get out of today?	I just want to get out of today!
What is the most important thing we should talk about?	How you can leave me alone and fix my wife!
What would you like to walk away with today?	Just walking away would be enough!

Get a Mandate on How to Work, What to Work on, or Whether to Work at All

Suggesting an honest and direct way of working is usually received well with therapy haters. This agreement can then be used to have the difficult conversations required to determine what the therapy hater wants to address and to help them address their definition of the problem. Like SST, NBT seeks to determine what the client wants to achieve as the motivator, not what the referring agent defines as the goal; however, the realities of the referral are raised and addressed honestly and directly.

Marry Honesty and Directness With Warmth and Care

Judicious amounts of warmth and care, presented in a businesslike and somewhat dispassionate way, tend to facilitate the working relationship, but in the early stages of engaging someone who is cynical about therapy, a greater focus on honesty and directness is usually more effective in building trust than well-meaning positivity.

Make a Feature of Constraints

Making a feature of, rather than trying to hide, the elephant in the room also helps address the sensitivities and complexities that usually accompany engaging someone who has been pressured in some way to see you. Often, the constraints to the work are what connects therapist and therapy hater early in their encounter. Acknowledging any constraints to the work tends to soften them, makes them transparent, and helps build trust.

Avoid Jargon

Avoiding jargon is about avoiding obfuscation. Being explicit, specific, and practical helps build trust, especially where bad faith predominates. Combined with honesty and directness, avoiding jargon means the therapy hater does not have to focus on actively exploring hidden threats.

SST and NBT

Both SST and NBT tend to elicit a blue-collar-type exhilaration of rolling up your sleeves and getting into the work—leaning into what is important to the client or essential to helping the client get what they want. I love the excitement of talking about the most important things—if this talking is in the interest of the client—even if the topics are sensitive and risky.

Therapy lovers and therapy haters are two extreme points on a continuum of how the population feels about therapeutic help. I focus on these extremes for purposes of outlining how the approach to engagement is different, depending on how a person comes to therapy. The path to talking safely about the most important things to a client is very different for therapy lovers and therapy haters. SST is like NBT for therapy lovers,[7] and NBT is like SST for therapy haters.

In NBT, getting an agreement to work in an honest and direct way is powerful. In SST the one session focus provides a boundary in which to explore the most important issues full-heartedly and safely. Together, SST and NBT help us provide support that gets to the heart of the matter with a wide range of clients. Both can help us design new ways of providing efficient services.

Concluding Remarks

Innovation and improvements often occur in the face of crises. The mental health care system is currently in crisis, hence there is a real opportunity for single session thinking to influence how a wide range of services are provided. Accessible care when, where, and how clients want services has the potential to not only improve care but reduce pressures on waitlists and services. Let's not waste this crisis.

Notes

1 *Single session thinking* was coined as an inclusive title for the 3rd International Single Session Therapy and Walk-In Services Symposium in Melbourne (2019) by the organizers, Jeff Young, Pam Rycroft, and Tess McGrane.
2 *Editors' note:* See Chapter 11 (Stephenson) and Chapter 16 (Lewis) of this volume.
3 *Editors' note:* As Hoyt (Chapter 5, this volume) has noted: "And these mind-set beliefs are not only held by therapists. We've all seen cartoon images of therapy that depict a patient laying on a couch or television programs in which the patient is endlessly 'in treatment.' They teach the public long-term therapy prophecies."
4 Originally, about 60% of families decided they did not need to attend further sessions, but over the year about 10% returned for either a second single session or ongoing work. Whilst this was often for a different presenting problem, we did not include these families in the "one only session" category.
5 Ellen Welsh is currently doing her Ph.D. research on the self-help online service.
6 This pilot project has been running for two years.
7 "Therapy lovers" and "therapy haters" are two extreme points on a continuum of how the population feels about therapeutic help. I focus on these extremes for purposes of outlining how the approach to engagement is different, depending on how a person comes to therapy.

References

Bobele, M., & Slive, A. (2021). An open invitation to walk-in therapy: Opening access to mental health care. In M.F. Hoyt, J. Young, & P. Rycroft (Eds.), *Single Session Thinking and Practice in Global, Cultural, and Familial Contexts: Expanding Applications* (pp. 54–65). Routledge.

Boyhan, P.A. (1996). Clients' perceptions of single session therapy consultations as an option to waiting for family therapy. *Australian and New Zealand Journal of Family Therapy, 17*(2), 85–96.

Boyhan, P.A. (2014). Innovative uses for single session therapy: Two case studies. In M.F. Hoyt & M. Talmon (Eds.), *Capturing the Moment: Single Session Therapy and Walk-In Services* (pp. 157–175). Crown House Publishing.

Boyhan, P.A. (2021). Complex and challenging issues in SST: Reflections on the past and learnings for the future. In M.F. Hoyt, J. Young, & P. Rycroft (Eds.), *Single Session Thinking and Practice in Global, Cultural, and Familial Contexts: Expanding Applications* (pp. 173–181). Routledge.

Burnham, J. (2018). Relational reflexivity: A tool for socially constructing therapeutic relationships. In *The Space Between* (pp. 1–17). Routledge.

Cannistrà, F. (2021). The vital role of the therapist's mindset. In M.F. Hoyt, J. Young, & P. Rycroft (Eds.), *Single Session Thinking and Practice in Global, Cultural, and Familial Contexts: Expanding Applications* (pp. 77–88). Routledge.

Cornish, P. (2020). *Stepped Care 2.0: A Paradigm Shift in Mental Health.* Springer Nature.

Greenhalgh, T., Robert, G., Macfarlane, F., Bate, P., & Kyriakidou, O. (2004). Diffusion of innovations in service organizations: Systematic review and recommendations. *The Milbank Quarterly, 82*(4), 581–629.

Hartley, E., Moore, L., Knuckey, A., von Doussa, H., Painter, F., Story, K., Barrington, N., Young, J., & McIntosh, J. (2023). Walk-in together: A pilot study of a walk-in family therapy intervention *Australian and New Zealand Journal of Family Therapy, 44*(2), 127–144.

Hoyt, M.F., Bobele, M., Slive, A., Young, J., & Talmon (Eds.). (2018). *Single-Session Therapy by Walk-In or Appointment: Administrative, Clinical, and Supervisory Aspects of One-at-a-Time Services.* Routledge.

Hoyt, M.F., & Cannistrà, F. (2023). Mindset in brief therapy. In M.F. Hoyt & F. Cannistrà (Eds.), *Brief Therapy Conversations: Exploring Efficient Intervention in Psychotherapy* (pp. 52–69). Routledge.

Hoyt, M.F., Young, J., & Rycroft, P. (Eds.). (2021). *Single-Session Thinking and Practice in Global, Cultural, and Familial Contexts: Expanding Applications.* Routledge.

Moore, L., Knuckey, A., Barrington, N., Tsorlinis, K., George, E., Story, K., Hartley, E., McIntosh, J., & Young, J. (in press). Walk-in together: Online therapy for families when and where they want it. In M. Bobele & A. Slive (Eds.), *Implementing Single-Session Therapy in Open Access Services.* Routledge, forthcoming.

Rycroft, P., & Young, J. (2021). Translating single session thinking into practice. In M.F. Hoyt, J. Young, & P. Rycroft (Eds.), *Single Session Thinking and Practice in Global, Cultural, and Familial Contexts: Expanding Applications* (pp. 42–53). Routledge.

Schleider, J., & Weisz, J.R. (2017). Little treatments, promising effects? Meta-analysis of single-session interventions for youth psychiatric problems. *Journal of the American Academy of Child & Adolescent Psychiatry, 56*(2), 107–115.

Shelly, S., Lodge, E., Heyman, C., Summers, F., Young, A., Brew, J., & James, M. (2021). Mental health services data dashboards for reporting to Australian governments during COVID-19. *International Journal of Environmental Research and Public Health*, 18(19), 10–14.

Talmon, M. (1990). *Single Session Therapy: Maximizing the Effect of the First (and Often Only) Therapeutic Encounter*. Jossey-Bass.

Talmon, M. (1993). *Single Session Solutions: A Guide to Practical, Effective, and Affordable Therapy*. Addison-Wesley.

von Doussa, H., Tsorlinis, K., Cordukes, K., Beauchamp, J., & McIntosh, J.E. (2021). One- off sessions to address a waitlist: A pilot study. In M.F. Hoyt, J. Young, & P. Rycroft (Eds.), *Single Session Thinking and Practice in Global, Cultural, and Familial Contexts: Expanding Applications* (pp. 117–124). Routledge.

Young, J. (2018). Single session therapy: The misunderstood gift that keeps on giving. In M.F. Hoyt, M. Bobele, A. Slive, J. Young, & Talmon (Eds.). *Single Session Therapy by Walk-In or Appointment: Administrative, Clinical, and Supervisory Aspects of One-at-a-Time Services* (pp. 40–58). Routledge.

Young, J. (2024). *No Bullshit Therapy: How to Engage People Who Don't Want to Work with You*. Routledge.

Young, J., Rycroft, P., & Hoyt, M.F. (2020). Guest editorial special issue: Expanding applications of single session thinking and practice. *Australian and New Zealand Journal of Family Therapy*, 41(3), 218–230.

Young, J., & Stephenson, K. (2023, November 2). *Single Session Therapy & Walk-In Clinics: Addressing Overwhelming Service Demand in Ways That Improve Rather Than Restrict the Client Experience*. Hybrid face-to-face and online workshop, Exeter University Psychology Department.

Young, J., Weir, S., & Rycroft, P. (2012). Implementing single session therapy. *Australian and New Zealand Journal of Family Therapy*, 33(1), 84–97.

Chapter 7

Single Session Thinking in Elite Sport Contexts

Considerations for a Practitioner's Mindset

Sam Porter, Tim Pitt, and Owen Thomas

Modern elite sport can be a spectacular but highly unstable, fast-paced, and unforgiving industry. It is far removed from normal life, which is to be expected given the sheer amount of investment devoted to eliciting high sporting performance (Nesti, 2010). This investment allows for the employment of large numbers of staff, state-of-the-art facilities, and sophisticated commercial and business arms (McDougall, Nesti, & Richardson, 2015). Fundamentally, these resources are deployed in pursuit of unlocking and executing individual and team performance, with the ultimate focus on medals, trophies, and world rankings. Evidently, this places numerous demands on the athletes, coaches, and support staff who operate within this sphere (Fletcher, Hanton, Mellalieu, & Neil, 2012; McDougall et al., 2015; Olusoga, Maynard, Hays, & Butt, 2012; Sly, Mellalieu, & Wagstaff, 2020). To help athletes and teams manage these pressures, Olympic, Paralympic, and professional sports will often employ sport psychologists as part of their sport science support team. Their work can occur at a one-to-one, team, and organizational level to help enhance performance (McDougall et al., 2015; Wagstaff, 2019). Typical areas of work focus on pressure management, developing confidence, managing emotions, developing communication skills, improving team dynamics, and developing more effective relationships. In summary, a sport psychologist's work largely centers on helping people develop optimal mindsets to meet differing contexts and challenges. It is therefore somewhat surprising that although sport psychologists often work on facilitating an athlete's performance mindset, limited attention has been given toward understanding how practitioners develop their performance mindset.

While the techniques used by sport psychologists are grounded in a variety of different therapeutic models (Hill, 2001), there are notable differences between the role and context in which sport psychologists operate compared to those of therapy. These differences include: the performance focus of a sport psychologist's work (as opposed to only managing/improving general functioning and well-being); that sport psychologists are often

DOI: 10.4324/9781032693828-9

employed as part of a team where they are required to travel with and support multiple stakeholders such as coaches, athletes, and other support staff (as opposed to the client being a single individual or family); that conversations sport psychologists have are often held in one-off informal settings such as training halls, hotel lobbies, and cafeterias (as opposed to only formal office settings); and that sport psychologists' interactions with athletes are often spontaneous in the time afforded to them (as opposed to having a set period of time). Working in the context of these elite sport environments, where time is pressured and tangible returns on investment are required, *brief* approaches for creating change are desirable (see Høigaard & Johansen, 2004; Pitt, Thomas, Lindsay, Bawden, & Hanton, 2015). In fact, brief approaches are particularly relevant for such performance environments, given their focus on solutions, growth, and practical improvements that can be operationalized quickly. In consideration of this context, there has been recent growing interest in the application of single session thinking and therapy within the sport psychology community (see Bowman & Turner, 2022; Pitt, Thomas, Hanton, & Cropley, 2023; Pitt, Thomas, Lindsay, Hanton, & Bawden, 2020, Pitt et al., 2015).

Herein, we discuss research that has explored the application of single session thinking in elite sport.[1] Through our work (e.g., Pitt, 2017; Pitt et al., 2015, 2020, 2023), we have come to recognize the critical importance of the practitioner's mindset in delivering effective single session work—much like that of an athlete's mindset in being able to execute their skills in key moments. We therefore also outline some of our more recent work that has focused on the single session mindset of practitioners (e.g., Porter & Pitt, 2023; Porter, Pitt, Thomas, Butt, & Eubank, in press). Finally, we discuss strategies for helping practitioners develop a single session mindset. Here, our focus is on the application of sport psychology to help practitioners mentally prepare themselves for being effective in a single session. We expect that therapist-readers will see many connections to the mindset shifts required for work in clinical therapeutic settings.

Single Session Thinking in Elite Sport

Perhaps the earliest consideration of single session thinking in sport psychology was Giges and Petitpas's (2000) discussion on brief contact interventions within sport psychology contexts. In their overview, Giges and Petitpas offered a framework designed to help sport psychologists implement one-off and often informal conversations with athletes. They suggested adopting targeted, goal-orientated, and action-focused conversation strategies to help inform brief contact interventions (i.e., single, unplanned professional interactions of short duration between practitioner and client) in field settings (e.g., at the side of the competitive arena prior to major events) where time constraints are present (e.g., no more than 10–20-minute time contacts). The authors shared case examples of the strategic strategies they used in such brief, impromptu, and informal encounters with athletes. These strategies included: trying to facilitate a small shift in the athlete's perception of their current situation; highlighting strengths and qualities conducive to their present circumstances; instructing relaxation techniques; introducing cue words to prime behavioral or attitudinal adjustments; and providing a supportive space for emotional ventilation ahead of significant competitive events. Consequentially, Giges and Petitpas's framework not only acknowledged the constraints of time-limited interactions but also emphasized the potential impact of strategic brief interventions to help optimize an athlete's mindset ahead of critical moments.

The first formal and empirical exploration of single session thinking in sport psychology rested within the doctoral work of Tim Pitt (2017). Initially, Pitt et al. (2015) reviewed the characteristics of single-session approaches across therapeutic settings (e.g., by-appointment or walk-in therapy) and discussed the potential for a systematic exploration of Single Session Therapy (SST) within the discipline of sport psychology. Through their review, Pitt et al. identified:

- SST was an effective model of practice that is well-suited to being adapted to different domains, including sport;
- Although a range of theoretical models guided SST delivery, solution-focused techniques were mostly adopted; and
- Common characteristics of single session thinking applications included pre-session questionnaires, consultancy teams, consultations that were goal-directed, and interventions that incorporated the client's strengths and resources.

Pitt et al. (2015) concluded that single session thinking could provide sport psychologists with well-suited, effective, and efficient means to solve problems in performance-driven environments.

In response, Pitt et al. (2020) developed a framework of single-session problem-solving across a series of empirical studies at a world-leading national institute of sport science and medicine. A 3.5-year ethnography established the essential features of a single-session approach to problem-solving in elite sport. Their approach integrated several reframing techniques to help change the client's initial description of their problem until it was described in a solvable frame. These techniques aligned with a range of existing brief therapeutic methods (e.g., de Shazer, 1985; Watzlawick, Weakland, & Fisch, 1974) and also included other new questioning approaches aimed at helping clients renegotiate the description of their problem until they had gained insight into how they could resolve their challenge(s). The authors described these questions as "problem cleaning" techniques as they allowed clients to consider the assumptions they were making about their problem that were preventing them from solving it. Overall, Pitt et al. (2020) illustrated that SST could be an effective form of problem-solving within an elite sport context. They also noted that developing a single-session mindset required a critical focus on the client's use of language, because the language clients used to describe their concerns contributed to both the maintenance of their problem and possible options for resolution (cf. see Lindsay, Pitt, & Thomas, 2014; Lindsay & Bawden, 2018).

Elsewhere, Bowman and Turner (2022) demonstrated that a single-session application of rational emotive behavior therapy (REBT) effectively reduced social anxiety and irrational beliefs and improved well-being and performance in amateur golfers. And Britton and colleagues (in press) furthered the application of cognitive behavioral approaches to Single Session Therapy (SST-CBT) and examined the needs and conditions where adopting SST-CBT might be most fruitful within a sport psychology context. Finally, Pitt et al. (2023) recently highlighted how single session thinking could be integrated into sport psychology practice using a series of case vignettes. Collectively, therefore, a growing number of publications and interest is evident within the sport psychology community on the application of single session thinking in sporting contexts.

Despite an emerging evidence base in sport psychology, single session thinking often does not feature as a curriculum requirement in most training pathways (e.g., British Psychological Society, 2019) and remains a novel concept to many practitioners (Pitt et al., 2020). For example, when first introducing single session thinking to the sport psychologists in the national institute of sport science and medicine, some practitioners experienced challenges when attempting to understand, learn, and make sense of single session thinking against the backdrop of their previous training regarding practice methods (Pitt, 2017; Pitt et al., 2020). These challenges often centered on how single session thinking did not align with the core beliefs and values sport psychologists held at the center of their professional philosophy (Pitt, 2017; Poczwardowski, Sherman, & Ravizza, 2004). Detailed exploration of these challenges was not a primary aim of Pitt and colleague's original research; but we have remained interested in exploring how sport psychology practitioners develop their applied knowledge and skills related to SST and a single session mindset. In response, our latest research focused on empirically investigating our interest in the single session mindset. To do so, we built upon Cannistrà's (2022) review and interviewed ten leading figures[2] from the world of SST to understand what they believed to be the essence of the single session mindset. The outputs of this study resulted in the conference presentation given at the 4th International Single Session Therapy Symposium (Porter & Pitt, 2023) with a full publication in progress (Porter et al., in press). Herein, a summary of the findings of Porter et al.'s (in press) work is given.

The Single Session Mindset

Our interviews with SST leaders aimed to define single-session mindset and capture the common mindset characteristics these practitioners described, despite differences in how they applied SST (see Figure 7.1).

Our data analysis (Porter et al., in press) led us to define the *single session mindset* as:

> A core set of beliefs and attitudes (about people, therapy, and change), which are intentionally embraced and enacted, before and during single session work, in order to align the practitioner and the client toward the possibility of creating change within a single session.

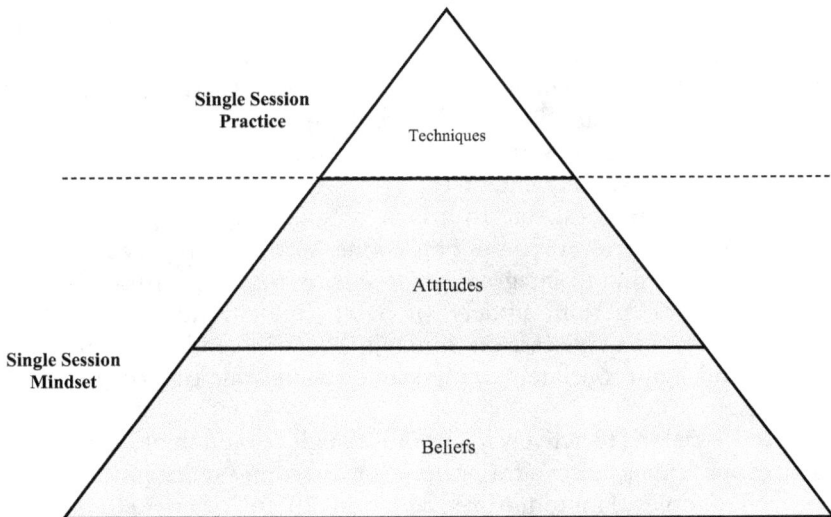

Figure 7.1 The distinction between the single session mindset and single session practice.

Source: (Porter et al., in press)

To enact this mindset before therapy, participants described the need to set themselves and their clients practically, something Cannistrà (2022) and Hoyt and Cannistrà (2023) termed "mind-setting." The suggested goal of mind-setting was to foster a shared understanding between the client and therapist regarding the nature and process of therapy. Several participants described how contextual pragmatics enabled them to achieve this alignment via organizational structures (e.g., intake team) and processes (e.g., pre-session questionnaire), as well as a series of individual strategies for mentally preparing for a single session, which we will discuss in greater detail later.

Nine core beliefs and 17 core attitudes (about *people*, *therapy*, and *change*) were identified as sitting at the heart of a single session mindset (see Table 7.1). Here, readers will appreciate their interconnected nature and the development of a structured framework for facilitating the adoption of a single session mindset, regardless of context or therapeutic orientation. Table 7.1 may highlight how adopting a single session mindset could challenge more traditionally held beliefs and assumptions of many therapeutic models and forms of training (e.g., one session can be enough versus real change happens gradually and requires multiple sessions). Hence, to work in this manner, practitioners may have to unlearn many things learned in traditional therapeutic training and be open to accommodating the beliefs and attitudes of the single session mindset. This may prove challenging given that a practitioner's beliefs are the most stable and enduring aspects of their professional philosophy (Poczwardowski et al., 2004). Such suggestions were also evident in Pitt's (2017) work, where he found three key challenges for practitioners when seeking to adopt SST approaches. These were: (1) difficulties in swiftly and adeptly incorporating single session thinking (and subsequent alterations to focus, goals, role of therapist/therapy, and techniques) due to a lack of sport psychology experience; (2) struggles to not revert to the practitioner's original approach to practice when attempting to integrate single-session thinking (caused by transitional/cognitive friction, anxiety, or habit), thereby hindering effective implementation of single session thinking; and (3) a tendency to misjudge contexts and inappropriately apply single session thinking to unsuitable situations.

For those seeking to actively incorporate single session thinking into their practice, our findings offer a framework for fostering a reflection-for-action approach (Cropley, Hanton, Miles, & Niven, 2010; Porter et al., in press). By contemplating the questions outlined next, alongside the beliefs outlined in Table 7.1, practitioners can systematically reflect on their professional philosophy (Anderson, Knowles, & Gilbourne, 2004) and perhaps question some of the implicit assumptions in their beliefs about people,

Table 7.1 Core beliefs and attitudes of a single session mindset (Porter et al., in press)

Core Beliefs	Core Attitudes
About People	• Take a collaborative stance.
• Clients are the experts in their own lives.	• Co-create and agree on an obtainable focus.
• Clients have strengths and resources to make things better.	• Look for what is working.
• People are always changing.	• Connect clients to their strengths and resources.
About Therapy	• Expect good things to happen.
• One session can be enough.	• See every interaction as whole and complete in itself.
• The therapist just needs to get the client moving.	• Leave the door open.
• The therapist should play an active role in creating a sense of hope within the client and for maximizing each therapeutic encounter.	• Aim small and simple.
	• Get clients moving in the right direction.
	• Roll up your sleeves.
• Every session should have a beginning, middle, and end.	• Use your own skills and resources.
• Treat the person and their situation, not their diagnosis.	• Be pragmatic and use time wisely.
	• Be laser focused and keep on track.
About Change	• Focus on the now.
• Change occurs in different forms.	• Be concrete not categorical.
	• Don't let your ego get in the way.
	• Remain hopeful and trust the client.

change, therapy, and their role as the therapist. This deliberate process is designed to enhance self-awareness and professional development, enabling practitioners to identify specific steps for integrating single session thinking into their practice (Cropley et al., 2010; Poczwardowski, Aoyagi, Shapiro, & Van Raalte, 2014).

- What do I currently believe about change? How does change happen? When and where does change tend to happen?
- What evidence or experiences (personal or professional) do I have that support my beliefs? What evidence or experiences (personal or professional) do I have that contradict my beliefs?
- What are my fundamental beliefs about the purpose/goals/aims of therapy and why?
- How similar or different are the core beliefs of the single session mindset to my current beliefs that underpin my professional philosophy?
- What evidence or experiences (personal or professional) do I have that support or contradict each of the core beliefs of the single session mindset?

Table 7.2 provides a detailed description of the single session mindset attitudes offered by Porter et al. (in press). The attitudes act as strategies for practitioners to adopt before and during therapy. Notably, our experience with athletes underscores the potential for rapid mindset shifts, something that can be facilitated by purposefully adopting attitudes tailored to different circumstances (e.g., an athlete recognizing when to be aggressive and take risks or when to be cautious and ensure a more pragmatic approach to competing). We suggest these strategies can be more readily integrated into single-session work via deliberate reflection-for-action (i.e., creating quick, actionable strategies for shifting mindset ahead of a session; for example, adopting an attitude of "rolling up your sleeves" and bringing a positive energy to make things happen) and reflection-in-action (i.e., helping the practitioner and/or the client shift their mindset during practice quickly toward the session goal; for example, being "laser focused and keeping on track"), compared to the more profound introspection needed when challenging one's beliefs (Schon, 1983). Practitioners are urged to find personalized approaches to embody and apply these attitudes congruently with their own styles.

Table 7.2 Summarizing the core attitudes of a single session mindset (Porter et al., in press)

Core Attitudes	Summary of the Attitude
Take a collaborative stance.	It is your job to work *with* the client to work out what they want and how they can move forward.
Co-create and agree on an obtainable focus.	Work with the client to define a tangible and realistic outcome for the current session.
Look for what is working.	Purposefully notice positive aspects of the client's situation that are problem free or where their strengths and resources are preventing their situation from being worse than it currently is.
Connect clients to their strengths and resources.	Be explicit in highlighting the client's inherent strengths, resources, and capabilities and how they can utilize them right now.
Expect good things to happen.	Anticipate that the session will lead to positive outcomes and keep an optimistic outlook (of progress being made).
See every interaction as whole and complete in itself.	See each conversation with the client as an opportunity to create change.
Leave the door open.	Explicitly ensure clients are made aware they can return for further sessions if they so wish.
Aim small and simple.	Break down complex and overwhelming problems into a manageable frame on the current issue. Then ensure clients have a realistic and tangible step they can take that can move them forward in the right direction.

(Continued)

Table 7.2 (Continued)

Core Attitudes	Summary of the Attitude
Get clients moving in the right direction.	Leave clients with a realistic and tangible step they can take that can move them forward in the right direction.
Roll up your sleeves.	Bring a positive energy to each session with a real desire to make progress and move the problem forward in one.
Use your own skills and resources.	Be willing to draw upon your own skills and resources to mobilize change.
Be pragmatic and use time wisely.	Make sure you have your own structure for a session that allows you to have a beginning (co-create a clear focus), middle (mobilize change), and end (action planning).
Be laser focused and keep on track.	Keep focused on the agreed-upon aim of the session and don't allow yourself or the client to move too far off this track. When noticing this, respectfully direct the client (and yourself) back on track.
Focus on the now.	Be interested in the client's current situation and what brings them to the session now. Get into their world view and put yourself in their shoes.
Be concrete not categorical.	Focus on extracting clear, contextual, and functional descriptions that describe the current nature of the problem.
Don't let your ego get in the way.	Do not attach your worth as a therapist to client outcomes or to the cleverness of your interventions.
Remain hopeful and trust the client.	Remember that clients, and not therapists, create the change they seek. So, keep an optimistic outlook and ensure clients feel empowered to take their first step.

Developing a Single Session Mindset

Working with athletes to develop a pre-performance routine is a common strategy used by sport psychologists to help athletes optimize their pre-competition mindset (Cohn, 1990; Winter & Collins, 2013). These routines often include a range of psychological strategies to help the athlete mentally "warm up" and be in their optimal mindset for performing (Yao, Xu, & Lin, 2020). Congruent with such an approach, provided next are three suggestions for how therapy practitioners might develop their own mental "warm-up" prior to a session to help them adopt an optimal single session mindset going into and during sessions. These are not exhaustive; they are illustrative to encourage practitioners to purposefully consider ways of priming some of the attitudes described in Table 7.2.

Chunking the Session

The attitudes outlined in Table 7.2 emphasize the need to stay focused in a practical and purposeful way within the session (e.g., be pragmatic and use time wisely, be laser focused and keep on track, focus on the now). Application of these attitudes centers around the belief that single session work should have a beginning, middle, and end. Sport psychologists commonly work with athletes and performers around creating a structured, well-planned approach to performance (e.g., breaking down races/games) into key compartmentalized phases. In a similar way, we encourage clinical practitioners to consider ways to purposefully compartmentalize or chunk their single session so that it has: (1) a beginning phase (focused on attaining a clear and obtainable goal for the session); (2) a middle phase (focused on ways of obtaining this goal); and (3) an end phase (focused on next steps and actions).

Possible techniques to help with compartmentalizing could include practitioners having pre-set boxes or structure to their notebooks, mentally assigning time to each phase (e.g., 10 minutes for the beginning phase, 45 minutes for the middle phase, 5 minutes for the end phase), or other strategies that encourage this structure to each session. This can help empower practitioners to guide clients purposefully, ensuring they help the client move in the right direction by design rather than by chance.

Mental Priming

Mental priming involves the purposeful use of a small behavior to influence how we then approach a subsequent task. We suggest that practitioners prime themselves to "look for what is working" and to embody the attitude of "connecting clients to their strengths and resources" (Porter et al., in press). As a practical example of this, practitioners can proactively enhance their preparedness for single session work by systematically writing down their clients' skills, strengths, and resources before each session. By undertaking this type of preparation, practitioners not only gain understanding of the client's potential assets but also lay the groundwork for maximizing each therapeutic encounter, which in turn should enhance client outcomes. This practice has shown a substantial impact on influencing client outcomes, with evidence demonstrating a 35% increase in client outcomes after therapists listed the client's strengths and resources before therapy (Flückiger, Caspar, Holtforth, & Willutzki, 2009; Flückiger & Grosse Holtforth, 2008; Porter et al., in press). We do, however, suggest possible caution with such an approach in that this technique requires the practitioner to have met or have some tangible information about the client before the session begins—which may be a challenge in a lot of single session work. One advocate from our study recommended that in situations where practitioners do not have any information on the client, you may consider how you can enjoy yourself in the upcoming session with a client (i.e., writing down three things you will enjoy about the upcoming session), a strategy that can prime a resource focus and also aid collaborative problem solving (e.g., quickly find something on which you can complement the client).

Mental Cues

Athletes frequently utilize physical and psychological cues to self-regulate emotions, arousal, and activation levels before competitive events (e.g., Meijen, Brick, McCormick, Lane, & Marchant, 2023). These "cues" help trigger a specific focus, emotion, or attitude that is helpful to them when performing and are often in the form of either: (1) cue words or phrases carefully chosen to elicit a specific mental state at a certain moment or (2) physical or behavioral cues designed to trigger a specific response (e.g., a golfer placing a dot on their glove as a reminder to take a breath before playing their shot). Such strategies may be adopted by therapy practitioners before a session to encourage the attitudes outlined in Table 7.2. For example, consider the attitude of "roll up your sleeves," which is about the practitioner bringing a positive energy to each session with a real desire to make progress and move the problem forward in one session. Cues could include a literal (physical) rolling up your sleeves or, alternatively, a meaningful cue word or phrase to trigger this attitude in a timely manner (e.g., "Let's go"). Readers are invited to find their own language that may help them embody the single session attitudes.

Summary

We have sought herein to bring to life the application of single session thinking in the world of elite sport. In doing so, we shared some of our work in this space, which has recently culminated in empirically grounding the concept of single session mindset. Crucially, practitioners should reflect upon the fundamental beliefs at the heart of a single session mindset and how this may align with their beliefs about people, therapy, and change. Furthermore, we outlined some suggestions for readers to consider on how they may adopt the attitudes of a single session mindset into their practice. In doing so, we hope to encourage therapy practitioners to consider themselves as performers in their own right and to embrace pre-performance routines and strategies ahead of single session work to optimize and prepare their practitioner mindset for SST.

Notes

1 Our practice in sport did not center on the direct implementation of Single Session Therapy with clients. Rather, our emphasis lay in employing single session thinking to address various challenges encountered within elite sport settings. In elucidating this contrast, we find the following quote from Hoyt, Young, and Rycroft (2021, p. 3) helpful: "The essence of single session thinking is to approach the first session as if it will be the only session, while creating opportunities for further work if it is requested by the client."
2 Participants included Arnie Slive, Bob Rosenbaum, Denise Fry, Flavio Cannistrà, Jeff Young, Jen McIntosh, Michael F. Hoyt, Monte Bobele, Moshe Talmon, and Pam Rycroft.

References

Anderson, A.G., Knowles, Z., & Gilbourne, D. (2004). Reflective practice: A review of concepts, models, and practical implications for enhancing the practice of applied sport psychologists. *The Sport Psychologist*, 18, 188–203. https://doi.org/10.1123/tsp.18.2.188

Bowman, A.W., & Turner, M.J. (2022). When time is of the essence: The use of rational emotive behavior therapy (REBT) informed single-session therapy (SST) to alleviate social and golf-specific anxiety, and improve wellbeing and performance, in amateur golfers. *Psychology of Sport and Exercise*, 60, 102–167. https://doi.org/10.1016/j.psychsport.2022.102167

British Psychological Society. (2019). *Standards for the accreditation of Masters and Doctoral programmes in sport and exercise psychology*. https://cms.bps.org.uk/sites/default/files/2022-07/Sport%20and%20Exercise%20Accreditation%20Handbook%202019.pdf

Britton, D., Wood, A. G., & Pitt, T. (2024). Having impact and doing it quickly: The place for brief and single-session cognitive-behavioral therapies in sport psychology practice. *The Sport Psychologist*, 38(2), 137–146. https://doi.org/10.1123/tsp.2021-0146

Cannistrà, F. (2022). The single session therapy mindset. *International Journal of Brief Therapy and Family Science*, 12(1), 1–26. https://doi.org/10.35783/ijbf.12.1_1

Cohn, P.J. (1990). Preperformance routines in sport: Theoretical support and practical applications. *The Sport Psychologist*, 4(3), 301–312. https://doi.org/10.1123/tsp.4.3.301

Cropley, B., Hanton, S., Miles, A., & Niven, A. (2010). The value of reflective practice in professional development: An applied sport psychology review. *Sports Science Review*, 19(3–4), 179–209. https://doi.org/10.2478/v10237-011-0025-8

de Shazer, S. (1985). *Keys to Solution in Brief Therapy*. Norton.

Fletcher, D., Hanton, S., Mellalieu, S.D., & Neil, R. (2012). A conceptual framework for organizational stressors in sport performers. *Scandinavian Journal of Medicine & Science in Sports*, 22, 545–557. https://doi.org/10.1111/j.1600-0838.2010.01242.x

Flückiger, C., Caspar, F., Holtforth, M.G., & Willutzki, U. (2009). Working with patients' strengths: A microprocess approach. *Psychotherapy Research*, 19(2), 213–223. https://doi.org/10.1080/10503300902755300

Flückiger, C., & Grosse Holtforth, M. (2008). Focusing the therapist's attention on the patient's strengths: A preliminary study to foster a mechanism of change in outpatient psychotherapy. *Journal of Clinical Psychology*, 64(7), 876–890. https://doi.org/10.1002/jclp.20493

Giges, B., & Petitpas, A. (2000). Brief contact interventions in sport psychology. *The Sport Psychologist*, 14, 176–187. https://doi.org/10.1123/tsp.14.2.176

Hill, K. (2001). *Frameworks for Sport Psychologists: Enhancing Sport Performance*. Human Kinetics.

Høigaard, R., & Johansen, B.T. (2004). The solution-focused approach in sport psychology. *The Sport Psychologist*, 18, 218–228. https://doi.org/10.1123/tsp.18.2.218

Hoyt, M.F., & Cannistrà, F. (2023). *Brief Therapy Conversations: Exploring Efficient Intervention in Psychotherapy*. Routledge.

Hoyt, M.F., Young, J., & Rycroft, P. (2021). Single session thinking and practice going global one step at a time. In M.F. Hoyt, J. Young, & P. Rycroft (Eds.), *Single Session Thinking and Practice in Global, Cultural, and Familial Contexts: Expanding Applications* (pp. 3–26). Routledge.

Lindsay, P., & Bawden, M. (2018). *Pig Wrestling: The Brilliantly Simple Way to Solve Any Problem . . . and Create the Change You Need*. Random House.

Lindsay, P., Pitt, T., & Thomas, O. (2014). Bewitched by our words: Wittgenstein, language-games, and the pictures that hold sport psychology captive. *Sport & Exercise Psychology Review*, 10(1), 41–54. https://doi.org/10.53841/bpssepr.2014.10.1.41

McDougall, M., Nesti, M., & Richardson, D. (2015). The challenges of sport psychology delivery in elite and professional sport: Reflections from experienced sport psychologists. *The Sport Psychologist*, 29(3), 265–277. https://psycnet.apa.org/doi/10.1123/tsp.2014-0081

Meijen, C., Brick, N., McCormick, A., Lane, A., Marchant, D., Marcora, S., & Robinson, D. (2023). Psychological strategies to resist slowing down or stopping during endurance activity: An expert opinion paper. *Sport and Exercise Psychology Review*, 18(1), 4–37. https://doi.org/10.53841/bpssepr.2023.18.1.4

Nesti, M. (2010). *Psychology in Football: Working with Elite and Professional Players*. Routledge.

Olusoga, P., Maynard, I., Hays, K., & Butt, J. (2012). Coaching under pressure: A study of Olympic coaches. *Journal of Sport Sciences*, 30, 229–239. https://doi.org/10.1080/02640414.2011.639384

Pitt, T. (2017). *Nudging' Sport Psychologists to Change: Developing a Framework of Single-Session Problem Solving Within Elite Sport* [Unpublished PhD Thesis, Cardiff Metropolitan University, UK].

Pitt, T., Thomas, O., Hanton, S., & Cropley, B. (2023). Brief and single-session therapy. In D. Todd, K. Hodge, & V. Krane (Eds.), *Routledge Handbook of Applied Sport Psychology* (2nd ed., pp. 145–154). Routledge. https://doi.org/10.4324/9781003173588-18

Pitt, T., Thomas, O., Lindsay, P., Bawden, M., & Hanton, S. (2015). Doing sport psychology briefly? A critical review of single session therapeutic approaches and their relevance to sport psychology. *International Review of Sport & Exercise Psychology*, 8(1), 1–31. https://doi.org/10.1080/1750984x.2015.1027719

Pitt, T., Thomas, O., Lindsay, P., Hanton, S., & Bawden, M. (2020). A framework of single-session problem-solving in elite sport: A longitudinal, multi-study investigation. *Frontiers in Psychology*, 11, 566721. https://doi.org/10.3389/fpsyg.2020.566721

Poczwardowski, A., Aoyagi, M.W., Shapiro, J.L., & Van Raalte, J.L. (2014). Developing professional philosophy for sport psychology consulting practice. In *Routledge Companion to Sport and Exercise Psychology* (pp. 895–907). Routledge.

Poczwardowski, A., Sherman, C.P., & Ravizza, K. (2004). Professional philosophy in the sport psychology service delivery: Building on theory and practice. *The Sport Psychologist*, 18(4), 445–463. https://doi.org/10.1123/tsp.18.4.445

Porter, S., & Pitt, T. (2023, November 10–12). *An Expert Opinion on the Application of the Single Session Mindset* [Conference Session]. Fourth International Single Session Therapy Symposium, Rome, Italy. https://www.singlesessiontherapies.com/single-session-therapy-symposium/

Porter, S., Pitt, T., Thomas, O., Butt, J., & Eubank, M. (in press). An expert understanding of the single session mindset. *Journal of Systemic Therapies* (forthcoming).

Schon, D.A. (1983). *The Reflective Practitioner: How Professionals Think in Action*. Basic Books.

Sly, D., Mellalieu, S.D., & Wagstaff, C.R.D. (2020). "It's psychology Jim, but not as we know it!": The changing face of applied sport psychology. *Sport, Exercise and Performance Psychology*, 9, 87–101. https://doi.org/10.1037/spy0000163

Wagstaff, C.R. (2019). A commentary and reflections on the field of organizational sport psychology. *Journal of Applied Sport Psychology*, 31(1), 134–146. https://doi.org/10.1080/10413200.2018.1539885

Watzlawick, P., Weakland, J.H., & Fisch, R. (1974). *Change: Principles of Problem Formation and Problem Resolution*. Norton.

Winter, S., & Collins, D. (2013). Does priming really put the gloss on performance? *Journal of Sport and Exercise Psychology*, 35(3), 299–307. https://doi.org/10.1123/jsep.35.3.299

Yao, Q., Xu, F., & Lin, J. (2020). A qualitative study on pre-performance routines of diving: Evidence from elite Chinese diving athletes. *Frontiers in Psychology*, 11, 193. https://doi.org/10.3389/fpsyg.2020.00193

Part III

Why, Where, and for Whom—Research, Applications, and Implementations

Chapter 8

The SST Model Developed in Canada and Texas for Walk-in, Drop-in, Open-Access, and Virtual Services

Monte Bobele and Arnold Slive

In this chapter, we will describe the unique features of what has been described as the "Canadian/Texan Model" of Single Session Therapy (SST). The primary distinguishing feature is that this model offers SST without an appointment. We will explain how the concept of open-access services has been applied in general healthcare settings, particularly in SST settings. For many mental health providers, open-access presents some implementation challenges, and we will address the most frequent ones we have encountered. Finally, many implementations of open-access/SST exist outside of Canada and Texas, mainly in North America. We will describe unique applications in Mexico and briefly mention some in Asia and Europe.

The description of the Canadian/Texan Model as a distinct mode of SST that initially appeared in Cannistrà and Piccirilli (2021; also see Piccirilli, 2023) differentiates our model of open-access/SST from what they identified as one of three models of SST. The other two are the Californian method of Hoyt, Rosenbaum, and Talmon (1992) and The Bouverie Centre's Australian method (Young & Rycroft, 1997). All three models share Talmon's single-session mindset (1990). SST generally occurs in one of three circumstances: (1) the client has made an appointment where the therapist and client understand that the visit may be the only visit that occurs, although the door is always open for return visits; (2) the client walks in or otherwise receives services without any pre-arranged appointment (Slive, MacLaurin, Oaklander, & Amundson, 1995); or (3) the therapist and client meet expecting that the current visit will be the first of many and either by mutual agreement or the client's subsequent decision not to return, a single episode of therapy occurs.

The difference among the different models that Cannistrà and Piccirilli (2021) have described lies in whether a prior appointment was required for the visit. Fortunately, the evidence favoring single sessions also opened another possibility: that services could be developed where clients could arrive for a single session with or without an appointment (Slive et al., 1995; Slive & Bobele, 2011). Slive and his colleagues developed Canada's

DOI: 10.4324/9781032693828-11

first walk-in, open-access model at the Eastside Family Centre in Calgary in the early 1990s. In Canada, SST is primarily delivered in walk-in or virtual environments. Bobele brought the Eastside open-access model to Texas in the late 1990s. So, although our model may be distinguished by open-access service delivery, by the end of this chapter, we hope to demonstrate that open-access forms of SST are practiced all over North America and have spread around the world, from Asia to Scandinavia.

What Is Open-Access?

These no-appointment services (referred to throughout this chapter as "open-access") were developed to meet the need for more accessible and rapid access to mental health services. In the broader health care industry, alternatives to by-appointment scheduling of patients and professionals have been explored for quite some time (Barit, 2019; Huff, 2017; Kaplan, 2015). In counseling agencies, a motivating factor leading to the development of an open-access option has been ever-lengthening waiting lists (Lamsal, Stalker, Cait, Riemer, & Horton, 2018; Shaffer, Love, Chapman, Horn, & Haak, 2017; Stalker et al., 2016; Young, Dick, Herring, & Lee, 2008). When Arnie started a traditional outpatient family and adolescent service at Wood's Homes in Calgary, Alberta, Canada, in the 1980s, they operated in the conventional appointment-making way. An intake coordinator interviewed prospective clients who asked for an appointment. They were then placed on a waiting list. When a clinician had an opening, often several months later, they contacted the client to make an appointment. Frequently, clients said they were no longer interested. Of the ones who accepted an appointment at that time, only about half who made a first appointment arrived for a therapy session.

As a result of these frequent cancellations and no-shows, Wood's Homes had a series of discussions within the organization and with stakeholders in the community. These discussions and subsequent planning led to the formation of the Eastside Family Centre's Walk-in/SST service that opened in 1990 and has continued to this day. The Eastside Walk-in/SST model was the first in Canada. Walk-in or open-access clinics have spread across Canada in the last 34 years (Duvall, Young, & Kays-Burden, 2012; Harper-Jaques & Leahey, 2011; McElheran, Harper-Jaques, & Lawson, 2020; Josling & Cait, 2018; Young, 2018).

When we began this work, we referred to it as "walk-in counseling" or "walk-in/single session therapy." This was an easy choice for us then because "walk-in" is a very commonly used term in English-speaking countries. In the USA and Canada, it's common to see "Walk-ins Welcome" signs for a variety of services (e.g., hair stylists or barber shops, oil change kiosks, mall optometry clinics). However, recently, there has been some question of the appropriateness of this term. Might this term be inadvertently offensive or disrespectful to those with mobility issues? We agree that the term "walk-in" could potentially raise diversity, equity, and inclusion (DEI) objections because it may be seen as insensitive or exclusionary toward individuals with physical disabilities or mobility challenges. To address these potential DEI concerns, we recommend using alternative terms such as "drop-in," "no appointment necessary," or "open-access." These terms are more neutral and do not make assumptions about an individual's physical abilities or mobility.

Synonyms for open-access are less problematic in other languages. For example, there is not a word for *walk-in* in Spanish. In Spanish-speaking countries, *sin cita previa*, or simply *sin cita* (without an appointment), is commonly used to describe such services. One of our colleagues in Mexico described how a collaboration with her local community resulted in a name for the service that suited them (Rodriguez, 2018). Initially, her service was called *Terapia Sesión Sola, Sin Cita* ("Single-session, no appointment needed"). However, shortly after the service began, few clients showed up, leaving her team puzzled. One of her clients, who also worked at the school that sponsored the clinic, told them she overheard a conversation between the receptionist and a local who had asked about the service. The gentleman declined a "single-session without an appointment," saying that one session would not be enough and preferred to make an appointment instead. Her team realized the term "single-session without an appointment" was confusing and unfamiliar to clients. They recognized that the name *"Terapia Breve, Sin Cita"* ("Brief Therapy, No Appointment") worked better because it conveyed the three key ideas they wanted to communicate: the therapy was short-term; clients could walk in without an appointment on designated days; and clients could attend one session at a time. The new name clarified the nature of the service for clients and staff, addressing the initial confusion caused by the "single-session" terminology. In our work in Canada, French speakers also use the without-an-appointment idea: *sans rendez-vous*. Open-access may be more universally understood when it makes a distinction that implies no appointment required, same-day services, or some form of virtual services.

Current Developments

The onset of the Covid-19 pandemic accelerated the development of open-access services to meet the increased demand for more accessible mental health services. In many countries, in-person meetings were discouraged. Newer forms of counseling became the norm, where clients could make immediate or same-day appointments for telephone and text-based services. Many existing walk-in services adapted to the pandemic by adopting these alternative formats.

Eastside Community Mental Health Services, formerly the Eastside Family Centre, at the start of the pandemic expanded their open-access service platforms. Services there now include in-person walk-ins as well as same-day virtual appointments, telephone, text, and live chat with mental health professionals.[1] Another recent development is the *Wellness Desk*. The Wellness Desk is in the Calgary Central Library and two other branch libraries. The Wellness Desk offers immediate mental health and addiction support, health information, and referrals to services. Through recent funding from a Canadian bank, the Central Library location now offers these services every day.

At the start of the pandemic, the Canadian government funded a nationwide initiative to provide free open-access/SST to all Canadian citizens (Cornish, Churchill, MacKay, & Jaouich, 2020; Cornish & Churchill, 2023; Basnet & Chaiton, 2024). Services were available seven days a week, 24 hours a day. The *Wellness Together Canada* (WTC) web portal provided information about the services and telephone numbers so children and adults could assess services by telephone or chat. Clients could call a phone number and be immediately connected with a qualified counselor. Callers were invited to call again as needed and were provided additional resources if desired. Now that the pandemic has come to an end, this WTC has closed, and local provinces have received funding to continue providing similar open-access services.

One Stop Talk (Strides Toronto, 2023), based in Toronto, is one such agency that began implementing these new open-access services just as the pandemic was winding down. This service is available in Ontario to any person age 17 or younger. A youngster calls a number or sends an email, answers some brief questions, and is immediately connected virtually with a qualified clinician in Ontario. One innovative feature of this service is that, when desired, a "navigator," located in a nearby part of Ontario, can be brought into the virtual conversation to assist the caller in connecting to additional mental health resources convenient to the youngster.

Many university counseling centers in the USA and Canada had already begun exploring the use of walk-in/SST as a way of making services more accessible to students and reducing their wait times by the beginning of the pandemic. Open-access/SST for university students has expanded (Cornish et al., 2017; Shaffer et al., 2017; Finch, Kleiman, Bentley, & Bernstein, 2023; Robinson, Harvey, McDonald, & Honegger, 2021; Zhu, Hu, Qi, Qin, & Chi, 2023). The pandemic accelerated university student counseling centers' adoption of open-access/SST. Clinicians in many of these settings have received training in open-access/SST and offer students both by-appointment and open-access single sessions.

Most online services, such as WTC, Strides, or BetterHelp, are made available to clients who can call, text, or email the service to ask for help. They are then provided with a link to an online platform for a confidential session with a therapist. Depending on the service provider, that session may begin immediately or be scheduled later that day. The prospective client can arrange for a telephone session by calling the service's number and being immediately connected with a clinician at a later designated time. Text-based services ordinarily begin when a client sends a text message to the service provider, which leads to an immediate text-based "conversation" with a clinician. Even though the pandemic has retreated, and in-person sessions are again available, many clients continue to prefer the online, telephone, and text-based options.

So far, no evidence exists that any of these formats is superior to another. Thus, giving clients a choice of format is a positive development because what will work best for a given client is what they think is the best fit for them. So, you can see that "walk-in" no longer captures the range of services we consider open-access/SST. This term can be applied to walk-in/SST, virtual online SST, over-the-phone SST, on-demand text-based SST, and same-day appointments for SST. We will now present some specific examples of how SST services have been expanded and implemented in open-access scheduling worldwide.

International Examples of Open-Access/SST

Open-Access/SST in Mexico

Several years ago, Monte began traveling to Mexico with graduate students to support our university's commitment to training culturally sensitive and culturally humble students. He was fortunate enough to have a couple of colleagues in Mexico interested in systemic, postmodern approaches to therapy. In the mid-2000s, a productive relationship with Jason Platt from Alliant University's Mexico City Campus led to multiple invitations to teach at Alliant and participate in cultural immersion programs for US students. Jason, already familiar with the walk-in/single session therapy (WI/SST) concept, expressed interest in collaborating to adopt the model for his training clinic at Alliant. Latin American liberation psychology significantly influenced Jason, notably Boal's Theatre of the Oppressed (ToO). ToO dramatically moved the performance and discussion of social and personal issues to the streets. Jason introduced Monte to his work in adapting ToO to street venues in Mexico City (Platt, 2016). Recognizing that ToO shared many characteristics with walk-in work as a single-session encounter, Jason and Monte began refining the merger of WI/SST with ToO (Platt & Bobele, 2022; Platt & Mondellini, 2014). This innovative approach aimed to move psychotherapy into public spaces, creating a more culturally relevant and meaningful client experience. This led to a model of service delivery where, following discussions with people on the street, they could be invited to visit the walk-in clinic right around the corner (Bobele, Cruz, Ceja, & Platt, 2018).

Helen Selicoff, a Mexico City psychologist, organized a workshop for Monte to present WI/SST to a group in Querétaro. There, he met Saúl Cruz-Valdivieso, a psychologist whose family founded *Armonía*, a charitable organization providing services to indigenous youth in rural Oaxacan villages. Beginning in 2010, Saúl had been building relationships specifically with Zapotec communities from Istmo de Huatentepec and from Sierra Juárez. Saúl, a psychologist by training, had been providing mental health services for several years to these indigenous peoples but felt constrained by the service delivery models he had been trained in. After attending the workshop, Saúl saw how the implementation of WI/SST fit perfectly with the mission of *Armonia*'s annual health clinics. Instead of the therapists working with a few people for several days in a row, they could see those needing mental health services only once during that visit. He began offering WI/SST services in the clinics, which allowed him to help more people and increased his competence. In 2017, Saúl invited Monte to one of *Armonia*'s medical missions in the small Oaxacan Zapotec mountain community of Santa Maria Zegache (Bobele & Ceja, 2020; Bobele et al., 2018; Bobele & Payne, 2022). Two years later, he was accompanied by another faculty member, four doctoral students, and some other volunteers from Texas to the remote town of Chichicaxtepec. During both visits, services were provided on a first-come/first-served, no-appointment-necessary basis. It is interesting that none of the people they helped during these medical clinics expected or requested that another session was going to be scheduled. The providers found that they were very busy. There were times when the makeshift waiting room, which consisted of metal folding chairs in the middle of the concrete basketball court that served as the area for the medical clinic, was occupied by 10 or more patiently waiting persons.

Other International Open-Access Examples

Finland: Despite its reputation for being the happiest country on Earth, Finland has also witnessed a decline in mental health in recent years that has seriously affected its young people. Two very enterprising therapists there have recently collaborated with the Evangelical Lutheran Church of Finland to provide open-access services to young people and young adults under the age of 29. From their beginning in 2021 until 2022 they established 14 new walk-in therapy services located in churches created in 12 communities (M. Mäkela & T. Perkiö, personal communication, November 2023).

Sweden: Söderquist (2018; 2023; Söderquist, Cronholm-Nouicer, Dannerup, & Wulff, 2021) has written extensively about SST with couples. He and his colleagues have recently introduced same-day and walk-in services to decrease the waiting time for couples to receive services (personal communication, 2023).

West Africa: An initiative to train hairdressers in mental health counseling is providing relief to hundreds of clients in a region with the world's least access to therapy. To meet those needs, mental health professionals are now providing hairdressers three days of training in which they learn basic counseling skills to talk with their customers, who ordinarily walk-in to get their hair done (Peltier, 2023).

Asia: Miller and his colleagues (Miller, Platt, & Conroy, 2018, 2021) have described their extensive work in adapting open-access/SST ideas in China and Cambodia. They have worked to understand and utilize the natural healing methods of the Khmer people and adapt these ideas in an open-access/SST context. In these contexts, therapy often occurs outside of offices and is rarely by appointment.

Challenges in Implementing Open-Access/SST

Therapists and clinic directors are often interested in how to adjust their procedures and policies when considering implementing open-access/SST. Here we will address some of the most common questions about implementation.

No Pre-Assessment

If people can arrive without an appointment and there is no pre-assessment, how do we start a session without information about the client/family? One of the main advantages of open-access/SST is its accessibility and ability to provide immediate support without lengthy waiting periods or intake processes. For many clients seeking help, pre-screening barriers can discourage them from seeking assistance altogether. Open-access/SST focuses on the client's presenting issues, and those goals drive the session, rather than adhering to a predetermined protocol driven by pre-assessments. Open-access/SST providers aim to meet the client in the moment and tailor interventions accordingly. Open-access/SST therapists adopt a strengths-based perspective, helping clients identify and build upon their existing resources and resilience. Most open-access services provide a brief intake form that can be quickly completed in less than 10 minutes. In many open-access services, pre-session information may consist of basic demographic information, perhaps with questions such as "What is the most critical concern you would like to address today?" At the Community Counseling Service, where Monte works, there is a scaling question about a client's current level of stress and a scaling question that asks the client how worried they are about harming themselves or someone else.

Follow-Up Session or Phone Call

Many open-access/SST services do not schedule follow-up sessions or phone calls. As a reminder to the reader, one definition of SST encourages us to treat each session as if it would be the last while *always making more sessions available.* Let us stress here that open-access/SST services routinely let clients know they are always invited to and may return for another SST session when they decide one is needed. So, it's true that we do not routinely schedule a follow-up. Instead, follow-up occurs if and when the client chooses. We believe this is empowering for clients. We trust that our clients are the experts in their lives and can decide when the next contact would be helpful for them. In some ways, we have begun to think that the subtle message we give our clients when we offer to schedule a follow-up appointment or even a phone call is that we don't have confidence they can decide for themselves when our next contact will be. We remind clients that the effects of the session may take a day or two to begin to be experienced. We also base this practice on the research that shows that most people don't return for a follow-up visit, even when it is scheduled at the end of the first visit. If a client needs reassurance that they are not being abandoned and that support will be easily available, we remind them how easy it was to access the current session.

Managing High Demand for Services

Some professionals questioned whether they would be overwhelmed by clients who took advantage of open-access scheduling. While this worried the Eastside Family Centre in the beginning, they soon realized it might be a sign that an open-access service was a good idea if lots of people were interested. It helped them rethink their staffing patterns. One of the things that frequently happens is that therapists who have cancellations and no-shows can fit walk-in or open-access clients into their schedules. We have found that it is unusual that we must turn someone away. When that happens, we inform the client that, should they arrive the next time the service is available, they will be the first one seen. In our experience, when open-access services begin, the demand is small and grows gradually over time. This slow startup gives an agency time to determine the optimal staffing and scheduling procedures.

Risk Issues

Some clinicians and administrators have asked about how to adjust their practices when clients arrive for an open-access/SST session presenting with serious risk issues. This, of course, does occur. As we described earlier, we find asking a simple question about risk on an intake form provides us a beginning to a risk assessment. One of the advantages we have found in asking about harm to oneself and/or others is that it provides a simple way for clients to alert us early on to potential suicidal issues along with domestic abuse. If the conversation requires, we address risk in open-access/SST sessions in the same ways as any other professional would in any other therapy session, and this could include extending the length of the session if necessary and arranging for additional resources to be contacted.

A meta-analysis by Franklin, Ribeiro, Fox, Bentley, and Kleiman (2017) examined research on risk factors associated with death by suicide. The analysis concluded that the current body of research is not sufficient to justify the common practices used to predict who is at risk of dying by suicide. Evidence suggests that suicide prevention strategies and screening in primary care settings have not been shown to reduce deaths by suicide (Zalsman, Hawton, Wasserman, van Heeringen, Arensman, Sarchiapone, & Purebl, 2016; Milner, Witt, Pirkis, Hetrick, & Robinson, 2017). Given the lack of empirical support for extensive suicide risk assessment, a brief one-question screening on an intake form, followed up by the clinician, may be a more efficient approach. On the other hand, this raises another issue about whether requiring clients to wait for a by-appointment session and delaying treatment with extensive pre-assessments may increase the risks associated with them. We think the mere existence of an open-access service reduces the risk in a community. The simple awareness of and availability to community members of easy access to a caring conversation may go a long way toward minimizing risk and increasing community mental health.

What Are the Advantages of Open-Access/SST?

We will elaborate on our previously offered advantages for providing open-access/SST (Slive & Bobele, 2018).

Open-Access/SST Seizes the Moment

When clients arrive for a session at a moment of their choosing without jumping through intake hurdles and waiting for an appointment, they will likely be highly motivated to address their issues with a mental health clinician. In fact, in our work, we find that clients frequently report that improvement has already begun once they have decided to contact our clinic. We can than begin the session by encouraging and planning for continued improvement. This increases the likelihood that the session will be productive, lead to positive outcomes, and address a client's highly important issue. Also, as a fortuitous byproduct, highly motivated and satisfied clients lead to happy and satisfied therapists (Borglum, 2014; Cohidon, Wild, & Senn, 2019).

Open-Access/SST Works!

An increasing number of researchers consistently find that clients report satisfaction with their SST sessions in community mental health centers (Boyhan, 1996; Ewen, Mushquash, Mushquash, Bailey, & Haggarty, 2018; Harris-Lane, Keeler-Villa, Bol, Burke, & Churchill, 2023; Harper-Jaques & Foucault, 2014; O'Neill, 2015) and in university counseling centers (Finch et al., 2023; Shaffer et al., 2017), reduction of distress by the end of their session, and positive outcomes immediately after the session and at follow-ups several months later (Barwick, Urajnik, Sumner, Cohen, & Reid, 2013; Harper-Jaques & Foucault, 2014; Riemer, Stalker, Dittmer, Cait, & Horton, 2018). A growing body of research in primary care settings confirms that people seeking healthcare are more satisfied with their care when some version of open-access scheduling is available to them (Huff, 2017; Richter, Downs, Beauvais, Huynh, & Hamilton, 2017).

Open-Access/SST Is Efficient

Open-access/SST reduces administrative costs associated with cumbersome intake processes, managing waitlists, and expensive emergency services use. It eliminates "no-shows." It also reduces overtreatment by inviting the client to focus on taking one small step to manage an immediate concern (Horton, Stalker, Cait, & Josling, 2012).

Other Advantages

Ezekiel Emanuel, an expert on the ethics of healthcare, and his team of researchers analyzed healthcare systems worldwide to arrive at several recommendations for improvement. Emanuel (2017) described the advantages of adopting open-access scheduling in healthcare clinics adopting open-access services. We think these advantages also apply to mental health services:

1. When patients are seen on the same day, wait times and waitlists are reduced (Ansell, Crispo, Simard, & Bjerre, 2017). He also cited a Kaiser Permanente study (Forjuoh, Averitt, Cauthen, Couchman, & Symm, 2001) that found that implementing open-access scheduling produced a 20% drop in no-shows.
2. A second advantage was that physicians and staff were happier because patients were more satisfied with the services they were receiving (Borglum, 2014; Cohidon et al., 2019).
3. Lastly, open-access benefits patients, lowers healthcare costs, and significantly reduces the use of emergency rooms and urgent care facilities (Ansell et al., 2017; Rust, Ye, Baltrus, Daniels, & Adesunloye, 2008).

Conclusion

In this chapter, we have described how the distinguishing feature of the Canadian/Texan Model of Single-Session, or One-at-a-Time, Therapy is the pathway clients follow from the point where they decide to get mental health services to the moment they begin talking with a therapist. The implementation of open-access scheduling practices significantly reduces many of the hurdles to get seen, increases choice for clients as to the timing of sessions, and perhaps most importantly, allows the client the opportunity to meet with a therapist at a moment in time that is meaningful. For the most part, although not exclusively, SST is provided in the appointment service delivery model. There is no question that by appointment SST is a valuable addition to the mental health service delivery system. However, the distinction between open-access and "by appointment" is not trivial.

Many practitioners have been curious about implementing open-access services such as those we have been developing. We have faced skeptical questions and comments about open-access/SST from the beginning of our work. For the most part, these were expressed by our mental health professional colleagues but not by other stakeholders in the community at large. These stakeholders (e.g., educators, medical professionals, and political representatives) have been universally positive about this new idea. A few wondered why, if there were already walk-in (open-access) medical clinics, shouldn't there also be walk-in mental health services? In this chapter, we have offered advice for the common implementation questions and concerns. We have provided examples of successful implementations of open-access/SST in North America, Europe, and Asia. We look forward to seeing the reports of more new implementations in print and at the next International Symposium on Single Session Therapy.

Note

1 *Editors' note*: See Chapter 14 (McElheran) in this volume.

References

Ansell, D., Crispo, J.A.G., Simard, B., & Bjerre, L.M. (2017). Interventions to reduce wait times for primary care appointments: A systematic review. *BMC Health Services Research, 17*, 1–9. https://doi.org/10.1186/s12913-017-2219-y
Barit, A. (2019). Appointment cancellations and no shows: To charge or not to charge? *South African Medical Journal, 109*(10), 733–735. https://doi.org/10.7196/SAMJ.2019.v109i10.14050
Barwick, M., Urajnik, D., Sumner, L., Cohen, S., Reid, G., Engel, K., & Moore, J.E. (2013). Profiles and service utilization for children accessing a mental health walk-in clinic versus usual care. *Journal of Evidence Based Social Work, 10*(4), 338–352. https://doi.org/10.1080/15433714.2012.663676

Basnet, S., & Chaiton, M. (2024). Effectiveness of the Wellness Together Canada Portal as a digital mental health intervention in Canada: Protocol for a randomized controlled trial. *JMIR Research Protocols, 13*, e48703. https://doi.org/10.2196/48703

Bobele, M., & Ceja, D. (2020). Érase una vez sin cita. (Once upon a time without an appointment). In A.T. Suck (Ed.), *Psicoterapia Integrativa: Una Aproximación a la Práctica Clínica Basada en Evidencias*. Editorial El Manual Moderno.

Bobele, M., Cruz, S., Ceja, D., & Platt, J.J. (2018). *Therapeutic Spaces in Public Places: Pláticas en la Plaza* [Conference Session]. Symposium Presented at the Annual Meeting of the American Psychological Association, San Francisco.

Bobele, M., & Payne, D. (2022). Once upon a walk-in (*Érase una vez sin cita*). *Journal of Systemic Therapies, 41*(1), 1–12.

Borglum, K. (2014). Five ways to optimize your patient schedule. *Urology Times, 42*(6), 25–25.

Boyhan, P.A. (1996). Client's perceptions of single session consultations as an option to waiting for family therapy. *Australian and New Zealand Journal of Family Therapy, 17*(2), 85–96. http://search.ebscohost.com/login.aspx?direct=true&db=psyh&AN=1997-02121-002&site=ehost-live

Cannistrà, F., & Piccirilli, F. (2021). *Single-Session Therapy: Principles and Practice*. Giunti.

Cohidon, C., Wild, P., & Senn, N. (2019). Practice organization characteristics related to job satisfaction among general practitioners in 11 countries. *Annals of Family Medicine, 17*(6), 510–517. https://doi.org/10.1370/afm.2449

Cornish, J., & Churchill, A. (2023). More than apps: Psychology's contribution to digital mental health. *Psynopsis: Canada's Psychology Newspaper, 45*(2), 34.

Cornish, P.A., Berry, G., Benton, S., Barros-Gomes, P., Johnson, D., Ginsburg, R., Whelan, B., Fawcett, E., & Romano, V. (2017). Meeting the mental health needs of today's college student: Reinventing services through Stepped Care 2.0. *Psychological Services, 14*(4), 428–442. https://doi.org/10.1037/ser0000158 (College Counseling Services)

Cornish, P.A., Churchill, A., MacKay, T.-L., & Jaouich, A. (2020). Wellness together Canada: Psychologists leading Canada's COVID-19 mental health response. *Psynopsis: Canada's Psychology Newspaper, 42*(3), 14–15.

Duvall, J., Young, K., & Kays-Burden, A. (2012). *No More, No Less: Brief Mental Health Services for Children and Youth*. Ontario Centre of Excellence for Child and Youth Mental Health. www.excellenceforchildrenandyouth.ca

Emanuel, E.J. (2017). *Prescription for the Future: The Twelve Transformational Practices of Highly Effective Medical Organizations*. Public Affairs.

Ewen, V., Mushquash, A.R., Mushquash, C.J., Bailey, S.K., Haggarty, J.M., & Stones, M. (2018). Single-session therapy in outpatient mental health services: Examining the effect on mental health symptoms and functioning. *Social Work in Mental Health, 16*(5), 573–589. https://doi.org/10.1080/15332985.2018.1456503

Finch, E.F., Kleiman, E.M., Bentley, K.H., & Bernstein, E.E. (2023). Helpful for all? Examining the effects of psychotherapy treatment history on outcomes of single session, transdiagnostic cognitive behavioral interventions for university students. *Psychological Services*. https://doi.org/10.1037/ser0000781

Forjuoh, S.N., Averitt, W.M., Cauthen, D.B., Couchman, G.R., Symm, B., & Mitchell, M. (2001). Open-access appointment scheduling in family practice: Comparison of a demand prediction grid with actual appointments. *Journal of the American Board of Family Practice, 14*(4), 259–265.

Franklin, J.C., Ribeiro, J.D., Fox, K.R., Bentley, K.H., Kleiman, E.M., Huang, X., Musacchio, K.M., Jaroszewski, A.C., Chang, B.P., & Nock, M.K. (2017). Risk factors for suicidal thoughts and behaviors: A meta-analysis of 50 years of research. *Psychological Bulletin, 143*(2), 187–232.

Harper-Jaques, S., & Foucault, D. (2014). Walk-in single session therapy: Client satisfaction and clinical outcomes. *Journal of Systemic Therapies, 33*(3), 29–49.

Harper-Jaques, S., & Leahey, M. (2011). From imagination to reality: Mental health walk-in at South Calgary Health Centre. In A. Slive & M. Bobele (Eds.), *When One Hour is All You Have: Effective Therapy for Walk-In Clients* (pp. 167–183). Zeig, Tucker, & Theisen.

Harris-Lane, L.M., Keeler-Villa, N.R., Bol, A., Burke, K., Churchill, A., Cornish, P., Fitzgerald, S.F., Goguen, B., Gordon, K., Jaouich, A., Lang, R., Michaud, M., Mahon, K.N., & Rash, J.A. (2023). Implementing one-at-a-time therapy in community addiction and mental health centres: A retrospective exploration of the implementation process and initial outcomes. *BMC Health Services Research, 23*(1), 1–13. https://doi.org/10.1186/s12913-023-09923-5

Horton, S., Stalker, C.A., Cait, C., & Josling, L. (2012). Sustaining walk-in counselling services: An economic analysis for a pilot study. *Healthcare Quarterly, 15*(3), 44–449.

Hoyt, M.F., Rosenbaum, R., & Talmon, M. (1992). Planned single session therapy. In S.H. Budman, M.F. Hoyt, & S. Friedman (Eds.), *The First Session in Brief Therapy* (pp. 59–86). Guilford Press.

Huff, C. (2017). To keep patients, some physicians get creative. *Health Affairs, 36*(12), 2040–2043. https://doi.org/10.1377/hlthaff.2017.1341

Josling, L., & Cait, C.-A. (2018). The walk-in counseling model: Research and advocacy. In M.F. Hoyt, M. Bobele, A. Slive, J. Young, & M. Talmon (Eds.), *Single-Session Therapy by Walk-In or Appointment: Administrative, Clinical, and Supervisory Aspects of One-at-a-Time Services* (pp. 91–103). Routledge. https://doi.org/10.4324/9781351112437-6

Kaplan, G.S. (2015). Health care scheduling and access: A report from the IOM. *JAMA: Journal of the American Medical Association, 314*(14), 1449–1450. https://doi.org/10.1001/jama.2015.9431

Lamsal, R., Stalker, C.A., Cait, C.-A., Riemer, M., & Horton, S. (2018). Cost-effectiveness analysis of single-session walk-in counselling. *Journal of Mental Health, 27*(6), 560–566. https://doi.org/10.1080/09638237.2017.1340619

McElheran, N., Harper-Jaques, S., & Lawson, A. (2020). Introduction to the special section: Walk-in single-session and booked single-session therapy in Canada. *Journal of Systemic Therapies, 39*(3), 15–20.

Miller, J.K., Platt, J.J., & Conroy, K.M. (2018). Single-session therapy in the majority world: Addressing the challenge of service delivery in Cambodia and the implications for other global contexts. In M.F. Hoyt, M. Bobele, A. Slive, J. Young, & M. Talmon (Eds.), *Single-Session Therapy by Walk-In or Appointment: Administrative, Clinical, and Supervisory Aspects of One-at-a-Time Services* (pp. 116–134). Routledge. https://doi.org/10.4324/9781351112437-8

Miller, J.K., Xing, D., Yaorui, H., & Yilin, X. (2021). Single session team family therapy (SSFT) in China: A seven-step protocol for adapting Western methods in Eastern contexts. In M.F. Hoyt, J. Young, & P. Rycroft (Eds.), *Single Session Thinking and Practice in Global, Cultural, and Familial Contexts: Expanding Applications* (pp. 245–254). Routledge. https://doi.org/10.4324/9781003053958-23-28

Milner, A., Witt, K., Pirkis, J., Hetrick, S., Robinson, J., Currier, D., Spittal, M.J., Page, A., & Carter, G.L. (2017). The effectiveness of suicide prevention delivered by GPs: A systematic review and meta-analysis. *Journal of Affective Disorders, 210*, 294–302.

O'Neill, I. (2015). What's in a name? Clients' experiences of single session therapy. *Journal of Family Therapy, 39*(1), 63–79. https://doi.org/10.1111/1467-6427.12099

Peltier, E. (2023). Need some therapy? In West Africa, hairdressers can help. *New York Times, 173*(59985), A4–A4.

Piccirilli, F. (2023). *How to conduct an SST: The Canadian—Texan model.* Retrieved July 31, 2022, from https://www.singlesessiontherapies.com/blog-post/how-to-conduct-a-sst-the-canadian-texan-model/

Platt, J.J. (2016). Pedestrians as professors: Theater of the oppressed in Mexico city. *Psychology International.* https://www.apa.org/international/pi/2016/09/pedestrians-professors

Platt, J.J., & Bobele, M. (2022). Therapeutic spaces in public places: Reflections on storytelling and antipropaganda dialogues in Mexico. *International Perspectives in Psychology: Research, Practice, Consultation, 11*(4), 238–245. https://doi.org/10.1027/2157-3891/a000042

Platt, J.J., & Mondellini, D. (2014). Single session walk-in therapy for street robbery victims in Mexico City. In M.F. Hoyt & M. Talmon (Eds.), *Capturing the Moment: Single Session Therapy and Walk-In Services* (pp. 215–231). Crown House Publishing.

Richter, J.R., Downs, L., Beauvais, B., Huynh, P.V., Hamilton, J.E., Kim, F., & Weigel, F. (2017). Does the proportion of same-day and 24-hour appointments impact patient satisfaction? *Quality Management in Health Care, 26*(1), 22–28. https://doi.org/10.1097/QMH.0000000000000121

Riemer, M., Stalker, C.A., Dittmer, L., Cait, C.-A., Horton, S., Kermani, N., & Booton, J. (2018). The walk-in counselling model of service delivery: Who benefits most? *Canadian Journal of Community Mental Health, 37*(2), 29–47. https://doi.org/10.7870/cjcmh-2018-019

Robinson, A.M., Harvey, G., McDonald, M., & Honegger, T. (2021). Introducing single session therapy at a university counseling center. In M.F. Hoyt, J. Young, & P. Rycroft (Eds.), *Single Session Thinking and Practice in Global, Cultural, and Familial Contexts: Expanding Applications* (pp. 143–152). Routledge.

Rodriguez, I.J. (2018). *Terapia Breve Sin Cita*: Colloboration with a marginalized community in Mexico City. In M.F. Hoyt, M. Bobele, A. Slive, J. Young, & M. Talmon (Eds.), *Single-Session Therapy by Walk-in or Appointment* (pp. 291–302). Routledge.

Rodriguez, I.J. (2022). Collaborative-dialogic practices in a single-session therapy format: A clinical example in an EAP. *Journal of Systemic Therapies, 41*, 13–27.

Rust, G., Ye, J., Baltrus, P., Daniels, E., Adesunloye, B., & Fryer, G.E. (2008). Practical barriers to timely primary care access: Impact on adult use of emergency department services. *Archives of Internal Medicine, 168*(15), 1705–1710. https://doi-org.ezproxy.ollusa.edu/10.1001/archinte.168.15.1705

Shaffer, K.S., Love, M.M., Chapman, K.M., Horn, A.J., Haak, P.P., & Shen, C.Y.W. (2017). Walk-in triage systems in university counseling centers. *Journal of College Student Psychotherapy, 31*(1), 71–89. https://doi.org/10.1080/87568225.2016.1254005

Slive, A., & Bobele, M. (Eds.) (2011). *When One Hour Is All You Have: Effective Therapy for Walk-In Clients.* Zeig, Tucker, & Theisen.

Slive, A., & Bobele, M. (2018). The three top reasons why walk-in/single-sessions make perfect sense. In M.F. Hoyt, M. Bobele, A. Slive, J. Young, & M. Talmon

(Eds.), *Single-Session Therapy by Walk-In or Appointment: Administrative, Clinical, and Supervisory Aspects of One-at-a-Time Services* (pp. 27–39). Routledge. https://doi.org/10.4324/9781351112437-2

Slive, A., MacLaurin, B., Oaklander, M., & Amundson, J. (1995). Walk-in single sessions: A new paradigm in clinical service delivery. *Journal of Systemic Therapies*, *14*, 3–11.

Söderquist, M. (2018). Coincidence favors the prepared mind: Single sessions with couples in Sweden. In M.F. Hoyt, M. Bobele, A. Slive, J. Young, & M. Talmon (Eds.), *Single-Session Therapy by Walk-In or Appointment: Administrative, Clinical, and Supervisory Aspects of One-at-a-Time Services* (pp. 270–290). Routledge. https://doi.org/10.4324/9781351112437-18

Söderquist, M. (2023). *Single Session One at a Time Counselling with Couples: Challenge and Possibility*. Routledge.

Söderquist, M., Cronholm-Nouicer, M., Dannerup, L., & Wulff, K. (2021). Making the leap with couples in Sweden: One-at-a- time mindset in action. In M.F. Hoyt, J. Young, & P. Rycroft (Eds.), *Single Session Thinking and Practice in Global, Cultural, and Familial Contexts: Expanding Applications* (pp. 163–172). Routledge. https://doi.org/10.4324/9781003053958-15-19

Stalker, C.A., Riemer, M., Cait, C.-A., Horton, S., Booton, J., Josling, L., . . . Zaczek, M. (2016). A comparison of walk-in counseling and the wait list model for delivering counseling services. *Journal of Mental Health*, *25*(5), 403–409. https://doi.org/10.3109/09638237.2015.1101417

Strides Toronto. (2023). *One stop talk expands access across Ontario this back-to-school season*. https://www.newswire.ca/news-releases/one-stop-talk-expands-access-across-ontario-this-back-to-school-season-844772919.html

Talmon, M. (1990). *Single Session Therapy: Maximizing the Effect of the First (and Often Only) Therapeutic Encounter*. Jossey-Bass.

Young, J., & Rycroft, P. (1997). Single session therapy: Capturing the moment. *Psychotherapy in Australia*, *4*(1), 18–23.

Young, K. (2018). Change in the winds: The growth of walk-in therapy clinics in Ontario, Canada. In M.F. Hoyt, M. Bobele, A. Slive, J. Young, & M. Talmon (Eds.), *Single-Session Therapy by Walk-In or Appointment: Administrative, Clinical, and Supervisory Aspects of One-at-a-Time Services* (pp. 59–71). Routledge. https://doi.org/10.4324/9781351112437-4

Young, K., Dick, M., Herring, K., & Lee, J. (2008). From waiting lists to walk-in: Stories from a walk-in therapy clinic. *Journal of Systemic Therapies*, *27*(4), 23–29.

Zalsman, G., Hawton, K., Wasserman, D., van Heeringen, K., Arensman, E., Sarchiapone, M., & Purebl, G. (2016). Suicide prevention strategies revisited: 10-year systematic review. *The Lancet Psychiatry*, *3*(7), 646–659.

Zhu, S., Hu, Y., Qi, D., Qin, N., Chi, X., Luo, J., Wu, J., Huang, H., Wu, Q., Yu, L., Ni, S., Hamilton, K., & Tse, S. (2023). Single-session intervention on growth mindset on negative emotions for university student mental health (U-SIGMA): A protocol of two-armed randomized controlled trial. *Trials*, *24*(1), 713. https://doi.org/10.1186/s13063-023-07748-5

Chapter 9

Bringing a Single-Session Mindset to Counselling in an Online Health Service in the UK

Windy Dryden

This chapter will outline my counselling work in the period March 2022–April 2023 for an online health service. This work can be described as single session by default rather than by design, as the modal number of my sessions is "1." At the same time, the service is advertised as providing between six and eight 30-minute counselling sessions annually. I will show how I bring a single-session mindset to this work and detail my experiences. This chapter is based on my experiences alone, and while there are more than 70 counsellors who work in a self-employed capacity for the organization, I know very little about how they work. I will describe my work with one of my clients, present another client's account of their session with me, and discuss some helpful and unhelpful aspects of working within the organization.

Introduction

"Scimitar Health" (a pseudonym) is a UK online health service offering online consultations to people with private health insurance with specific companies. These companies contract with Scimitar Health—through the insurance companies—to provide consultations that can be had with GPs, physiotherapists, nutritionists, mental health counsellors, and life coaches. The consultations are accessed and booked through a mobile phone application and conducted via video or phone. Depending on which company a person is insured with, they can have between six and eight 30-minute counselling sessions a year. When using the counselling part of the service, the person can choose to use their annual entitlement of sessions in any way they choose, although they are discouraged from seeing more than one practitioner at a time and having more than one session a week. It appears that the modal number of counselling sessions that people have is one. I have been a counsellor for Scimitar Health since March 2022 and typically offer between 25 and 50 half-hour sessions monthly.

DOI: 10.4324/9781032693828-12

The Process

When clients book a counselling session, they do so on the app on their phone. They can see the appointment times available for consultations and the counsellors that can be seen at those times. Each counsellor has a short biographical statement next to their name. Mine is:

> I am Emeritus Professor of Psychotherapeutic Studies at Goldsmiths University of London. I am a Fellow of the British Psychological Society (BPS) and the British Association for Counselling and Psychotherapy (BACP). I am the developer of ONEplus therapy. This means that I will work with you to help you take away something that will make a difference in your life due to our conversation (the 'ONE'). If you need more help, that is fine too, and you can always talk to me again or to one of my colleagues (the 'plus'). I aim to help you make the most out of every session we have together—one or more.

This indicates my interest in Single Session Therapy (which I refer to as *ONEplus therapy*—see Dryden, 2023a, 2023b) and makes clear that I will work to help the person to take away what they have come for from the session but that more help (up to six or eight sessions depending on the company with which they are insured) is available to them (Dryden, 2024a, 2024b)

Scimitar Health does not explicitly offer SST by design; its utilization patterns suggest that its work best be characterized as SST by default.

Problem Categories

When a booking is made, the counsellor can view the client's portal page, and here the client's issue is listed as being one of the following: "anxiety," "depression/low mood," "stress," "bereavement," and "other." Only individual counselling of adults is permitted in the service.

Preparing for an Online Counselling Session

I email the person when I receive a booking sent to my company email account as follows:

> Dear _____
> We have a 30-minute video counselling session booked through 'Scimitar Health' on (date and time), and I look forward to meeting you.
> You access the session through the app.
> I have found it helpful to ask clients to prepare for their session with me, and to that effect, I would be grateful if you would download and

complete the attached form. Let me emphasize that this is not mandatory; it is just something that will help you get the most from our session. If you decide to complete it, I would be grateful if you would share a copy with me by email attachment so I can prepare for our session too. Please send it back as a Word document or as a PDF.

Please be in an indoor, private space with no disruptions and a good internet connection. It does not work to have a counselling session in a coffee bar, in a car (even when stationary) or in an outside space. It is also not appropriate for you to be in your bedroom when having a counselling session.

Best wishes,
Windy Dryden

As the email clarifies, I outline the netiquette[1] of having an online session with me. I also invite the person who has booked a session with me to complete an attached form, which is the Pre-Session Questionnaire (PSQ)—see Table 9.1. I stress that the purpose of completing the PSQ is to

Table 9.1 Pre-session questionnaire sent to people who book a counselling session with me

---

Pre-Session Questionnaire

I invite you to fill in this questionnaire before your session with me. This will help you to prepare for the session so that you can get the most from it. It also helps me to help you as effectively as I can. Please return it by email attachment before our session. This will help me prepare for the session. Please be brief and concise in your answers.

Name: Date:

1. **What is the issue that you want to focus on in the session?**
   Be concise. In one or two sentences, get to the heart of the problem, if possible.

2. **Why is this significant?**
   What's at stake? How does this affect your life? What is the future impact if the issue is not resolved?

(Continued)

Table 9.1 (Continued)

3. What do you want to get from the session?

4. Specify briefly the relevant background information.
What do you think I need to know about the issue to help you with it? Summarise in bullet points.

5. How have you tried to deal with the issue up to this point?
What steps, successful or unsuccessful, have you taken so far in addressing the issue?

What are the strengths or inner resources that you have as a person that you could draw upon while tackling the issue?
If you struggle with answering this question, think of what people who really know you and who are on your side would say.

6. Who are the people in your life who can support you as you tackle the issue?
Name them and say what help each can provide.

7. What help do you hope I can best provide you in the session? Please check the main one.

☐ Help me to develop greater understanding of the issue

☐ Just listen while I talk about the issue

☐ Help me to express my feelings about the issue

☐ Help me to solve an emotional or behavioural problem; help me get unstuck

☐ Help me to make a decision

☐ Help me to resolve a dilemma

☐ Other (please specify):

Thank you.
Windy Dryden

help the person prepare for the session so that they get the most from it. I also invite them to send me the completed form so that I can prepare for the session. I stress that its completion is not mandatory. Approximately 80% of people complete and return the questionnaire. There is a high correlation between those who don't return it and those who cancel or fail to attend the session.

As far as I am aware, I am the only Scimitar Health counsellor to ask clients to prepare for what is probably the only session they will have (see the later section of this chapter "The Modal Number of My Sessions is '1'").

Type of Help Requested by Clients

Norcross and Cooper (2021) argue and provide data to support the contention that effective therapy is more likely to occur when the client receives the type of help they seek from the therapist than when they receive a different type of help. To provide clients with the help they want from the session, I ask them to specify this on the PSQ. Table 9.2 outlines the help requested by a sample of 300 people who booked a counselling session between March 2022 and April 2023. This shows clearly that the most frequent form of help requested by this cohort was for a specific emotional or behavioral problem with which the person had become stuck. However, as Table 9.2 also shows, a minority of clients sought a different form of help. As someone guided by single-session thinking (e.g., Cannistrà, 2022), I aim to offer each client the help they want rather than the help I think they need.

30-Minute Sessions

Scimitar Health only offers clients 30-minute counselling sessions. While this may be considered relatively short compared to the "standard"

Table 9.2 Type of help wanted (N = 300)—(pre-session questionnaire—select one)

Category	Number	%
Help me to solve an emotional or behavioural problem; help me get unstuck	163	54.3%
More than one category specified	58	19.3%
Help me to develop a greater understanding of the issue	37	12.3%
Other	13	4.3%
No category specified	9	3.0%
Help me to express my feelings about the issue	7	2.3%
Help me to make a decision	7	2.3%
Help me to resolve a dilemma	4	1.3%
Just listen while I talk about the issue	2	0.7%

50-minute therapy session, I find it quite ample given my experience con-ducting demonstrations of SST in training workshops (Dryden, 2018). In over 750 such sessions, the average session length was 22 minutes, 14 seconds. Thus, I am used to helping clients get what they want from a counselling session within the 30 minutes allotted to counsellors.

The Modal Number of My Sessions Is "1"

As I have already stated, while 70 counsellors work for Scimitar Health, I know very little about the nature of the work they do and what the modal number of their sessions is. The data I am now going to present concerns only the work I do for the organization.

From March 2022 to April 2023, I saw 463 Scimitar Health clients for 601 sessions. Figure 9.1 outlines the number of people I saw in that period and the number of sessions I had with them. As can be seen, the modal number of sessions that I had with clients is "1." However, I do not know if clients sought further help from other counsellors in the service because such data are not available to individual practitioners.

The Case of "George"

As an example of the counselling work I do for Scimitar Health, I will pre-sent the case of "George" (a pseudonym). George is a 31-year-old man who

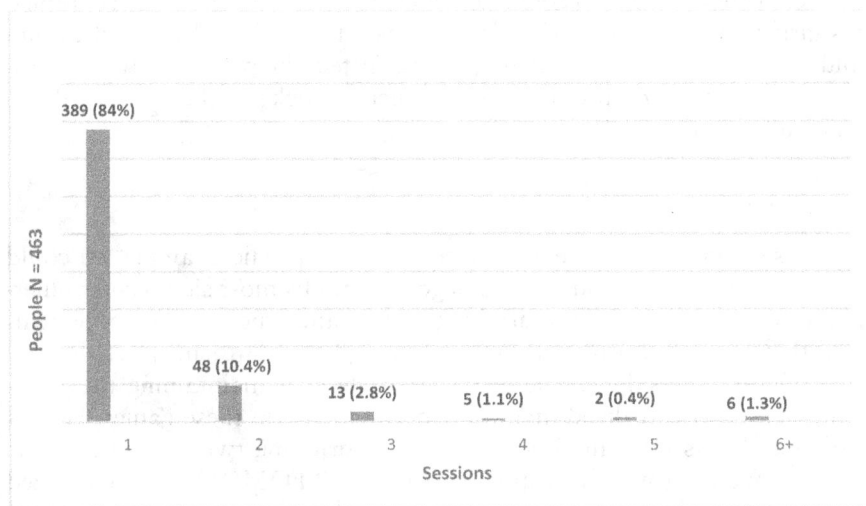

Figure 9.1 Modal number of sessions (N = 601) carried out by Windy Dryden for 'Scimitar Health' from March 2022 to April 2023.

listed his problem as "Other." As described earlier, I sent George an email requesting that he prepare for the session by completing the Pre-Session Questionnaire (PSQ) and returning it to me so I could also prepare for the session.

George's PSQ

George reported having an issue with binge drinking, which led him to neglect his friends and girlfriend. Occasionally, he drinks so much that he blacks out and cannot remember what happened to him. He has not yet gotten into trouble but recognizes that he is putting himself at risk by drinking the way he does. He wanted to discuss the issue with a neutral party to see if there was a reason for his behavior and to discover "good methods for dealing with this." He wanted to learn how to go out drinking with his friends without getting "blackout" drunk. He mentioned that he does not seem to have great self-control and struggles to say no to people. He also said that he used to be shy and is now more confident but has used alcohol to help him with his confidence.

In response to the question concerning what he had done to deal with the issue, George replied that he had tried tracking his use of alcohol on nights out and setting himself limits. When he did reduce his alcohol intake use, he later rewarded himself by drinking more on subsequent nights out.

Outlining the strengths he has that he could use to address the issue, George said that he has a scientific outlook and likes to know the why of things. He also said that he is competitive and does not like to lose. Listing the people in his life who could help him with the issue, George mentioned his girlfriend, three male friends, and his father, who all listened to him and tried to reassure him. Finally, George listed "help me to solve an emotional or behavioural problem; help me get unstuck" as the type of help he wanted from me.

The Session

In the session, I asked George to nominate a specific example we could work with to understand what was going on. His most significant vulnerability was to participate in drinking games, and when he did so, he realized that his competitive self believed he had to win them. Here, he saw that what he considered one of his strengths was maintaining the problem. George also realized that while participating in these games, he was ordering drinks for himself so that he was drinking twice as much as he wanted. We dealt with his fear of missing out ("FOMO"), and he realized he could enjoy himself without engaging in drinking games. Not wanting to disappoint others was another factor here, but I helped him see that his friends would still like him if he chose not to participate in drinking games or decided to drink less and that if any of his friends stopped liking him, they were not his true friends. He also concluded that he would not order drinks outside of the game if he chose to engage in a drinking game.

I distinguished between distal and proximal factors, which George thought was helpful. His distal factors were why he wanted to control his drinking—not wanting to worry his girlfriend and not wanting to be vulnerable when he is "blackout" drunk. However, while these factors were important, they did not help him deal with the proximal factors—the factors that he faced in the moment (e.g., dealing with disappointing his friends, not wanting to miss out and ordering drinks outside of drinking games while having drinking drinks in these games).

I helped him deal with these proximal factors in imagery so that he could practice assertion and self-control. For example, he imagined being invited to join a drinking game when he was out and rehearsed the idea that he didn't need to accept this invitation, even if his friends seemed disappointed. Then he pictured himself saying no to the game. He then pictured himself feeling uncomfortable about missing out on the fun but reminded himself that he was doing so to protect his well-being and repay the trust placed in him by his girlfriend. He resolved to rehearse this imagery method daily and at the beginning of an evening out.

Finally, I helped George see that while he had tried in the past to deal with logical factors (e.g., monitoring his alcohol intake and setting limits on his drinking), these had not been successful because he had not dealt with the psychological factors that we discussed in the session. This explanation, he said, appealed to his scientific nature. At the end of the session, George said that he had gotten what he had come for and would seek further help if he needed to in the future.[2]

Claire's Perspective

Claire was another client I saw through my work with Scimitar Health. What follows is her account of the session she had with me put into the context of her life.

> I myself am a counsellor, but I came to this single session model when I needed help personally. I reached out for help after a difficult interaction with my Mum left me shaken and was getting in the way of me reaching out to people professionally.
>
> I had been excited and confident about new business plans when I shared them with my Mum. We have a difficult relationship and she is often critical. On this occasion, I'd let myself believe she might be encouraging, so her evident disapproval and lack of support stung. It

left me feeling rejected and like a child again seeking validation. I needed to believe in myself to move forward, but her criticism had derailed me.

This became a problem on the work front when I noticed myself avoiding the influential people I wanted to reach out to. I was holding back and wanted to keep all my ideas safe inside me. I knew my relationship with my critical and opinionated Mum was at the heart of all this. But this insight wasn't helping me do things differently. I didn't want or have the capacity for long-term therapy. I wanted a shortcut back to "me" after this recent incident at a critical time had shaken my sense of self and identity. I was just tired, a bit lost, and needing a strategy.

I received the questionnaire[3] several days before my planned session with Windy and I. Filling it out saved me. Taking time to reflect on my problem prevented me from falling into an age-old trap. The trap of spending time and energy trying to make it "right" with my Mum, of desperately trying to change her mind and alter her perception of me. I still did this from time to time, even after years of boundary-setting and long-term therapy and knowing full well we can't change what others choose to see.

Under the question, "How have you tried to deal with the issue up to this point?" I wrote everything I knew helped (which was helpful), then lastly,

I've also tried engaging with and speaking with her about this.—This has never been successful!

Seeing this written down in black and white had a big impact. "Oh," I thought to myself, "I HAVE tried this endlessly and doggedly for years. Every time it fails to help and actually harms me." Clear that I shouldn't go there, this galvanised me to look for solutions elsewhere.

While I didn't relish the "work" involved in writing about my problems, it was helpful to list my resources and strengths and get things out of my head and onto paper. It brought lightness and clarity to something that had felt heavy and messy. I'm not one for journaling, even though I know it's helpful. Here I got the benefits of journaling but with helpful structured questions to help me pinpoint the problem and accountability. I felt ready for our session and hopeful about the change it promised.

I had already identified the crux of my problem and knew what I wanted via a questionnaire, so we had a productive start. Though I didn't know Windy, I immediately felt comfortable and knew he genuinely wanted to understand me and my problem in order to help. We didn't discuss my Mum, just what I wanted to achieve which was a simple strategy to shore me up and hold in mind as I reached out with my work. Using an upcoming real-life situation as an example, we imagined how I'd feel and what I could do differently. I felt supported yet challenged to stay focused. This didn't feel like a holding space. It felt like a safe space to imagine and do.

It became clear that I had a perspective problem. I saw myself as "less than" the "important" people I wanted to engage. I wanted a way to elevate my view of myself. Windy suggested something I couldn't see: I could change how I see others by humanising them, metaphorically bringing them down to size, too. I envisioned myself as a bit bigger AND others as essentially human like me. We also prepared for dismissal from some busy people because that was the likely reality. I realised dismissal itself wasn't a problem; it was linking rejection to feeling unworthy and small that hindered me. I could feel differently after any rejection, so be free to proceed confidently. Resizing my perception of myself and others would allow me to reach out effectively. As a therapist used to 50-minute sessions, I was struck that we hadn't even used our half hour. I left hopeful, with a clear plan to apply this perspective shift.

Professionally, it completely changed the way I work. I retrained to offer Single-Session Therapy to ensure more people aren't left waiting and get help at the time of need. My experience of being let down by a system that had promised to support led me to rethink what we need from the systems themselves. I do now believe that, sometimes, one session working in a focused and intentional way is all the support they need.

I now know that things go well for me when I feel an appropriate size in professional relationships. I know to mentally "right-size" people whenever things feel out of whack. This has helped hugely as I establish myself in my work and bring my ideas to the world. As I write, it's clear I should try this technique with my Mum now, too. Half an hour of therapeutic time well spent had a huge impact. And time spent in preparation and reflection has as well.

Organizational Factors

Jeff Young (2018) has pointed out that SST occurs in a given context. When that context is an organization, the "health" of that organization will impact whether the practice of SST will flourish or wither. So, let me end this chapter by discussing the aspects of Scimitar Health that facilitate the work I do for the organization and those that detract from that work.

Features of Scimitar Health That Facilitate My Work

One of the biggest drivers in my work life is autonomy. Most of the time, I know what I am doing and want to be left alone to do it. Given that all counsellors who work for Scimitar Health are self-employed, we are autonomous about how we practice, but, of course, we must work within organizational guidelines, which, in the period covered by this chapter is that we offer between six and eight sessions to each client annually depending upon which insurance company they are covered by. This means I can work as much or as little as I want and practice as I want (within the aforementioned constraints). On this latter point, I bring a single-session mindset to the work and clarify this in my biographical statement. My main aim is to help each client take away from the session the help they specified on my pre-session questionnaire (PSQ), which I have permission from the organization to send out to a person once I have received their booking (see Postscript).

The best aspect of my work for Scimitar Health is that I love it and would be loath to give it up (although see the following section for a discussion of factors that detract from my work). I consider that there is a lot I can do with a client who comes to the 30-minute session duly prepared to work with me to get the most from it. In short, being a counsellor for Scimitar Health allows me to help a range of people while bringing a single-session mindset to this work.

Features of Scimitar Health That Detract From My Work

However, my experience has taught me that there is also a downside to working for Scimitar Health. First, given that counsellors are self-employed, the organization does not supervise our counselling work, arguing that this is our responsibility given our self-employed status. They make no checks on whether counsellors seek clinical supervision and do not know if our supervisors are skilled at the work we do so that they can offer us informed supervision.

Second, in the period covered by this chapter (March 2022–April 2023), Scimitar Health did not provide counsellors with any access to a relevant clinical lead for our work. Clinical leads are typically responsible for overseeing the delivery of high-quality client care and implementing best practices and guidelines to ensure that clinical standards are maintained. The role of a supervisor is to give a counsellor *specific* feedback on their work with clients, while the role of a clinical lead is to provide *general* guidance on clinical standards. The company's clinical lead in this period was a medical general practitioner who was not professionally trained as a counsellor. Consequently, counsellors were left without the clinical guidance they could reasonably expect from an organization such as Scimitar Health. Subsequently, the organization appointed two counsellors to join a clinical oversight team whose duties have not been clarified for the counsellors.

Third, in the designated period, counsellors had no opportunity to talk to one another about therapeutic matters raised by working for the organization. This lack of an appropriate forum meant that counsellors were isolated and lacked the support that is, in my view, necessary for those working for an organization such as Scimitar Health.

Fourth, the 30-minute video sessions—or phone calls if there are connection issues—are recorded and are kept by the company for an unspecified period for safeguarding purposes or if there is a complaint. Clients give their informed consent for these recordings to be made. However, if they refrain from doing so, the session does not take place. These recordings could be used—with permission—for training and development purposes, but this is not done.

Fifth, the organization does not attempt to collect data from clients to assess the outcome of counselling, and there is no evaluation of individual counsellors' performance. Thus, if the organization is asked about the effectiveness of its counselling service or how it discriminates between effective and ineffective counsellors, it cannot answer such questions. That said, as a practitioner, I ask clients at the end of the session if they have gotten what they have come for and how they plan to implement their takeaways.

I have tried to address these five issues with the organization but have not had valuable responses, and in some cases, my questions have been unanswered. I am constantly wavering between continuing to do the work I love and working for an organization I am critical of. Despite these frustrations, it is a delight to be able to help clients often in one session.

Postscript

While I was attending the 4th International Symposium on Single Session Therapy in Rome in November 2023, I and other counsellors working for Scimitar Health received an email stating that given the changes that had been recently made to service provision, counsellors were only allowed to have contact with clients during counselling sessions or through the Silver Cloud portal.[4] This seemed to mean that I would no longer be able to send my welcome email to clients who had booked in to see me and the Pre-Session Questionnaire presented in Table 9.1, even though I had previous permission to do so and had done so for over a year. The newly appointed clinical lead confirmed this. This proved to be the tipping point for me, and I tendered my resignation in November 2023.

Scimitar Health's position on counsellor-client contact meant to me the following:

1. I could not welcome clients who had booked a session with me.
2. I could not outline the "netiquette" of online counselling to clients.
3. Most importantly, I could not ask clients to prepare to get the most from the session by completing my pre-session questionnaire.
4. I could not send clients any relevant information after the session.

While I loved the work, I had reached a point where the fit between myself as a practitioner and Scimitar Health as the host organization was not a sustainable one.

We can expect online SST to expand in the future, and I hope these experiences will help guide us towards what can make online SST optimally useful.

Notes

1 *Netiquette* describes the rules of conduct for respectful and appropriate online communication.
2 As I will discuss later, Scimitar Health does not attempt to gain outcome data from its clients, so at present I do not know what use George made of the session.
3 This refers to the pre-session questionnaire discussed earlier.
4 Silver Cloud is a digital mental health and well-being platform providing digital cognitive behavioral therapy (CBT) programs and tools.

References

Cannistrà, F. (2022). The single session therapy mindset: Fourteen principles gained through an analysis of the literature. *International Journal of Brief Therapy and Family Science, 12*(1), 1–26.

Dryden, W. (2018). *Very Brief Therapeutic Conversations*. Routledge.

Dryden, W. (2023a). *ONEplus Therapy: Help at the Point of Need*. Onlinevents Publications.

Dryden, W. (2023b). What's in a name? What to call therapy when a client may come once. *Inside Out, 100*, 12–14.

Dryden, W. (2024a). *Single-Session Therapy: 100 Key Points and Techniques* (2nd ed.). Routledge.

Dryden, W. (2024b). *How to Think and Intervene Like a Single-Session Therapist*. Routledge.

Norcross, J.C., & Cooper, M. (2021). *Personalizing Psychotherapy: Assessing and Accommodating Patient Preferences*. American Psychological Association.

Young, J. (2018). SST: The misunderstood gift that keeps on giving. In M.F. Hoyt, M. Bobele, A. Slive, J. Young, & M. Talmon (Eds.), *Single-Session Therapy by Walk-In or Appointment: Administrative, Clinical, and Supervisory Aspects of One-at-a-Time Services* (pp. 40–58). Routledge.

Chapter 10

Designing, Testing, and Disseminating Digital Single-Session Interventions for Youth Mental Health

Jessica L. Schleider

As a clinical psychology Ph.D., professor, and intervention scientist, I have spent over a decade studying and delivering mental healthcare for children, adolescents, and families—and growing convinced that existing treatment systems are largely built to fail. My journey to leading a clinical research laboratory focused on highly scalable, single-session interventions did not emerge out of early training experiences or exposure to mentors in this subfield. (In fact, it was not until several years into studying single-session interventions did I realize that a community of single-session therapy practitioners existed at all!) Rather, my path has stemmed from total frustration with the failures of status-quo mental health infrastructures—and an overwhelming desire to help build something better. In this chapter (also see Schleider, 2023), I will share how I came to single-session interventions (SSIs) as a promising path to improving access treatment; developed and studied *self-guided, digital single-session interventions* for youth mental health problems, which expand traditional professional-delivered single-session therapies; how my research team, the Lab for Scalable Mental Health, has studied and disseminated digital SSIs to date; and how, moving forward, digital SSIs might bridge gaps within and beyond formal systems of care.

Status-Quo Mental Health Systems Will Never Be Enough

There is a breathtaking chasm between need and access to youth mental health care. Between 50% and 80% of youth who need support access no treatment at all (Costello, He, Sampson, Kessler, & Merikangas, 2014).

And this gap is a feature, not a bug, of how care is delivered. Most mental health treatment happens in brick-and-mortar, hard-to-access clinics; it is carried out by highly trained professionals over long periods of time (often months to years) (Kazdin, 2019). If the number of licensed child therapists were to miraculously double overnight, provider shortages

DOI: 10.4324/9781032693828-13

would still be insurmountable. Treatment would still be unaffordable, clinics out of reach, and insurance coverage unreliable. Perhaps most damningly: Even among youth who do access therapy, the most common number of sessions they receive is just one. The average is fewer than four. Yet, most evidence-based therapies for child depression, anxiety, and behavior problems are meant to last between twelve sessions and twenty.

Existing mental health treatments are structurally incompatible with how people access treatment. The youth mental health crisis will keep getting worse without radical changes to where, when, and how mental health support can be delivered.

How I Came to Study Single-Session Interventions

When I began my clinical psychology Ph.D. training at Harvard University in 2012, I already had a primary interest in "nontraditional" approaches to providing mental health treatment, mainly by offering psychotherapies through schools and community-based settings. I hoped to "meet youth where they are" by embedding evidence-based treatments, such as cognitive behavioral therapy, into the settings where young people already were. However, my early practical experiences as a Ph.D. student revealed the challenges of these approaches: multi-session therapies were incredibly challenging to embed into school and community settings, and the problems of early patient dropout and provider shortages were just as bad (if not worse) in these settings as in traditional mental health clinics and hospitals. Time after time, I saw youth and clients who were unable to return for session two, regardless of how much they wanted help. By midway through my training, I had grown deeply interested in strategies to maximize the odds that a young person's first session—and often their *only* session, especially in lower-resource service settings like schools and community centers—could sustainably help them. So, I launched a systematic review project to learn whether single-session interventions could benefit children and teens at all, and more generally, whether anyone had tried to find out. I had not heard of SSIs in my graduate training, so I was delighted to learn that I was far from the first person to ask this question! Our resulting meta-analysis compiled results from fifty RCTs spanning a forty-year period and including 10,508 young people across Asia, North America, South America, Europe, and Australia (Schleider & Weisz, 2017). We saw that SSIs significantly reduced a wide range of youth mental health problems, compared to various controls, with only slightly smaller effects on symptom levels than multi-session (on average, sixteen-session) treatments (Weisz, Kuppens, Ng, Eckshtain, & Ugueto, 2017). SSIs' positive effects were *no different* for youth with more- or less-severe symptoms, or for youth with or without a formal diagnosis. In other words, SSIs seemed to benefit youths with mild, moderate, and more severe mental health challenges. This meta-analysis also supported the promise of *online* SSIs: positive SSI effects emerged even for self-guided programs (digital interventions that did not involve any therapist). Given my early and sustained interested in "meeting youth where they are," this finding was particularly striking to me. Young people lead rich, active digital lives, and the dominance of online communication is only growing. Studying SSIs that could be delivered online—especially those that were self-guided, seemed like an enormously promising path toward improving youths' support access at scale.

A quick note on my use of the term "single-session interventions," or SSI: I use this term to be maximally inclusive as to what one-session supports can look like and how they can be delivered. The term single-session *therapy*, or SST, is ostensibly specific to treatments that require a trained clinician—and since single-session supports can be delivered outside the confines of formal treatment settings and do not necessarily require a provider, my team has adopted the term SSI as a broader alternative. In this vein, we have offered an updated definition of SSIs (including therapist-delivered SST and self-guided single-session tools) as "specific, structured programmes that intentionally involve just one visit or encounter with a clinic, provider or program" (Schleider, Burnette, Widman, Hoyt, & Prinstein, 2020).

The Lab for Scalable Mental Health's Work on Digital SSIs to Date

Over the past six years, my research team and I have built and tested digital, self-guided SSIs for adolescents with depression, anxiety, body image difficulties, and self-harm, among other common mental health difficulties. Several of these SSIs—all twenty-minute, interactive activities completable from any internet-equipped device—have been tested in multiple clinical trials. (These SSIs are also freely available online if you would like to try them yourself or share with others: www.schleiderlab.org/ YES). Collectively, they have served >50,000 youth to date (Schleider & Weisz, 2018; Schleider, Mullarkey, Fox, Dobias, & Shroff, 2022; Schleider et al., 2020; Schleider, Dobias, Sung, Mumper, & Mullarkey, 2020; Dobias, Morris, & Schleider, 2022; Shen, Rubin, Cohen, Hart, & Sung, 2023; Cohen, Dobias, Morris, & Schleider, 2023; Shroff, Roulston, Fassler, Dierschke, & San Pedro Todd, 2023; Smith, Ahuvia, Ito, & Schleider, 2023; Dobias, Schleider, Jans, & Fox, 2021). Here, I will overview our digital SSI research specifically in the realm of adolescent depression—among the leading causes of youth disability worldwide, and where much of my research on youth mental health began.

Two of our digital SSIs have shown promise in reducing youth depression. One, called Project Personality, teaches that personal traits (like shyness, sadness, or likeability) and mental health problems (like depression and anxiety) are *malleable* through a combination of personal effort and support (this is often called a "growth mindset"). The other, the Action Brings Change (ABC) Project, teaches how and why doing activities in line with your personal values—such as friendship, learning, or generosity—can disrupt and reverse "negative mood spirals" linked to depression.

In a 2019 *Atlantic* article on our team's digital SSIs, reporter Olga Khazan described her experience trying Project Personality herself "to see how teens might use it to essentially perform therapy on themselves, without the aid of a therapist":

> The strange little PowerPoint asks me to imagine being the new kid at school. I feel nervous and excluded, its instructions tell me. Kids pick on me. Sometimes I think I'll never make friends. Then the voice of a young, male narrator cuts in. "By acting differently, you can actually build new connections between neurons in your brain," the voice reassures me. "People aren't stuck being shy, sad, or left out." In the middle of my new-kid scenario, the program tells me the story of Phineas Gage, the 19th-century railroad worker whose behavior changed radically after a metal spike was driven through his skull. [. . .] The program uses Gage's experience to suggest that personality resides at least partly in the brain. If a metal spike can change your disposition, Project Personality reasons, so can something less violent—such as a shift in your mind-set. [. . .] Project Personality finds a way to make [this] uplifting: "By learning new ways of thinking, each of us can grow into the type of person we want to be." Toward the end, the activity asks me to reassure a friend who was snubbed by another friend in high school. What would I tell the friend about how people can change? It encourages me to apply what I just learned about personality and the brain. The total program takes me less than an hour to complete.

The reporter summarized her understanding of the program's main takeaway in a few simple statements: "Your story isn't over till it's over. Your character's plot is still unfolding; there's still time to escape. Sometimes, it can take hours and hours on a therapist's couch to understand that. Maybe, just maybe, it could start to take less."

In our first RCT of Project Personality with ninety-six high-symptom teens, the SSI increased teens' sense of control over their own emotions and actions. It also led to clinically meaningful reductions in teens' depression and anxiety symptoms nine months later. For this trial, it's worth noting that we created an "active" comparison program: a single-session online activity that encourages teens to share their emotions, without teaching specific skills (we call it the Sharing Feelings Project). Comparing Project Personality to the Sharing Feelings Project helps us make sure that our

SSI isn't just better than *nothing*—but that it's better than *something* that seems, on its face, like it might help.

Project Personality has also prevented increases in depression symptoms in a school-based clinical trial, which included 222 high school girls in a low-income, rural U.S. town (Schleider et al., 2020). And in an open trial (meaning that everyone got an SSI right away, with no control group), we saw that high-symptom teens who completed the ABC Project (as well as another SSI, Project CARE, teaching how and why self-compassion can help us reach our goals) showed boosts in their perceived problem-solving abilities, along with feelings of agency and hope (Schleider et al., 2020). We've seen the same pattern of results for SSIs adapted for Spanish-speaking youth in San Antonio, Texas (Dobias et al., 2022).

When the COVID-19 pandemic hit, given skyrocketing mental health needs, we decided to put our digital SSIs to the most rigorous test yet: in a large, diverse teen sample, and in an incredibly high-stress context, could our digital SSIs *still* help alleviate depression symptoms? We secured grant funding from the National Institute of Health to find out. For this randomized clinical trial, we took to social media (specifically, Instagram) to recruit a nationwide sample of 2,452 teens (50% youth of color; 80% sexual and gender minority youth; across all fifty U.S. states). Results indicated that *both* Project Personality and the ABC Project outperformed the Sharing Feelings control. That is, they both led to meaningful three-month reductions in depression symptoms, hopelessness, and restrictive eating in teens experiencing depression (Schleider & Weisz, 2018). Project Personality also helped reduce anxiety and COVID-related trauma symptoms three months later. With these results, we finally felt confident in asserting that our digital SSIs really *could* help reduce teen mental health challenges, even amidst unprecedented global stress.

Understanding Theories of Change in Digital SSIs to Streamline Adaptation and Dissemination

By understanding *how* digital SSIs work, or identifying their "active ingredients," we can streamline different groups' efforts to adapt and implement these tools within specific communities and contexts. Broadly, the digital SSIs we have designed target theory-driven principles and proximal factors that underlie general behavior change—regardless of the distal outcome of interest. Our group has outlined a four-component process to designing digital SSIs capable of spurring behavior change, grounded in basic research in social psychology, education, and marketing. These design features involve (1) including scientific evidence and social-norming data to normalize the users' experiences and boost message credibility; (2) empowering users as "experts"; (3) allowing users to share back what they learn during the intervention to help others in their community navigate similar challenges; and (4) including lived experience narratives from others facing similar challenges. Many SSIs also guide users to develop an "action plan" for using the new skill, to strengthen motivation and self-efficacy in future strategy use (Schleider & Weisz, 2018; Schleider et al., 2022; Schleider, Burnette, et al., 2020; Schleider, Dobias, et al., 2020). These design principles reflect insights from participatory action research, which highlights the benefits of empowering individuals to "expert" positions (Baum, MacDougall, & Smith, 2006), consistent with effective implementation approaches; self-determination theory, which suggests that boosting feelings of competence, agency, and relatedness can motivate adaptive behavior change (Berg, Coman, & Schensul, 2009); as well as meta-analyses suggesting that narratives increase persuasiveness of health-related messaging (Shen, Sheer, & Li, 2015; van Laer, Feiereisen, & Visconti, 2019). It is also consistent with the notion of creating what Hoyt (2014) has termed a "context of competence" promoted within a provider-delivered SST session: both digital and human-facilitated SSIs aim to strengthen clients' feelings of strength, hopefulness, expectancies that change is possible, and a sense of agency to make meaningful changes in their lives. Indeed, evidence from digital SSI trials suggests that short-term changes in these outcomes (e.g., perceived control and agency) predict larger improvements in long-term clinical outcomes (e.g., depression, anxiety), suggesting these targets as likely mechanisms of the programs' effects (Schleider, Abel, & Weisz, 2019). Notably, all four of these design principles may be integrated into even the briefest of digital SSIs, including those that have required just five to eight minutes of users' time (e.g., via inclusion of a single peer quotation, a single free-response item, or a two-sentence description of a psychoeducational concept). The SSI design features highlighted here reflect recommendations for framing SSI content, which may be built-out as briefer or longer interventions, per context-specific needs. At the same time, it is not necessarily required that an SSI encompass all four design features; they are presented as one of potentially many approaches to constructing digital SSIs that spur improvements in relevant outcomes.

The Future of Digital SSIs for Youth Mental Health: Targeted Dissemination and Implementation

Digital, self-administered SSIs have potential to catalyze dissemination of evidence-based treatments on a population and global level, reaching individuals who may not otherwise have access to care (Ghosh, McDanal, & Schleider, 2023). To realize this potential, demonstrating that they can benefit young people is only the first step. The next (far more challenging) steps involve building sustainable pathways for youth to actually access them, outside of federally funded clinical trials, both in and beyond systems of care. Our team members (and many others!) are testing the promise of several such pathways, evaluating SSIs' promise as both stand-alone and adjunctive supports and for youth with and without acute mental health difficulties. Implementation efforts to date have shown particular promise in three contexts: online (via social media), in healthcare settings (in both specialty and non-specialty mental health settings), and in schools.

Disseminating Digital SSIs Online

In digital forums, posts, and direct messages, young social media users routinely share their mental health symptoms and experiences, including those related to depression (De Choudhury, Gamon, Counts, & Horvitz, 2013), eating disorders (Fitzsimmons-Craft, Krauss, Costello, Floyd, & Wilfley, 2020), and self-harm (Kruzan, Bazarova, & Whitlock, 2021), to find support from peers with shared experiences. Critically, social media users often belong to the groups that are least likely to access traditional mental health treatment (e.g., LGBTQ+ and racial/ethnic minority young people; McInroy & Craig, 2015). This makes social media platforms an ideal setting for bridging gaps in existing avenues to care.

Despite the potential for SSI delivery through social media, popular platforms have rarely been used for this purpose (Rideout, Fox, Peebles, & Robb, 2021). However, our team did establish a now-ongoing partnership with Koko—a nonprofit, online mental health organization—to test whether "in-the-moment" SSIs might be helpful, and acceptable, to users of Tumblr, a popular social media platform with more than 130 million monthly active users (Dobias et al., 2022). Users searching for mental health–related topics on the platform received a direct message with links to crisis resources and SSIs, presented within Koko as "mini-courses." Each of these three SSIs was self-guided, five to eight minutes in length, and targeted a core idea or skill (e.g., "taking action can help improve your mood") drawn from multi-session, evidence-based therapies (e.g., behavioral activation). Not only were youth very willing to try (and complete!) the SSIs, but they seemed to concretely help. The 6,179 Tumblr users who finished an SSI showed meaningful drops in their hopelessness and self-hate, along with increased motivation to stop self-harm. And the magnitude of these improvements matched the benefits of SSIs we had seen previously, in our randomized trials—suggesting that our digital SSIs appeared immune to what treatment researchers have termed the "voltage drop" effect, or the tendency for the impact of evidence-based interventions to shrink when delivered within real-world contexts (as opposed to well-controlled research studies). Our lab's SSIs are now permanent offerings provided by

Koko, which has delivered in-the-moment social media–based support to more than two million people to date.

Disseminating Digital SSIs in Healthcare Settings

Within non-specialty medical settings (e.g., primary care, emergency departments), self-administered SSIs may be offered alongside standard referrals to mental healthcare clinics, allowing youths presenting with elevated symptoms the opportunity to receive immediate care, while still pursuing longer-term treatment if desired (Eyllon, Dalal, Jans, Sotomayor, & Peloquin, 2023). Within the extant literature, primary care clinics have offered digital SSIs focused on positive parenting practices (Bailin & Bearman, 2022), growth personality mindset (Ching, Bennett, Morant, Heyman, & Schleider, 2023), and preventing cannabis use (Walton, Resko, Barry, Chermack, & Zucker, 2014). Additionally, emergency departments have implemented SSIs targeting alcohol use and peer violence (Ranney, Goldstick, Eisman, Carter, & Walton, 2017; Walton, Chermack, Shope, Bingham, & Zimmerman, 2010).

Digital SSIs may also have utility within more specialized healthcare settings, such as mental health clinics. Specialty clinics often have waiting lists of up to several months, which may lead to clinical deterioration of youth waiting for psychiatric services (Reichert & Jacobs, 2018). The availability of digital SSIs during these waiting periods may allow treatment-seeking youths and young adults to capitalize on their motivation and receive evidence-based care the moment they seek it. While digital SSIs have not been formally investigated in this context, promising results from open trials indicate that provider-delivered SSIs may facilitate clinically and improve later treatment attendance (Perkins, Bowers, Cassidy, Meiser-Stedman, & Pass, 2021). Given that the effectiveness of digital SSIs is comparable to that of provider-delivered SSIs (Schleider & Weisz, 2017), digital SSIs for youth mental health may serve as an especially scalable option to connect treatment-seeking youth in specialized healthcare settings with low-intensity, in-the-moment support.

Disseminating Digital SSIs in Schools

While medical settings may serve as a logical path for offering digital mental health SSIs to high-acuity youth, school settings have more commonly been used to evaluate digital SSIs (Perkins et al., 2021). School-based SSI delivery confers several pragmatic benefits, including reducing stigma (e.g., by normalizing SSIs as tools available and helpful for all students) and decreasing access barriers to youth with resistance toward formal help-seeking. Within school settings, digital SSIs have often been tested as stand-alone supports, showcasing their potential for improving mental health outcomes for young people who may not otherwise have sought out or accessed traditional care. Trials of SSI delivery in middle and high schools have targeted youth depression symptoms and suicidal ideation (Miu & Yeager, 2015), anxiety symptoms (Schleider & Weisz, 2018), and overall emotional well-being (Perkins et al., 2021). Despite these studies' promising results, efforts to *sustain* digital SSIs within school settings after clinical trials end—and to create accessible on-ramps to students to access these supports—remain scarce. Moving ahead, cross-sector collaborations involving school staff and administrators, clinical scientists, and students will be crucial to identifying opportunities to move beyond clinical trials and into systemic sustainment.

Conclusion

Status-quo mental health systems will never be sufficient to meet youth mental health needs worldwide. Thus, it is essential to embrace out-of-the-box, evidence-grounded approaches to bridging gaps in ecosystems of care. As work from within and well beyond our lab has demonstrated, digital single-session interventions (SSIs) offer a scientifically supported means of expanding youths' access to in-the-moment mental health support—but there is considerable work to be done, particularly in cross-system integration, toward realizing their promise as a force for public health. That is, the existence of evidence-based digital SSIs does not guarantee uptake or sustainment. Long-term implementation of digital SSIs will require thoughtful integration and partnership within existing clinical and non-clinical workflows. This includes offering SSIs as an option to young people in diverse settings and ensuring that youths can equitably and securely access them on internet-equipped electronic devices. Ultimately, digital SSIs' promise to complement and extend mental healthcare systems and increase treatment access will only be realized through intentional, sustained deployment efforts involving communities (youth), multi-sector stakeholders, and clinical researchers alike. Regardless of the challenges ahead, evidence affirms that strategic dissemination of digital SSIs will be a worthwhile investment of time, expertise, and creativity, ultimately presenting an opportunity for a paradigm shift in the field of mental health.

References

Bailin, A., & Bearman, S.K. (2022). Brief, digital, self-directed, and culturally adapted: Developing a parenting intervention for primary care. *Children and Youth Services Review, 132*, 106314.

Baum, F., MacDougall, C., & Smith, D. (2006). Participatory action research. *Journal of Epidemiological Communications in Health, 60*, 854–857.

Berg, M., Coman, E., & Schensul, J.J. (2009). Youth action research for prevention: A multi-level intervention designed to increase efficacy and empowerment among urban youth. *American Journal of Community Psychology, 43*, 345–359.

Ching, B.C., Bennett, S.D., Morant, N., Heyman, I., Schleider, J.L., Fifield, K., Allen, S., & Shafran, R. (2023). Growth mindset in young people awaiting treatment in a paediatric mental health service: A mixed methods pilot of a digital single-session intervention. *Clinical Child Psychology and Psychiatry, 28*(2), 637–653.

Cohen, K., Dobias, M.L., Morris, R., & Schleider, J.L. (2023). Improving uptake of mental health crisis resources: Randomized test of a single-session intervention embedded in social media. *Journal of Behavioral and Cognitive Therapy, 33*, 24–34.

Costello, E.J., He, J., Sampson, N.A., Kessler, R.C., & Merikangas, K.R. (2014). Services for adolescents with psychiatric disorders: 12-month data from the national comorbidity survey–adolescent. *Psychiatric Services, 65*(3), 359–366.

De Choudhury, M., Gamon, M., Counts, S., & Horvitz, E. (2013). Predicting depression via social media. In *Proceedings of the Seventh International AAAI Conference on Weblogs and Social Media* (p. 10). Association for the Advancement of Artificial Intelligence.

Dobias, M.L., Morris, R., & Schleider, J.L. (2022). Single-session interventions embedded within Tumblr: A test of acceptability and utility. *JMIR Formative Research, 6*(7), e39004.

Dobias, M.L., Schleider, J.L., Jans, L., & Fox, K.R. (2021). An online, single-session intervention for adolescent self-injurious thoughts and behaviors: Results from a randomized trial. *Behaviour Research and Therapy, 147*, 103983.

Eyllon, M., Dalal, M., Jans, L., Sotomayor, I., Peloquin, G., Yon, J., Fritz, R., & Schleider, J. (2023). Referring adolescent primary care patients to single-session interventions for anxiety and depression: Protocol for a feasibility study. *JMIR Research Protocols, 12*, e45666. https://doi.org/10.2196/45666

Fitzsimmons-Craft, E.E., Krauss, M.J., Costello, S.J., Floyd, G.M., Wilfley, D.E., & Cavazos-Rehg, P.A. (2020). Adolescents and young adults engaged with pro-eating disorder social media: Eating disorder and comorbid psychopathology, healthcare utilization, treatment barriers, and opinions on harnessing technology for treatment. *Eating and Weight Disorders: Studies on Anorexia, Bulimia and Obesity, 25*(6), 1681–1692.

Ghosh, A., McDanal, R., & Schleider, J.L. (2023). Digital single-session interventions for child and adolescent mental health: Evidence and potential for dissemination across low- and middle-income countries. *Advances in Psychiatry and Behavioral Health, 3*(1), 129–138.

Hoyt, M.F. (2014). Psychology and my gallbladder: An insider's account of a single session therapy. In M.F. Hoyt & M. Talmon (Eds.), *Capturing the Moment: Single Session Therapy and Walk-In Services* (pp. 53–72). Crown House Publishing.

Kazdin, A.E. (2019). Annual research review: Expanding mental health services through novel models of intervention delivery. *Journal of Child Psychology and Psychiatry, 60*(4), 455–472.

Khazan, O. (2019, August 21). The quick therapy that actually works. *The Atlantic.* https://www.theatlantic.com/health/archive/2019/08/can-you-just-got-therapy-once/

Kruzan, K.P., Bazarova, N.N., & Whitlock, J. (2021). Investigating self-injury support solicitations and responses on a mobile peer support application. *Proceedings of the ACM on Human-Computer Interaction, 5*(CSCW2), 1–23.

McInroy, L.B., & Craig, S.L. (2015). Transgender representation in offline and online media: LGBTQ youth perspectives. *Journal of Human Behavior in the Social Environment, 25*(6), 606–617.

Miu, A.S., & Yeager, D.S. (2015). Preventing symptoms of depression by teaching adolescents that people can change: Effects of a brief incremental theory of personality intervention at 9-month follow-up. *Clinical Psychological Science, 3*(5), 726–743.

Perkins, A.M., Bowers, G., Cassidy, J., Meiser-Stedman, R., & Pass, L. (2021). An enhanced psychological mindset intervention to promote adolescent wellbeing within educational settings: A feasibility randomized controlled trial. *Journal of Clinical Psychology, 77*(4), 946–967.

Ranney, M.L., Goldstick, J., Eisman, A., Carter, P.M., Walton, M., & Cunningham, R.M. (2017). Effects of a brief ED-based alcohol and violence intervention on depressive symptoms. *General Hospital Psychiatry, 46,* 44–48.

Reichert, A., & Jacobs, R. (2018). The impact of waiting time on patient outcomes: Evidence from early intervention in psychosis services in England. *Health Economics, 27*(11), 1772–1787.

Rideout, V., Fox, S., Peebles, A., & Robb, M.B. (2021). *Coping With Covid-19: How Young People Use Digital Media to Manage Their Mental Health.* Common Sense and HopeLab. https://www.commonsensemedia.org/sites/default/files/research/report/2021-coping-with-covid19-full-report.pdf

Schleider, J.L. (2023). *Little Treatments, Big Effects: How to Build Meaningful Moments That Can Transform Your Mental Health.* Robinson.

Schleider, J.L., Abel, M.R., & Weisz, J.R. (2019). Do immediate gains predict long-term symptom change? Findings from a randomized trial of a single-session intervention for youth anxiety and depression. *Child Psychiatry and Human Development, 50,* 868–881.

Schleider, J.L., Burnette, J.L., Widman, L., Hoyt, C., & Prinstein, M.J. (2020). Randomized trial of a single-session growth mindset intervention for rural adolescents' internalizing and externalizing problems. *Journal of Clinical Child and Adolescent Psychology, 49,* 660–672.

Schleider, J.L., Dobias, M.L., Sung, J.Y., & Mullarkey, M.C. (2020). Future directions in single-session youth mental health interventions. *Journal of Clinical Child & Adolescent Psychology, 49*(2), 264–278.

Schleider, J.L., Dobias, M.L., Sung, J., Mumper, E., & Mullarkey, M. (2020). Acceptability and utility of an open-access, online single-session intervention platform for adolescent mental health. *Journal of Medical Internet Research: Mental Health, 7,* e2013.

Schleider, J.L., Mullarkey, M.C., Fox, K.R., Dobias, M.L., Shroff, A., Hart, E.A., & Roulston, C. (2022). A randomized trial of online single-session interventions for adolescent depression during COVID-19. *Nature Human Behaviour, 6,* 258–268.

Schleider, J.L., & Weisz, J.R. (2017). Little treatments, promising effects? Meta-analysis of single-session interventions for youth psychiatric problems. *Journal of the American Academy of Child & Adolescent Psychiatry, 56*(2), 107–115.

Schleider, J.L., & Weisz, J.R. (2018). A single-session growth mindset intervention for adolescent anxiety and depression: Nine-month outcomes of a randomized trial. *Journal of Child Psychology and Psychiatry, 59,* 160–170.

Shen, F., Sheer, V.C., & Li, R. (2015). Impact of narratives on persuasion in health communication: A meta-analysis. *Journal of Advertising, 44,* 105–113. https://doi.org/10.1080/00913367.2015.1018467

Shen, J., Rubin, A., Cohen, K., Hart, E.A., Sung, J., McDanal, R., Roulston, C., Sotomayor, I., Fox, K.R., & Schleider, J.L. (2023). Randomized evaluation of an online single-session intervention for minority stress in LGBTQ+ adolescents. *Internet Interventions, 33*, 100633.

Shroff, A., Roulston, C.A., Fassler, J., Dierschke, N.A., San Pedro Todd, J., Rios, Á., Plastino, K., & Schleider, J.L. (2023). A digital single-session intervention platform for youth mental health: Cultural adaptation, evaluation, and dissemination. *JMIR Mental Health, 14*(10), e43062.

Smith, A.C., Ahuvia, I., Ito, S., & Schleider, J.L. (2023). Project body neutrality: Piloting a digital single-session intervention for adolescent body image and depression. *International Journal of Eating Disorders, 56*(8), 1554–1569.

van Laer, T., Feiereisen, S., & Visconti, L.M. (2019). Storytelling in the digital era: A meta- analysis of relevant moderators of the narrative transportation effect. *Journal of Business Research, 96*, 135–146.

Walton, M.A., Chermack, S.T., Shope, J.T., Bingham, C.R., Zimmerman, M.A., Blow, F.C., & Cunningham, R.M. (2010). Effects of a brief intervention for reducing violence and alcohol misuse among adolescents: A randomized controlled trial. *JAMA, 304*(5), 527.

Walton, M.A., Resko, S., Barry, K.L., Chermack, S.T., Zucker, R.A., Zimmerman, M.A., Booth, B.M., & Blow, F.C. (2014). A randomized controlled trial testing the efficacy of a brief cannabis universal prevention program among adolescents in primary care: Efficacy of a brief cannabis universal prevention program. *Addiction, 109*(5), 786–797.

Weisz, J.R., Kuppens, S., Ng, M.Y., Eckshtain, D., Ugueto, A.M., Vaughn-Coaxum, R., Jensen-Doss, A., Hawley, K.M., Krumholz Marchette, L.S., Chu, B.C., Weersing, V.R., & Fordwood, S.R. (2017). What five decades of research tells us about the effects of youth psychological therapy: A multilevel meta-analysis and implications for science and practice. *American Psychologist, 72*(2), 79–117.

Chapter 11

Single Session Approach

How It Can Be Beneficial to Early Intervention and Youth Mental Health Services in the United Kingdom

Katy Stephenson

This chapter will focus on how a single session mindset in Early Intervention and Youth Mental Health Services in the United Kingdom, when introduced effectively, sensitively, and in a timely manner, can lead to positive outcomes. While there are numerous evidence-based interventions and approaches that demonstrate effectiveness in how we assist youth mental health presentations, a fundamental issue for our complex world is that they are often expensive, unobtainable, and time consuming. Single session thinking can enable us to utilize our resources promptly and efficiently and gives the client tangible ideas or resources to implement from the moment they enter the service.

Post-pandemic there has been an increase in the need for support in our communities due to unique challenges with global crises and cost-of-living increases as well as young people attempting to developmentally and academically catch up. Resuming normality has led to an increase in anxiety, social difficulties, and has impacted their mental health. The demand on public-sector services with limited resources and government cutbacks has led to skilled professionals leaving the profession or being burnt out. This ultimately has had a significant impact on the public, who are unable to access treatment or support in a timely manner. Child and Adolescent Mental Health Services (CAMHS) are often seen as the only option to obtain assistance for young people who are struggling, and those who are accepted into the service are often placed on a waiting list for two years or longer in some areas around the UK. This post-pandemic context requires us to think differently about how traditional public systems respond in a timely manner, utilizing resources in the most efficient and effective way.

In the United Kingdom, Young Minds (2023) reports that yearly referrals to young people's mental health services have risen by 53% since 2019. This data supports the evidence that due to youth public services being disbanded or significantly reduced by the government since 2010 young people requiring assistance has increased but they have no sufficient supports to access. We are also aware that a large percentage of vulnerable

DOI: 10.4324/9781032693828-14

young people who die by suicide may never access or be known to services, and therefore it is essential that as professionals we develop or consider other approaches that are easily accessible for our evolving generations.

How I Got Involved With SST

As described in Stephenson (2023), I had worked with young people in the public sector for 20 years in the UK and Australia. Whilst I was undertaking my Masters in Family Therapy training at The Bouverie Centre in Melbourne, Australia, in 2012 I had the privilege of meeting Moshe Talmon, one of the founders of Single Session Therapy (SST), who identified that the most common number of sessions a client will attend is *one* "no matter what their therapist's orientation or approach."

Talmon (1990) conceptualized SST—also known as Single Session Work (SSW; see Young & Rycroft, 2012; Hoyt, Young, & Rycroft, 2021, pp. 11–15)—as a process rather than an event that assists workers to make the most of the first, and what may be the only, session for clients. In Talmon's formulation, the process typically includes:

- initial phone contact between clinician and client(s) and/or the completion of a pre-session questionnaire
- one face-to-face session
- a follow-up phone call booked in by the clinician at the end of the session, which functions both as a clinical contact and a means to determine future treatment or referral options.

The initial phone contact supports buy-in from families to participate in the single session; describing the concept, evidence of effectiveness, what is expected, and giving hope to the family that this is an opportunity to meet with a clinician to help them navigate and understand how they might be able to help their situation. The clinician would make it clear if further intervention or specialist input through specific referral pathways should be considered and discussed following the session depending on their needs.

In collaboration with Robert Rosenbaum and Michael F. Hoyt (see Talmon, 1990; Rosenbaum, Hoyt, & Talmon, 1990/1995; Hoyt, Rosenbaum, & Talmon, 1992[1]), Talmon had researched the effectiveness and frequency of SST, and together they have influenced many practices globally. Further SST research (some cited later in this chapter) has demonstrated that it is particularly helpful to utilize a systemic approach in mental health services with the child and adolescent cohort. This led me to explore whether SST could be utilized in CAMHS, given the increase in demand and limited services.

Family and systemic psychotherapists in CAMHS settings in the UK usually work with the whole system involved in the child or young person's life and are traditionally positioned to work with young people and their families at the acute end of CAMHS services. This has always left me wondering whether our skill set would be better utilized earlier on; preventing long-term dependency and enabling families to take agency on their situation, building on their resources both internal and external to assist their situation.

Single session has been utilized in public health settings within Australia for over 20 years. Alfred CYMHS (Child & Youth Mental Health Services) in Melbourne (e.g., see Barbara-May, Denborough, & McGrane, 2018; Renkin, Alexander, & Wyder, 2021; McDonald, Hickey, & Wyder, 2021; Mildred, Hunter, Goldsworthy, & Brann, 2021) has documented that involving all family members, utilizing a reflecting team, and working systemically from the beginning can lead to positive outcomes for children and young people. Work (e.g., see Fuzzard, 2021) done at headspace, Australia's early intervention national youth mental health service, also has provided an opportunity to positively intervene at the right time and has been received favorably by the community, resulting in this being offered as a stand-alone treatment.

Kessler, Amminger, Aguilar-Gaxiola, Alonso, and Lee (2007; quoted in Edbrooke-Childs, Hayes, Lane, Liverpool, & Jacob, 2021) report that children and young people have the highest levels of mental health difficulties across the lifespan yet do not necessarily engage in traditional mental health services. In their research they explored different characteristics of young people and complexities to understand who attends for one session. They acknowledge that a large proportion of young people only attend for one session and note that further research is required to examine and identify the reason why high numbers only present for one session and do not sustain or require long-term treatment.

However, when single session has been introduced to clinicians in the UK there often appear to be concerns that there is a political agenda in trying to utilize this method as a way of cost-cutting services or reducing the number of sessions offered. Traditionally CAMHS services has not had a specific time limit on how or when services should cease. This often is left up to the discretion of the clinician and young person or family. This has therefore led to inconsistencies in how services are offered, and it can appear unfair to those who have been waiting for lengthy periods of time without any intervention. Furthermore, the title "single session" can raise anxiety in some clinicians due to concerns that it implies that children's mental health problems are simple to resolve and that the extensive training of family therapists and other professionals is unnecessary. When I was first introduced to the approach in 2010, I too was skeptical about how useful it would be. Only when I experienced this approach in practice and saw how effective it could be with families who were reporting positive feedback did I begin to explore how this approach could be utilized in all aspects of my work.[2]

Single Session Mindset

One of the primary advantages of a single session mindset is increased accessibility. Traditional therapeutic models often involve extended commitments, deterring some individuals from seeking help. Single Session Therapy offers immediate support. Swift accessibility is particularly crucial for youth mental health where timely intervention can prevent escalation or high-risk presentations that may require acute interventions.

Often young people's symptoms are a natural human response to their situation. When we reframe their symptoms in ways that promote resilience, self-awareness, and skill building, this prevents us from feeling the need to pathologize, which can at times be detrimental to a person's well-being and keep them in a state of mental unwellness. As clinicians we are realistically only involved in a client's life for a very short period of time. Therefore, it is essential to adopt a mindset from the onset that gives the client, their families, and carers hope that they have the resources internally and externally to manage, ultimately encouraging our role to become unneeded.

When I Think About Single Session Mindset These Are the Key Principles That Stand Out

Reducing Stigma and Encouraging Engagement

The stigma surrounding mental health can be a significant obstacle to seeking help. We know that young people who die by suicide are often not known to services, which suggests that there were barriers to them accessing support. Single session, which is brief and focused in nature, helps reduce this stigma. As noted earlier, individuals and families may find it less daunting to engage in single session rather than committing to longer-term therapy. The SST approach also aligns with evolving societal attitudes toward mental health, promoting a more open and accessible environment.

Relinquishing the Expert Stance and Encouraging Agency in Decision-Making

Encouraging agency in decision-making involves relinquishing the expert stance, fostering empowerment, and respecting individuals' autonomy to make choices that align with their values and goals. This approach acknowledges that individuals are the ultimate experts in their own lives and experiences and emphasizes collaborative and respectful partnerships between clients and practitioners.[3] By empowering individuals to actively participate in decision-making processes, they can take ownership of their choices and actions, leading to greater self-awareness, motivation, and positive outcomes.

In youth mental health services, it is essential that we enable the young person's voice to be heard regardless of age. They often are overlooked or unintentionally undermined. Enabling the young person's voice in a safe, respectful, and meaningful way empowers them to feel heard and understood in their context. In my own practice, when I have creatively brought in the young person's voice, it has enabled a much more positive outcome.

Empowering Individuals With Coping Strategies

The one-at-a-time (OAAT) mindset equips people with tangible coping strategies. By focusing on specific challenges and symptoms during a session, therapists can work collaboratively with clients to develop tailored strategies for managing challenges. This empowerment fosters a sense of control and self-efficacy, which are often essential components in maintaining well-being.

Collaborating With the System

As a systemic family therapist, I understand that it is important from the onset to explore the whole system that is involved in the child or young person's life. We are not born nor do we live in isolation. If we take a systems approach to understand the young person's symptoms, we often discover, particularly in early intervention youth mental health services, that many young people's issues and difficulties are relational in nature and all family members are affected. It also assists in helping family members who are crucial in the young person's life to attend. Parents are under significant pressures and do not always have the means (nor interest) to attend therapy on an ongoing basis, but a one-off session for some families is appealing.

Fostering a Preventative Approach

Beyond addressing current concerns, an OAAT mindset contributes to a preventative approach. By intervening early and providing timely support, single session therapies have the potential to prevent the development of more severe mental health issues.

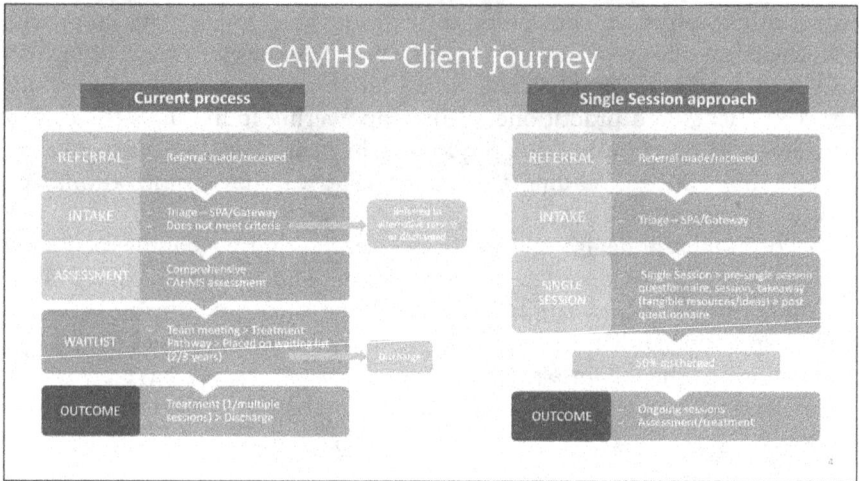

Figure 11.1 The CAMHS client journey.

If we adopt single session in CAMHS settings, could we shift the paradigm, preventing young people from being overly assessed, pathologized, and diagnosed when—as noted earlier—what they may be experiencing are natural human emotions for the situation or circumstance they are placed in? As Hoyt (2025, p. 33) has noted, " 'I'd be surprised and worried if you *didn't* feel that way, given what you've been through' can be a normalizing and very useful statement."

Figure 11.1 shows how services might look if we adopted a single session approach.[4]

Implementing Single Session in CAMHS Contexts in the UK

After my time in Australia, back in the UK I shared with CAMHS colleagues my experience of Single Session Family Therapy from the work of Jeff Young and his colleagues (e.g., see O'Hanlon & Rottem, 2021; von Dousa, Tsorlinis, Cordukes, Beauchamp, & McIntosh, 2021; Westwater, Murphy, Handley, & McGregor, 2020) at The Bouverie Centre in Melbourne. Young, then-director at The Bouverie, carried out research to explore length-of-term approaches to psychological treatment. He reported (Young, 2018, p. 44[5]):

1. The most common number of service contacts that clients attend, worldwide, is one, followed by two, followed by three—irrespective of diagnosis, complexity, or the severity of the problem.

2. 70–80% of people who attend only one session, across a range of therapies, report the single session was adequate given their current circumstance.
3. It is impossible to accurately predict who will attend only one session and who will attend more. Given this, why not approach the first session "as if" it might be the last?

Initially I introduced this to Sussex Partnership in 2018, and since then other trusts are utilizing this approach—although some might say they have been utilizing variants of this method for years. Single session was offered within four weeks of receiving the referral, and we also trialed using this after a spontaneous suicide attempt with positive outcomes. Clinicians are responsive to what the client wants by sharing ideas or thoughts with them. Single session may be all the client requires, but if they need more intervention or a different treatment pathway this can be discussed. The approach allows the clinicians to be direct in the moment and check in with the family to ensure it is proceeding in the right direction.

Single session is not necessarily the panacea for every presentation that we see in mental health settings. However, it provides a service model which assists to identify those that would benefit from an intervention over one, two, or even three sessions and makes availability for those that require longer-term treatment who will ultimately be treated more efficiently.

Single session doesn't necessarily suit everyone. We need to be mindful that it suits families that do have a reasonable level of insight or support. One-off sessions may not be appropriate when there are ongoing safeguarding concerns, which may not be clear until meeting with a family. Single session, however, does attend to risks immediately; by quickly meeting with children and young people and their families or carers, it gives us the time and space to ensure the appropriate response is carried out. If it is evident that single session is not appropriate, it is important to be transparent in a sensitive manner to ensure they get the right support.

Case Examples

In the United Kingdom, I have worked in two Child and Adolescent Mental Health Services (CAMHS); at Hampshire (run by Sussex Partnership Trust) and at Dorset Healthcare University Foundation Trust (DHUFT). CAMHS is a free National Health Service (NHS) helping children and young people from 0–18 years old with emotional, behavioral, and mental health difficulties. The service is broad and provides support and treatment, including individual and family therapy, medication, inpatient care, and parenting support courses. CAMHS teams only diagnose neurodevelopmental conditions (such as autism and ADHD) if there are significant co-morbid mental health difficulties.

Single session was first introduced at the Single Point of Access stage in Hampshire (known as Gateway in Dorset) when it was identified that a systemic and one-by-one approach may offer assistance or determine whether CAMHS treatment or other services were required. Sussex Partnership piloted this framework and now offers it as a stepped-care intervention.

When I worked in Dorset I was working as a family therapist in Tier 3 services, which is long-term acute stage of treatment. Children and young people had often undergone long extensive assessments and placed on a treatment pathway that had been identified to support their needs or symptoms. Often children and young people had been placed on a waiting list for a significant period of time before accessing treatment, therefore their presentations or symptoms had changed. I was always curious about why systemic psychotherapists weren't positioned at the entrance of CAMHS services, given that children and young people are not born in isolation and their system is crucial, as we know from the evidence to aid recovery. I presented Single Session Family Therapy (SSFT; Fuzzard, 2021; O'Hanlon & Rottem, 2021) to the leadership team to commence offering as an intervention from when a referral was received.

SSFT was identified by clinicians as a possible option for young people and their families from the onset. A phone call was made by either the intake worker or clinician receiving the referral to discuss this as a possible intervention, and a letter was sent with a leaflet that had been created by a previous service user. A questionnaire was also sent with the letter, and it explained that this assisted the clinician meeting with them in understanding the presenting concerns/problem. Autonomy was given over whether they wanted to accept SSFT or whether they wanted to wait for their child/young person to be assessed. It was also made clear that if they required more than SSFT that this would be discussed and should they not require any further SSFT interventions they could re-refer to CAMHS at any time. The majority of families were keen to engage with SSFT given the current waitlist times and lack of resources to assist in the community. The majority of families seen within SSFT expressed their gratitude and were pleased to be given guidance and support in helping their child.

Dorset Healthcare has trained clinicians and clinical services managers to adopt this approach. They are supportive and looking to use the concepts of SST to improve and transform the services to benefit young people. It is also recognized that this approach is not the panacea to all mental health presentations.

Here are three cases typical of what I have seen:

Case #1. "Tim," a 16-year-old young person who identified as he/him was referred to CAMHS after attending the Accident and Emergency (A&E) following an impulsive overdose. Tim and his mum were offered this session two weeks after being referred. He attended the session with his mum, Sally. Tim was one of three siblings. The parents' relationship had been conflictual since they separated some years ago. Single session was introduced to Tim and his mum, who had initial reservations about how one session would assist, given the risk concerns and Tim's suicidal thoughts. My colleague (another CAMHS clinician who was shadowing me) and I revisited the idea that one session may be enough to assist but that if they required more, we could explore next steps.

Tim was initially reluctant to engage, but when we explored his situation and what led to the overdose he began to soften and open up. I sensed Tim realized we were not viewing him as the problem and instead were viewing his overdose as an expression of his feelings.

"It sounds like you have been dealing with a lot recently. I am just wondering if your actions were more in response to how you were feeling and you didn't know how to express yourself or were worried about how this would be viewed by your parents?" Tim spoke of finding it hard to understand and talk about difficult emotions he was experiencing in fear of upsetting his mum and disappointing his dad, whom he was close to. Tim was completing his end of school exams and felt pressure to academically excel like his siblings; however, he acknowledged he was not academically minded and preferred sports. During the session I was able to be more direct and check in with him about alternative ideas or possibilities about his situation. "Tim, I am wondering if it would be okay to share some thoughts that have come up for me and as I hear you talk about your situation? It sounds like you are worried about your relationship with your parents and you worry about upsetting them?" I learned he had withheld his feelings to protect his family from upset and disappointment. Once Sally became aware of how he felt she attended to him in a nurturing way and apologized that he felt that way. The session evoked a lot of emotion and new information, which led to them deciding they could build on their communication and relationship by spending more time together and increasing his time with his dad. His dad was not involved in the session but was later contacted by me and collaboratively agreed to the plan. I checked in with the family to ensure they were satisfied with how the session had gone, and they agreed they did not feel the need to return.

Comment: This young person had been initially assessed by a number of different professionals due to the alarming information reported by the professionals. When I met with him I learned that he was engaged in education and functioning well in all areas of his life. I noticed how quick adults around him had reacted in a pathologized way when the reality for this young man was that he was struggling with his family context (parents' separation), sibling reactions to the situation, and also peer relationships. His emotive response and the language used, although initially alarming, was clearly a reaction given his personal context, and he was unaware of the consequences of what he was saying. The young man was embarrassed and felt very concerned about how he was perceived.

Case #2. "Annie," a 13-year-old female who identified as she/her, was referred to CAMHS by her school due to concerns in relation to social isolation, anxiety, and her parents' concerns about her diet. Annie related well throughout the session, although she did not engage in eye contact and did not have any concerns herself. She acknowledged that she did have difficulties socializing with her peers and that she often felt misunderstood. Her parents described Annie as highly intelligent, committed to learning but isolated. They were concerned that although she was engaged in physical activities, she was eating unhealthily. English was Annie's parents' second language, and when they reported their concerns to the school they felt that it may have gotten lost in translation. Annie had been spending a significant amount of time in her bedroom, playing computer games, which is how she preferred to interact with her peers. She was keen for her dad to engage in gaming to help her feel understood and connected. Her mum was concerned that she was eating unhealthily, and when this was explored further it was acknowledged that this was more in the context of how this was impacting Annie's emotional and mental well-being. Annie did not have any concerns about food; she did not understand why this had been mentioned. Annie's mother acknowledged that she may have used language that could be misunderstood or deemed as inappropriate and realized the importance of how this may make Annie feel. Annie wasn't concerned and realized her mother may have used incorrect language to express concerns.

Comment: Toward the end of the session we explored the idea that a neurodevelopmental assessment might be helpful for Annie to gain a better understanding of how she functions, but only if Annie was in agreement and felt this would help her to feel understood. Annie and her parents were keen to explore this further. Annie did not present anxious, although she did report feeling socially anxious at school. It was decided that the family did not want further SSFT sessions, and they felt satisfied with what the session had provided, which was in relation to how Annie functions and the importance of language.

Case #3. "Chloe," a 12-year-old female who identified as she/her, had been seen at Accident and Emergency (A&E) on a number of occasions within a four-month period due to taking significant overdoses. Chloe's parents had been separated for some time, but she typically had overnight contact with her father on a regular basis, which had recently stopped due to reasons Chloe was unaware of. Chloe had an older brother who had decided to reside with her father and new partner. Her brother had ceased all contact with her; this was also contributing to the decline in Chloe's mental health, as she was unsure why.

When I met with Chloe she was keen to be understood. She engaged really well and expressed her frustration with her family situation, which she was finding difficult to understand. I met with her parents separately utilizing an attachment-based family therapy (Diamond, Siqueland, & Diamond, 2003) approach to rebuild an emotionally safe and secure parent-child relationship. It became apparent that communication had broken down between Chloe's parents, which resulted in Chloe and her brother feeling torn in their loyalties between parents. Chloe was feeling distressed by what was happening within her family situation, and her suicidality was a way of her expressing her distress. Some questions we explored:

- "I understand you haven't seen your dad and older brother for a while, is this contributing to how you feel?"
- "Do you find it hard to tell your parents how you feel?"
- "What response do you get from your parents when you attempt to talk to them?"

Chloe's parents both worked full-time and therefore had limited time to attend sessions, therefore SSFT was more appealing, and it allowed for her parents to both engage. When her parents became aware that her suicidality could be understood as a way of her trying to express how distressed she feels, in an attempt to be seen and hope that her parents would communicate or contact with her dad would resume, her parents opened up about their own challenges.

Comment: SSFT enabled the systems in Chloe's life to communicate and understand her situation better. Measures were put in place to safely enable Chloe to have contact with her dad again, and although her brother was reluctant to see Chloe there was a decline in Chloe taking any further overdoses or re-presenting at A&E. It was recognized that further SSFT sessions would be required to support Chloe and her family to prevent further declines.

Outcomes

In a three-month period, I saw 11 families utilizing a SSFT approach, similar to The Bouverie Centre's Single Session Family Consultation (SSFC; see O'Hanlon & Rottem, 2021), which works with the child and their family/carer and wider system to aid recovery. I received referrals at different stages of service provision within CAMHS. Although the sample is small, the data support the finding that early intervention enables positive outcomes and prevents long-term intervention (e.g., see Perkins & Scarlett,

2008). A post-SST questionnaire has enabled us to gain immediate feedback; checking in to ensure they are happy with how the session went. Some typical responses:

One Thing You Liked About the Session Was:

- "A wonderful opportunity to sit with someone and talk about our concerns."
- "I was surprised at how quickly we were seen."
- "How sensitive they were to the awkward situation."
- "Trying to understand my past."
- "Many thanks for everything. You have been beyond amazing and we have always felt safe when speaking as a family and individually."

When One Session Wasn't Enough:

- "Knowing that if we needed further support, we could make contact was reassuring."
- "Knowing that we could re-refer in the future if things didn't work out."
- "We were hoping to get medication for our son but understand that we may need to explore alternative ways of responding."
- "It was disappointing that we could no longer see the clinician who we had developed a positive rapport with and felt comfortable talking to."
- "Understanding and identifying with further contextual information that our daughter may require a neurological assessment to assist her at school. The information provided help us to better understand her presentation and way of functioning."

Expanding Applications

The feedback from families continues to motivate and inspire me in ensuring this approach is considered across other services. I am passionately driven by the idea that NHS England (see NHS England, 2023) and public services working with children and young people adopt this framework nationally. I also wonder if a walk-in clinic or youth hubs could adopt the SST approach in the UK to provide immediate assistance and am also now exploring the possibility of utilizing a single session intervention approach to guide and support one-off mental health workshops within school settings and communities within Australia.

Ideas arising from SST are developing globally in mental health settings—walk-in clinics and/or online SSFT sessions are being offered and are being received favorably. The network has gone global (Hoyt & Talmon, 2014; Hoyt, Bobele, Slive, Young, & Talmon, 2018; Hoyt et al.,

2021; Stephenson, 2023).[6] Clinicians report that this approach represents a metaphor of dandelion seeds dispersing across our field and are reporting that the approach has re-energized them, provided solutions in challenging times, helped them to think differently about how to offer services in other public sectors, validated their approach, and enabled them to maximize their clinical skills and provide tangible outcomes.

Notes

1 *Editors' note*: See Chapters 3, 4, and 5 in this volume.
2 *Editors' note*: For more discussion about the use of SST in the UK's National Health Service, see Chapter 16 (Lewis) in this volume.
3 For more on the importance of helping clients to trust their own internal wisdom rather than relying predominantly on the expertise of professionals, see www.theholisticpsychologist.
4 *Editors' note*: see P. Rycroft (Chapter 20 this volume) for a related "map" from The Bouverie Centre.
5 *Editors' note*: See J. Young, Chapter 6 in this volume.
6 For more information, please contact the author at kathystephensonsystemic1@gmail.com.

References

Barbara-May, R., Denborough, P., & McGrane, T. (2018). Development of a single-session family program at Child and Youth Mental-Health Services, Southern Melbourne. In M.F. Hoyt, M. Bobele, A. Slive, J. Young, & M. Talmon (Eds.), *Single-Session Therapy by Walk-In or Appointment: Administrative, Clinical, and Supervisory Aspects of One-at-a-Time Services* (pp. 104–115). Routledge.

Diamond, G., Siqueland, L., & Diamond, G.M. (2003). Attachment-based family therapy for depressed adolescents: Programmatic treatment development. *Clinical Child Family Psychology Review*, 6, 107–127.

Edbrooke-Childs, J., Hayes, D., Lane, R., Liverpool, S., Jacob, J., & Deighton, J. (2021). Association between single session service attendance and clinical characteristics in administrative data. *Clinical Child Psychology and Psychiatry*, 26(3), 770–782.

Fuzzard, S. (2021). Embedding Single Session Family Consultation in a national youth mental-health service: Headspace. In M.F. Hoyt, J. Young, & P. Rycroft (Eds.), *Single Session Thinking and Practice in Global, Cultural, and Family Contexts: Expanding Applications* (pp. 133–139). Routledge.

Hoyt, M.F. (2025). *Single Session Therapy: A Clinical Introduction to Principles and Practices*. Routledge.

Hoyt, M.F., Bobele, M., Slive, A., Young, J., & Talmon, M. (Eds.). (2018). *Single-Session Therapy by Walk-In or Appointment: Administrative, Clinical, and Supervisory Aspects of One-at-a-Time Services*. Routledge.

Hoyt, M.F., Rosenbaum, R., & Talmon, M. (1992). Planned single-session psychotherapy. In S.H. Budman, M.F. Hoyt, & S. Friedman (Eds.), *The First Session in Brief Therapy* (pp. 59–86). Guilford Press.

Hoyt, M.F., & Talmon, M. (Eds.). (2014). *Capturing the Moment: Single Session Therapy and Walk-In Services*. Crown House Publishing.

Hoyt, M.F., Young, J., & Rycroft, P. (Eds.). (2021). *Single Session Thinking and Practice in Global, Cultural, and Familial Contexts: Expanding Applications.* Routledge.

Kessler, R.C., Amminger, G.P., Aguilar-Gaxiola, S., Alonso, J., Lee, S., & Ustan, T.B. (2007). Age of onset of mental disorders: A review of recent literature. *Current Opinion in Psychiatry, 20*(4), 359–364.

McDonald, J., Hickey, P., & Wyder, M. (2021). Implementing Single Session Thinking in a public mental health setting in Queensland: Part II—Adapting and integrating Single Session Therapy into an acute care setting. In M.F. Hoyt, J. Young, & P. Rycroft (Eds.), *Single Session Thinking and Practice in Global, Cultural, and Familial Contexts: Expanding Applications* (pp. 110–116). Routledge.

Mildred, H., Hunter, L., Goldsworthy, B., & Brann, P. (2021). Embedding the "Family Oriented Collaboration Utilising Strengths" (FOCUS) clinic in a child and youth mental health service and university partnership. In M.F. Hoyt, J. Young, & P. Rycroft (Eds.), *Single Session Thinking and Practice in Global, Cultural, and Familial Contexts: Expanding Applications* (pp. 278–286). Routledge.

NHS England. (2023). *Mental health of children and young people in England, 2023 wave 4 follow up to the 2017 survey.* https://digital.nhs.uk/data-and-information/publications/statistical/mental-health-of-children-and-young-people-in-england/2023-wave-4-follow-up

O'Hanlon, B., & Rottem, N. (2021). Single Session Family Consultation (SSFC). In M.F. Hoyt, J. Young, & P. Rycroft (Eds.), *Single Session Thinking and Practice in Global, Cultural, and Familial Contexts: Expanding Applications* (pp. 66–76). Routledge.

Perkins, R., & Scarlett, G. (2008). The effectiveness of single session therapy in child and adolescent mental health. Part 2: An 18-month follow-up study. *Psychology and Psychotherapy: Theory, Research, and Practice, 81,* 143–156.

Renkin, C., Alexander, K., & Wyder, M. (2021). Implementing Single Session Thinking in public mental health settings in Queensland: Part I—Introducing Single Session Family Consultations into adult inpatient and community care. In M.F. Hoyt, J. Young, & P. Rycroft (Eds.), *Single Session Thinking and Practice in Global, Cultural, and Familial Contexts: Expanding Applications* (pp. 101–109). Routledge.

Rosenbaum, R., Hoyt, M.F., & Talmon, M. (1990). The challenge of single-session therapies: Creating pivotal moments. In R.A. Wells & V.J. Giannetti (Eds.), *Handbook of the Brief Psychotherapies* (pp. 165–189). Plenum. Reprinted in Hoyt, M.F. (1995). *Brief Therapy and Managed Care: Readings for Contemporary Practice* (pp. 105–139). Jossey-Bass.

Stephenson, K. (2023, December). Single session thinking: Its global impact and role in therapeutic services. *Context, 190,* 29–31.

Talmon, M. (1990). *Single-Session Therapy: Maximizing the Effect of the First (and Often Only) Therapeutic Encounter.* Jossey-Bass.

von Dousa, H., Tsorlinis, K., Cordukes, K., Beauchamp, J., & McIntosh, J.E. (2021). One-off sessions to address a waitlist: A pilot study. In M.F. Hoyt, J. Young, & P. Rycroft (Eds.), *Single Session Thinking and Practice in Global, Cultural, and Familial Contexts: Expanding Applications* (pp. 117–124). Routledge.

Westwater, J.J., Murphy, M., Handley, C., & McGregor, L. (2020). A mixed-methods exploration of single session family therapy in a child and adolescent mental health service in Tasmania, Australia. *Australian and New Zealand Journal of Family Therapy, 41,* 258–270.

Young, J. (2018). SST: The misunderstood gift that keeps on giving. In M.F. Hoyt, M. Bobele, A. Slive, J. Young, & M. Talmon (Eds.), *Single-Session Therapy by Walk-In or Appointment: Administrative, Clinic and Supervisory Aspects of One-at-a-Time Services* (pp. 40–58). Routledge.

Young, J., & Rycroft, P. (2012). Single session therapy: What's in a name? *Australian and New Zealand Journal of Family Therapy, 33*(1), 3–5.

YoungMinds. (2023). *Monthly referrals to children's mental health services highest on record.* https://www.youngminds.org.uk/about-us/media-centre/press-releases/monthly-referrals-to-childrens-mental health-services-highest-on-record

Chapter 12

Can Work Add More to Life With SST?

Online Single Session Therapy in the Corporate World in the Netherlands

Helen van Empel and Rita Zijlstra

"What makes a good life?" is a pretty big question to start with, but it makes perfect sense to ponder this, especially in the context of mental health interventions. Our ultimate goal with any form of psychological therapy or support is to assist individuals in living their best lives. While we might not find a definitive answer here to this age-old question that has always intrigued humanity, we were introduced to a sustainable health model (Bohlmeijer & Westerhof, 2021) that offers insightful perspectives in this area.

Work and a Good Life

A good life is a life where work fuels us, not consumes us. We should be aiming to see work as something that adds to our well-being, rather than something we have to be protected from. Work should be a place that positively contributes to employees' sense of meaning, purpose, relatedness, life satisfaction, performance, productivity, and well-being. A place that nourishes our mental health and helps people do more than just get by, making them thrive (Infinite Potential, 2024).

The State of Workplace Burnout 2024 Report (Infinite Potential, 2024) shows that despite increased focus on employee well-being, burnout persists. Chronic workplace stress has become the narrative of modern life. In the past three years there was a steady growth in workplace burnout rate, but now it seems to have stabilized at 38%. Work is an important source of stress, with symptoms of powerlessness, exhaustion, and feeling overwhelmed. Chronic workplace stress is being normalized despite the abundant evidence of corrosive impact on individuals, teams, and organizations.

To break free from this cycle, employees and employers need to rewrite the script of work and take more control over their well-being at work. Single Session Therapy (SST), provided in our online service previously

DOI: 10.4324/9781032693828-15

called One Session and now called Yet, is a helpful tool in rewriting the narrative and focusing on work that adds to life and mental health instead of making us ill. The reason for this name change is that we wanted the focus to be on growth and not on the tool. At the heart of Yet's ethos lies a commitment to fostering a culture of growth and development. Employees aren't merely workers; they're explorers, constantly seeking new horizons and pushing the boundaries of what's possible. Failure isn't met with scorn but viewed as a stepping stone on the path to success—a valuable opportunity for learning and improvement. Ergo, Single Session Therapy to make the first step in what you can't do . . . yet.

What Is Mental Health?

According to the World Health Organization (2022), mental health is

> [A] state of mental well-being that enables people to cope with the stresses of life, realize their abilities, learn well and work well, and contribute to their community. It is an integral component of health and well-being that underpins our individual and collective abilities to make decisions, build relationships and shape the world we live in.

In this definition it is important to notice that mental health is not the same as the absence of mental illness. The Sustainable Mental Health model (Bohlmeijer & Westerhof, 2021; Kloos, Kraiss, ten Klooster, & Bohlmeijer, 2023) stresses this concept, and it played a significant role in guiding us toward the single session mindset. The model involves five important aspects:

1. Mental health isn't just about not being ill. It involves both *mental well-being and mental illness* as separate but related aspects. It shows that people can feel well and function well even while facing mental health issues. It's crucial to look after our mental well-being, not only to avoid future problems but also because it has a positive impact on our lives right now. This aligns with the World Health Organization's definition of mental health as "a state of mental well-being that enables people to cope with the stresses of life, to realize their abilities, to learn well and work well, and to contribute to their communities." Mental well-being means more than just feeling happy, it's also how you function in life. On a personal level, it's about things like setting goals, feeling confident in dealing with problems, and being productive in a way that's meaningful to you. Socially, it's about feeling connected, getting and giving support, and making your contribution.

2. The second component focuses on *adaptation processes*, which can either hinder or enhance our mental health. While we often view the absence of mental health issues and the presence of well-being as ideal states, it is much more complex. Life is a mix of both struggles and successes, and our mental health naturally fluctuates over time. Understanding how people adjust their mental health in response to life's ups and downs is crucial for developing effective psychological treatments. The ways we adapt to challenges can vary greatly. Traditionally, mental health research has concentrated on handling stress and symptoms, aiming to solve problems, returning to previous functioning levels, or bouncing back from hard times. However, recent trends in positive psychology focus on boosting well-being (Jankowski, Sandage, Bell, Davis, & Porter, 2020; Waters, Algoe, Dutton, Emmons, & Fredrickson, 2021). This means nurturing positive emotions, using personal strengths, and increasing psychological flexibility. It's about more than just overcoming difficulties; it's about building and keeping well-being, even when facing challenges.

3. We all have *barriers and resources* in dealing with life's ups and downs. Barriers could be unhelpful thoughts about ourselves or trying to push away our feelings. On the other side, we've got resources—our tools and supports. Keeping a positive attitude and having good friends can make a huge difference. These factors shape the way we deal with life, how we feel, and how we act day to day. Effective mental health management involves addressing challenges and also building on our strengths and resources.

4. *Context* is key. We need to look beyond just the individual in therapy and understand we're part of something bigger. Our mental health is always changing, influenced by various factors. Think about the different groups we're part of—our close friends and family, our school or workplace, and the wider community. All of these factors can either help boost our mental health or make it harder for us to stay well.

5. And sometimes, we might need additional support to manage. This is where the fifth part of the model comes in, offering a range of *psychological treatments*. The Sustainable Health Model shows that there are many ways to work on our mental health and that all the different interventions have their own place and can impact the whole system. This aligns with a flexible and practical SST mindset, with the aim to provide the right help at the right time along the life course. Another key point from this model is that dealing with mental health challenges doesn't mean you can't feel good or be productive. You don't have to wait on the sidelines until everything is perfect. In fact, actively participating and being able to contribute is essential for our well-being. For the workplace it means you don't have to be healthy to start working but the other way around: work helps you to improve your mental health.

Engaging in work or meaningful activities is not just about financial stability; it's also closely tied to our sense of purpose, accomplishment, and well-being.

Interventions in the Workplace

Workplaces play a big role in our lives. If we're lucky, we spend a lot of time at work. It's not just about earning money; work can also boost or hurt our mental health. Things like daily structure, meaningful work, and social support contribute to well-being. But factors like work overload, poor communication, and the "always on" culture can harm our well-being. It's a complex, dynamic system with a lot of factors that can either help or hinder us, and there are many potential strategies for improvement.

All of these factors emphasize the importance of focusing on enhancing well-being in the workplace. Providing individual interventions is one promising approach, as highlighted by a recent umbrella review of meta-analyses (Miguel, Amarnath, Akhtar, Malik, & Baranyi, 2023) that looks at different types of mental health support at the workplace. Universal interventions, like online mindfulness training, aim to support all employees. Selective interventions focus on high-risk groups, such as informal caregivers. Indicated interventions are for those showing signs of mental health issues, like stress or anxiety, aiming to address issues early on. Specific single session interventions, however, have not yet been included in these studies.

SST in the Corporate Sector in the Netherlands

Let's explore the application of online SST in the corporate sector in the Netherlands. We will illustrate our approach to aiding employees in overcoming challenges and obstacles in their professional and personal lives, aiming to convert uncertainties, concerns, and stress into positive transformations. As this chapter forms part of a broader book on SST, with excellent introductions to the SST method available elsewhere, we will not delve into the basics of SST.

We just want to highlight two things concerning SST in the workplace:

- SST empowers employees to decide when and what issue they need help with. This makes it a democratic, non-stigmatizing, accessible intervention that saves time and effort by eliminating unnecessary steps in assessing severity and appropriate intervention by HR (Human Resources) and managers.
- In a work setting, it can be especially important to emphasize confidentiality because employees may be concerned about HR and managers keeping an eye on them. That's why we've made it very easy to set up

a meeting anonymously and within 48 hours online. We aim to reduce the barriers to a minimum and make the whole process very simple and transparent.

Yet Platform

The Yet platform (Yet.nl) has been established to provide a tailored approach to mental health support within the corporate sector. It facilitates one-hour video-call sessions that employees can book online 24/7, offering flexibility with availability within 48 hours and including evenings and weekends. For organizations wishing to provide these services, a subscription model is available, granting employees access via a unique code for confidential, direct, and free booking on our website.

Yet's distinctiveness lies in its diverse range of professionals, encompassing not just psychologists but also other professionals such as career coaches, life counselors, and leadership coaches. All are highly experienced in their respective fields and trained in the SST method, ensuring employees receive support that is best suited to their current needs. To help users select the right professional, our platform features a simple two-question process:

1. *What do you want to talk about?* This question helps pinpoint the discussion topic. Users can select one or more topics from the following list or proceed to the next question:

   - High workload
   - Mismatched work content
   - Unpleasant working environment
   - Lack of fun at work
   - Conflicts
   - Dilemmas
   - Transgressive behavior
   - Relationship problems
   - Loneliness
   - Informal caregiving
   - Mourning
   - Leadership

2. *What do you want to improve?* This question targets areas for personal and professional growth, including:

   - Feeling mentally healthy
   - Managing stress
   - Adapting to change

- Living a healthy, meaningful life
- Finding meaningful work
- Setting career goals
- Improving leadership skills

Based on the answers provided, individuals will receive one to three suggestions for the most suitable professional. To assist in making a selection from these recommendations, or to enable a direct choice without responding to any questions, we offer the following brief description of each professional's expertise.

Psychologist. Insights and development. Obstacles, challenges, or struggling? This expert will listen, ask poignant questions, and offer the right advice to help you move forward.

Work-Life Coach. Balancing work and home life. Events at work or at home can throw you off balance. This expert can offer practical advice to help you restore the balance in your life.

Confidential Adviser. Feel safe at work. You want to feel safe at work. This expert is a first point of contact for questions about transgressive behavior.

Leadership Coach. A dedicated coach for executives and managers, specialized in addressing issues related to management, team dynamics, and leadership.

Career Coach. Toward the future. Your job should align with your ambitions and competencies. This expert helps you discover more job satisfaction and supports your personal development.

Life Counselor. Meaningful life. We understand that this can be an ongoing challenge. Our life counselor is here to help you get back to feeling good again, both at work and beyond.

This straightforward process ensures that you receive support tailored to your unique needs and goals.

The booking procedure is efficient and user-friendly. Employees can select a date and time that works best for them, provide basic contact information, and receive a confirmation email. This email not only confirms their appointment but also includes the link for the video call and a set of optional preparatory tips. These tips aim to help clients prepare for their session by encouraging them to think about what they wish to discuss, reflect on their current challenges, identify any patterns in their behavior that may be contributing to these challenges, consider their strengths and resources, and think about the kind of support they feel would be most helpful to them. We also suggest creating a quiet, private space for the session to minimize interruptions and enhance focus. This guidance is designed to make the session as productive and beneficial as possible by encouraging clients to come prepared and engaged. It reflects our approach to facilitating sessions that are not only insightful but also empowering for clients, enabling them to take an active role in their own change process. This structured yet flexible system is designed to provide accessible, professional support tailored to individual needs in the corporate environment.

Professionals

In our approach, we don't rely on a fixed protocol but rather on the expertise of seasoned professionals who utilize their skills and tools to make a meaningful impact in just one session. A critical aspect of our process is the careful selection of professionals. Our key selection method involves a trial session. We provide basic information about SST to our candidates and then pair them up. They engage in two half-hour sessions, alternating between the roles of client and therapist. These sessions are recorded and sent to us for evaluation, ensuring a good fit for the job. Additionally, experiencing SST from both the therapist's and client's perspective is invaluable, as it provides a well-rounded understanding of the method and its suitability.

Our Principles

We aim to simplify access to support for corporate employees, eliminating the need for an immediate commitment to a long-term program. This framework fosters quick, fully confidential discussions on sensitive topics not yet ready to be shared with managers or partners, yet significantly influencing performance and communication. Additionally, we emphasize viewing stress as an inherent part of life and a vehicle for learning. Given the ubiquity of stress due to rapid changes, information overload, work pressures, and personal challenges, we advocate for a reevaluation of stress perception and management. Seeing stress as a chance for personal development can improve performance, elevate confidence, and bolster overall health, equipping clients to tackle their obstacles with greater resilience and autonomy.

Some Examples

Each session is unique and can't be scripted, although we do follow certain guidelines.

- Clarify the session's purpose: Begin by ensuring that both the professional and the client understand the session's purpose, what can be achieved, and the role each will play. This is also the moment to discuss the method, privacy, and practical matters if they're not yet clear.
- Identify the issue: Understand the reason behind the session from the client's perspective, focusing on the current situation and concerns without seeking explanations.
- Clarify the objective: Find out what the client aims to achieve during the session and discuss what can be accomplished in the session regarding the issue at hand. This encourages the client to think critically and helps focus the session.
- Establish the desired professional role: Understand how the client wishes the professional to assist, whether through advice, information, or simply listening.
- Maintain focus and structure: The collaboration should be equal yet directed, with the professional helping to keep the session focused on the client's priorities, asking for feedback, and being ready to adjust as necessary.
- Leverage client expertise: Engage clients in utilizing their own knowledge and skills by exploring past attempts to address the issue, identifying their strengths, and considering who in their support network can assist. Discuss how these insights can be applied moving forward, making plans more tangible and specific. Encourage reflecting on what worked before, enhancing awareness of their strengths, and actively seeking help from their environment or external resources.
- Collaborate on solutions: Together, explore possible solutions, drawing from both the client's insights and the therapist's expertise. This may involve internal changes (like cognitive techniques or mindfulness), improving communication, or external adjustments (such as changing jobs). Aim to select one thing to help to initiate change without overwhelming someone; you just want to help someone to get started. If possible, practice this solution within the session—whether through visualization exercises or role-playing—to concretize it, adjust as needed, and enhance the client's confidence and readiness to overcome anticipated challenges.
- End positively: Encourage summarization and generalization of the session's insights. The goal is for clients to depart with a clearer vision for moving forward, increased self-confidence, and a positive outlook. Conclude the session on an uplifting note, strengthening hope, trust, and enthusiasm for moving forward.

Let's consider several case examples.

Case Example 1: Reframing

Client's Initial Statement: "Three years ago, I started a company with two
  partners. It's now more successful than I could have ever hoped for.
  I should be happy about the success and feel confident. However, the
  strange thing is, I can't enjoy it. I'm always worried. It's never good
  enough. I'm never good enough."
Client's Initially Stated Goal: "I want to understand why I'm always so
  worried and insecure, so I can hopefully do something about it."
Our SST Process: Digging deeper into this goal and what achieving it could
  bring him, it becomes clear that he fears his two partners might want to
  part ways with him. He's always serious and negative. He puts on the
  brakes, while they only see opportunities and a bright future. They meet
  with external parties as a duo, making grand promises. And he's the bit-
  ter one left to execute these promises. He often feels left out and angry.
  "They're ruining the company with commitments we can't keep. They
  should damn well listen to me once. They make these lovely promises.
  But I say nothing, because I want them to value me. How pathetic is
  that?"

Discussing his anger, he acknowledges that someone needs to take on his
role. They are engaging, outward- and forward-looking, while he is realistic, responsible for execution, the products. They need each other. He
couldn't do what they do, and that frustrates him. Could they do what he
does? He ponders this for a long time. He has never considered that what
he does is also a quality.

What if he flips the perspective? Instead of being a nagging brake,
dragged through the mud behind proud horses, he could be a wise coach-
man on the box. He steers, maintains oversight and control. That is his
quality. He sees that. But he also wishes he could run freely sometimes and
not always sit alone on the box. He thinks for a moment. But that's not
realistic. He couldn't do what they do.

And indeed, they can't do what he can. For a moment, he looks very
satisfied. And then worried again.

"Now, I think, 'Am I good enough to steer?'"
"Who's steering now?"
"I am."
"And how is your company doing?"

We discuss that, unfortunately, our expectations often don't match
reality. You think that if you perform enough, do enough, feelings of

appreciation and self-worth will naturally follow. But that's not the case. It doesn't help if you constantly think you should be different, that things should be different, that you should be the great sales talent, the extravert hitting the gas instead of the brakes. And some people naturally worry more than others. And that can be difficult, but it also has positive sides. This seems obvious in his organization. He usually bears the burden of worries. It can work really well and still be a burden.

This realization matters, he concludes. "I have indeed always been worried and always thought I could change that if I just achieved enough. But perhaps, I achieve precisely because I'm worried. Not just for myself but also for others. I still find it unfair, but well, that's just how it is."

Case Example 2: A Single Session, a First Step

Client's Initial Statement: "I often find myself agreeing with others, trying to please, and diminishing my presence. Sometimes, I completely shut down. For example, during important presentations, even though I'm well-prepared, I can't share my opinions or knowledge, contribute, or take responsibility, which is crucial for me as a consultant."

Client's Initially Stated Goal: "I am looking for advice and practical tools to learn how to express myself more clearly and assertively."

Our SST Process: We discuss what is most important to her right now, which is the shutting down that sometimes happens. Upon examining specific examples, it becomes clear that this occurs not only in certain situations, like presentations and meetings, but especially with, as she puts it, "dominant people." To better understand what exactly is happening, I ask what could help her in those situations. She mentions the desire for the presence of a kind, empathetic person, a colleague or coach, who would ask her, "What's happening to you?" and give her that moment of attention. Ideally, she wishes for the "dominant boss" to show vulnerability. What she truly desires is genuine contact—not to win an argument or to put someone in their place, but to have a real conversation.

I ask her to imagine the situation she's currently dreading: a presentation for her boss next week. How his behavior could optimally trigger her reaction: not listening to what she says, interrupting her, giving his own opinion, speaking loudly, making remarks about her work that others laugh at. As she describes it, her reaction is visible and palpable in the moment, which she acknowledges, "I just fall into it." I suggest an unusual exercise, which she agrees to. I ask her to close her eyes (and say I will close mine, too) and instruct her to let go of the situation and hold on to the unpleasant feeling, then to let a memory from the past come up, no matter what or from what age.

A memory surfaces of the school library, where she used to hide during breaks from the bullying kids, who were never in the library. She still feels good among books. She is surprised by this memory, having never made the connection before. We briefly discuss how such old memories can suddenly shift the entire system into a different mode and what she could potentially do with this insight, such as exploring schema therapy, should she feel the need.

But more importantly, what she can immediately do with this insight: certain situations, and especially certain behaviors and demeanors, can trigger an old reaction in her. This is not foolish or weak; it's a fact. And we discuss how she could deal with it.

She now realizes she can predict the situations "where the 13-year-old girl takes over." The link is clear and consistent with past examples. "Good, then you can prepare," I say. "Can't I just leave her at home?" she asks. "No, you can't."

We return to the image of the library, at school. What if she, as the adult woman she is now, goes with her, stays by her side? What would you say to that girl? "It gets better, it passes." And what would you do? "Comfort her, sit next to her. Yes, that would help."

"Ah, so I become the coach or colleague I would want with me," she says as she opens her eyes. It is a profound moment, and I have to force myself to stay realistic. I ask about her doubts.

"That it won't work, that I'll still shut down or start pleasing. That would stress me out, and it would be my fault, ruining it for myself even though I know this now. Once is okay, but it shouldn't happen too often. Hmmm, no, that would make it worse. I don't know, can you help me?"

"Perhaps. I would say, 'Your sensitivity and openness are also what make you so beautiful and special, allowing you to connect with others. Those who don't act like bullies—and you're not responsible for educating everyone. It's not your fault you have this reaction. I'm here for you now, and I'll stay with you. I want to help you suffer less from this reaction, and we'll do it together, for you, not for anyone else. And it takes as long as it takes.'"

"Oh, that does touch me. That's going to take some practice. I'm going to ask my GP for a referral for schema therapy. And next week? I can do the presentation with a very nice colleague, I don't have to tell her everything. She also finds him very unpleasant but doesn't get affected by him like I do. She offered to do it together last week, but I felt I had to be able to do it myself. But that is not necessary yet."

Case Example 3: The Importance of Individualizing Help: "Do You Have Some Relaxation Exercises for Me?"

The client's needs and inquiries are central to our approach. However, it's not just about directly answering their questions. The true value of a personal session lies more in tailored questions than in a tailored answer. It's about clarifying what the client truly seeks to achieve in the session, which may differ slightly from what they initially had in mind. This difference can be the key to why someone feels stuck. They're caught in a cycle of repeating the same actions and perspectives. Stepping back is hard because we're creatures of habit and naturally shy away from confronting difficult or uncomfortable issues.

For example, a seemingly straightforward request like, "Do you have some relaxation exercises for me?" can often lead to different questions and a variety of solutions, showing how a single query can branch out into multiple directions. Consider these two scenarios:

Scenario #1: "Do You Have Some Relaxation Exercises for Me?"

Client's Initial Statement: "My shoulders ache, I'm unable to sleep, and I can't seem to let go of certain issues. I've previously reported that things are not going well in our department, leading to unmanageable pressure. Although my concerns were acknowledged, no effective action followed. My efforts to communicate these issues are perceived as troublesome, leaving me feeling unheard and invisible. Consequently, I've resorted to just doing my job, trying not to worry about the rest."

Client's Initially Stated Goal: "I aim to be less affected by this situation, hoping that you have some effective relaxation exercises."

Our SST Process: Listening to her, it's clear there's a significant issue in her department. Without addressing this, relaxation exercises might just prolong her stay in an unwanted situation.

She's relieved that I (HvE) see it that way. This makes me realize how crucial and sensitive the idea that she's nagging is and that it's a relief for her that I acknowledge that we need to take this situation seriously.

We talk about the specific issue she's facing: in their team of four, one person consistently fails to complete their tasks. The rest of the team, not wanting things to fall apart, picks up the slack. The manager is aware but insists they handle it internally. When she shares this with friends and family, they suggest she should just stop covering for the absentee team member to make the problem more obvious. But that's not a viable option for them. The manager advises them to work it out and improve communication, yet agreements they make keep falling through. This situation leaves her feeling hopeless and insecure, as they're unfairly labeled as troublesome women who can't resolve their own conflicts. As time goes on, this not only sours their work environment but also makes it harder for her to communicate their needs effectively.

We focus on the message she wants to convey: "We need a manager to step in and enforce consequences for failing to uphold agreements, or we should be empowered to do so ourselves." We practice how she can communicate this effectively. At first, she finds it challenging, but with a bit of practice, she gets better and more confident. From this exercise, she gains not just a practical skill but also a subtle shift in how she sees herself. She starts to see herself as someone who is capable of speaking up for herself and her colleagues, and she moves away from seeing herself as a whiner to someone who is assertively taking a stand.

By the end of our 60-minute session, she feels confident about her next steps. She says that the meeting has been very helpful and agrees to recontact me as needed. Per our standard practice, she agrees to receive and complete an anonymous feedback/evaluation questionnaire.

Scenario #2: "Do You Have Some Relaxation Exercises for Me?"

Client's Initial Statement: "I'd like to feel less bothered by the pressure at work. It's not always there, but when it spikes, I don't always handle it the way I wish to. I become short with colleagues, and they notice that I'm struggling. They start to wonder, 'What's wrong with her?'"

Client's Initially Stated Goal: "I don't want to burn-out, I want to relax, maybe you have some relaxation exercises?"

Our SST Process: To get a clearer understanding, we look at a recent, concrete example from this morning. She works in a department handling customer complaints, like flooding incidents. After a weekend with bad weather, like the recent one, they get a surge of complaints, often from irate customers. "We're not available on weekends, and of course, they want everything resolved immediately," she says. She's learned to manage this better now. When dealing with such calls, she takes a deep breath, looks at a smiley sticker (a suggestion from a coach, which she finds surprisingly helpful), and puts on a smile. While invisible to the callers, it's audible in her voice.

She's also become more open to asking for help, especially since a critical colleague left the department. It wasn't just her; the whole department was strained under that colleague's constant criticism and inability to take feedback. Now, she leaves her work at the office and sleeps well. Yet, there's still an underlying issue, she says. We delve deeper. I ask her to explain as if I were an alien unfamiliar with stress, how she physically and mentally puts herself in that state. This leads us to the trigger: the thought, "Oh no, we're not going to make it; things won't work out today." This thought sets off a cascade—her breathing quickens, her shoulders tense, and she has thoughts about not being so stressed, which paradoxically only makes her feel worse and act brusquely. But she acknowledges it always works out in the end with teamwork, delegation, and focus, even if it means temporarily keeping other tasks and colleagues at bay.

Hearing this, I wonder aloud whether her stress response is actually inappropriate or if it's a natural preparation to adapt to challenging environments. Maybe it's appropriate and meaningful, particularly if she can strip away the negative thoughts about the reaction. I propose this perspective to her.

She instantly gives a brilliant example that illustrates this better than anything I could have thought of. She mentions that she's gone parachuting twice. I comment that parachutists shouldn't be too relaxed before a jump; a certain level of tension is necessary for the right focus. "Exactly," she agrees.

Her next step? She decides to print a photo of herself in mid-jump, capturing that exhilarating free-fall moment. She plans to place it on her desk as a reminder of that feeling and mindset.

Case Example 4: Learning From Mistakes

Generally, the feedback on our sessions has been overwhelmingly positive, with an average rating of 4.8 out of 5 across 521 cases. However, there have been a few cases of lower ratings, with the lowest being 3. The first instance of such a rating happened in a session I (HvE) conducted. I'll admit, my first thought was somewhat ashamedly: "I'm not going to tell anyone about this."

This experience highlighted the critical importance of a client-centered approach and the necessity of offering flexible options for support, whether that be a single session or a different type of assistance.

This particular session began under less-than-ideal conditions. The client was dealing with poor internet connectivity, which caused a delayed start and forced her into an uncomfortable setting within her home. Her irritation was evident, both with the technical difficulties and with the appointment itself. She mentioned that HR had suggested this single conversation approach, but she was skeptical about its effectiveness. She wasn't keen on having just an isolated session. Looking back, I realize I should have acknowledged her reluctance and possibly reconsidered our approach. However, eager to convince her and not disappoint HR, who recommended us, I pushed forward, saying, "Let's see how far we get."

The reason she was seeking help through HR was due to the criticism she receives, mainly anonymous and online. Her work involves making frequent public appearances and statements that would generate a lot of feedback, which bothered her. She dismisses the suggestion from her circle to not read these comments as nonsense; she wants to be informed about what's being said, so she warned me not to propose ignoring them. She also made it clear that she was not interested in relaxation exercises, mindfulness, or anything like that. Her goal was not to simply ignore the criticism but to read it without it affecting her. If I had felt that she had genuinely chosen this session and wanted to use it to make progress, I probably would have told her I couldn't help with her specific request, and we might have explored a different objective together. Instead, being defensive and out of balance, I tried to persuade her that her desire was unattainable. Rather than having an open conversation, it turned into an unpleasant tug-of-war about what's possible and what's not, where I was too focused on convincing her and not enough on hearing her.

What I value in SST conversations is their openness and equality, but that was missing from the start here. I think I could have corrected this by immediately acknowledging her reluctance for this conversation. I could have offered her the option to either end the session right away, continue to see if we could achieve something, or reschedule for a better time with a more stable connection. Laying out these options and allowing her to choose would have been more effective than timidly picking a direction and trying to pull her along. This is especially important in settings where employees are given a session by the organization, which might create an impression that they have to make do with just one session and not make a fuss, feeling short-changed with just one conversation.

Toward the Future

As noted earlier, based on 521 cases, our internet SST service has received an average rating of 4.8 out of 5. At the end of each session, we also ask clients a few open-ended questions like: "What helped me most during the session was . . ." and "The session would've been even better for me if . . ." The responses were collected and ChatGPT was used to find out, based on all the reviews, which words really capture what we do. These are the words that came up: EMPOWERMENT, CLARITY, RELIEF. These results encourage us to continue providing and studying online SST.

References

Bohlmeijer, E., & Westerhof, G. (2021). The model for sustainable mental health: Future directions for integrating positive psychology into mental health care. *Frontiers in Psychology, 12*. https://doi.org/10.3389/fpsyg.2021.747999

Infinite Potential (2024, February). *Infinite potential.* https://infinite-potential.com.au/the-state-of-burnout-2024

Jankowski, P.J., Sandage, S.J., Bell, C.A., Davis, D.E., Porter, E., Jessen, M., Motzny, C.L., Ross, K.V., & Owen, J. (2020). Virtue, flourishing, and positive psychology in psychotherapy: An overview and research prospectus. *Psychotherapy, 57*(3). https://doi.org/10.1037/pst0000285

Kloos, N., Kraiss, J., ten Klooster, P., & Bohlmeijer, E. (2023). First validation of the model of sustainable mental health: Structural model validity and the indirect role of adaptation. *Journal of Clinical Psychology, 79*(11), 2650–2667. https://doi.org/10.1002/jclp.23574

Miguel, C., Amarnath, A., Akhtar, A., Malik, A., Baranyi, G., Barbui, C., Karyotaki, E., & Cuijpers, P. (2023). Universal, selective and indicated interventions for supporting mental health at the workplace: An umbrella review of meta-analyses. *Occupational and Environmental Medicine, 80*(4), 225–236. https://doi.org/10.1136/oemed-2022-108698

Waters, L., Algoe, S.B., Dutton, J., Emmons, R., Fredrickson, B.L., Heaphy, E., Moskowitz, J.T., Neff, K., Niemiec, R., Pury, C., & Steger, M. (2021). Positive psychology in a pandemic: Buffering, bolstering, and building mental health. *Journal of Positive Psychology, 17*(3), 1–21. https://doi.org/10.1080/17439760.2021.1871945

World Health Organization. (2022). *Health and Well-Being.* World Health Organization. https://www.who.int/data/gho/data/major-themes/health-and-well-being

Chapter 13

Single Session Therapy
Exploring Research Evidence and Frontiers

Giada Pietrabissa

As we enter the 21st century, psychologists and other mental health professionals face many new challenges and opportunities shaped by social changes, technological advancements, and emerging research findings. An increasing number of studies have convincingly demonstrated the general effectiveness of psychological therapies for a wide range of mental health conditions in specific contexts and populations (Gaskell, Simmonds-Buckley, Kellett, Stockton, & Somerville, 2023; Hansen, Lambert, & Forman, 2002). However, nearly 70% of people with mental disorders in the world do not receive treatment (Mongelli, Georgakopoulos, & Pato, 2020).

This chapter provides a comprehensive exploration of the various aspects related to SST research, including methodology, effectiveness, client satisfaction and characteristics, limitations, potential applications, and future directions. As Jay Haley wrote in his back cover endorsement of Moshe Talmon's (1993) *Single Session Solutions*: "We used to think long-term therapy was the base from which all therapy was to be judged. Now it appears that therapy of a single interview could become the standard for estimating how long and how successful therapy should be."

There are several reasons why mental health is one of the most neglected areas of health globally. Among these, social stigma still represents one of the main barriers to care, together with fragmented and outdated service models and a lack of resources and trained health workers. The treatment gap is even broader in low- and middle-income countries, where 76% to 85% of people suffering from mental disorders lack access to care (World Health Organization, 2022). Structural inequalities related to income, geography, and race continue, indeed, to represent significant obstacles to addressing the increasing burden of mental health problems worldwide. In particular, the historical dependence on lengthy and costly treatments, as well as the absence of a commercial incentive to promote psychological

DOI: 10.4324/9781032693828-16

therapies, also contributes to the difficulties in engaging patients (Singla, Schleider, & Patel, 2023).

In this scenario, however, low-intensity psychotherapies are short and prioritize patient empowerment over complex treatment plans (Singla et al., 2023). Among these, Single Session Therapy (SST) offers a unique approach to providing rapid and focused support to the client within the confines of a single encounter. It can be defined as a systemized set of maneuvers intended to address a specific client's problem or concern in a single session, where any therapeutic approach can be applied (Campbell, 2012; Schleider, Dobias, Sung, & Mullarkey, 2020).

The core principle of SST lies in its ability to engage clients in a goal-oriented conversation, emphasizing the importance of well-defined objectives, exploring the client's concerns, offering insight or coping strategies, and collaboratively working toward a resolution or plan of action within the limited time frame, thus maximizing the use of the available resources from clients (Slive & Bobele, 2013; Young & Dryden, 2019).

By understanding the definition and principles of SST, researchers can delve deeper into assessing the efficacy and applicability of this time-limited intervention. Indeed, since SST is a self-contained approach, it has the potential to be effective by offering pragmatic intervention for many of those clients seeking assistance who otherwise might not receive treatment or be termed "dropouts." SST challenges traditional notions of the duration of therapy and opens venues for novel investigations in the field of low-intensity psychotherapies. Indeed, existing literature examining the relationship between the number of treatment sessions and the rate of change suggests that greater improvement occurs at the beginning of therapy to decrease over the treatment course (Hansen, Lambert, & Forman, 2002) and that longer treatments do not always translate to superior clinical results (Weisz, Kuppens, Ng, Eckshtain, & Ugueto, 2017).

Evolution of Single Session Therapy Research Findings and Methodology

The rationale for SST is based on findings from the first study ever conducted on the topic revealing that the most common number of therapeutic sessions people attended was one and that the vast majority (68–88%) of those attending a single session reported they have solved their problem or were satisfied with that session (Talmon, 1990). A further prospective investigation conducted by Talmon and his colleagues concluded that 58.6% of the clients attending SST registered a noticeable improvement in their presented difficulties after the intervention and that the results were maintained at 3–12 months of follow-up. This challenged the idea that clients who only attend one session are unmotivated dropouts, suggesting instead that their decision to not return for a second encounter might stem from perceived improvements after the initial session (Hoyt, Rosenbaum, & Talmon, 1992).

Since the publication of Talmon's research, there has been a notable evolution and growing interest in exploring the potential and opportunities of SST throughout the world.

Studies conducted in Australia, Canada, and North America have indicated that clients are generally satisfied with SST services (Boyhan, 1996; Brooks, Chambers, Lauby, Byrne, & Carpenedo, 2016; Harper-Jaques & Simms, 2015; Hoyt & Talmon, 2014; Hymmen, Stalker, & Cait, 2013; O'Neill, 2015; Perkins & Scarlett, 2008; Rodda, Lubman, Cheetham, Dowling, & Jackson, 2015; Toneatto, 2016). Positive results on the application of SST have also been found in investigations carried out in Colombia (Urrego, Abaakouk, Roman, & Contreras, 2009), Israel (Kutz, Resnik, & Dekel, 2008), Indonesia (Situmorang, 2022), Mexico (Schmulson, Ortiz-Garrido, Hinojosa, & Arcila, 2006), South Korea (Eom, Kim, Kim, Bang, & Chun, 2012), Peru (Church, Piña, Reategui, & Brooks, 2012), and Turkey (Basoglu, Salcioglu, & Livanou, 2007), among others. In Europe, SST research has been mainly conducted in the United Kingdom (Ellis, Cushing, & Germain, 2015; Lamprecht, Laydon, McQuillan, Wiseman, & Williams, 2007; Tantirangsee, Assanangkornchai, & Marsden, 2015; Whicher, Utku, Schirmer, Davis, & Abou-Saleh, 2012) and Sweden (Andreasson, Hansagi, & Osterlund, 2002; Berman, Forsberg, Durbeej, Kallmen, & Hermansson, 2010; Boman, Lindqvist, Forsberg, Janlert, & Granasen, 2018; Falkenstrom, Ekeblad, & Holmqvist, 2016; Hellstrom & Ost, 1995; Holst, Willenheimer, Martensson, Lindholm, & Stromberg, 2007; Oar, Farrell, & Ollendick, 2015; Ollendick, Halldorsdottir, Fraire, Austin, & Noguchi, 2015; Ollendick, Ost, Reuterskiöld, Costa, & Cederlund, 2009; Söderquist, 2018), but evidence for the efficacy of this approach also comes from other countries, including, but not limited to, Germany (Martin, Rauh, Fichter, & Rief, 2007; Thom, Sartory, & Johren, 2000), Finland (Luutonen, Santalahti, Makinen, Vahlberg, & Rautava, 2019), Norway (Haukebo, Skaret, Ost, Raadal, & Berg, 2008), Switzerland (Zehnder, Meuli, & Landolt, 2010), and Italy (Bertuzzi, Fratini, Tarquinio, Cannistrà, & Granese, 2021; Cannistrà, Piccirilli, D'Alia, Giannetti, & Piva, 2020). Conducting studies in different countries allowed researchers to determine whether brief interventions are universally effective or if modifications are needed to address specific cultural or contextual factors. Investigations were conducted in a variety of settings, as SST can be offered by appointment or by walking in without a scheduled appointment, in person or by telephone or virtual platforms, thus further improving the accessibility (Barwick, Urajnik, Sumner, Cohen, & Reid, 2013; Young & Jebreen, 2019).

Some of the highlights of the research on potential changes resulting from SST include:

1. Client Satisfaction

Satisfaction rates ranged from 74% to 100% across studies (Harper-Jaques & Simms, 2015; Miller & Slive, 2004; Perkins & Scarlett, 2008; Slive & Bobele, 2013), indicating that clients perceived SST as useful for addressing their mental health needs. In particular, clients were satisfied with the service in terms of feeling heard, understood, and respected; working on or talking about the issues they wanted to talk about; and feeling that the approach and the overall session were a good fit (Hoyt et al., 1992; Hymmen et al., 2013).

2. Symptom Improvement

A significant number of clients reported improvements in their functional status and quality of life as a result of attending a single session, although these changes were smaller compared to the decrease in severity (Ewen, Mushquash, Mushquash, Bailey, Haggarty, & Stones, 2018). This may be due to the relatively short follow-up period and the lack of longitudinal studies on the topic, as functional improvement generally occurs at a slower rate than symptom decrease. Results may also be affected by the use of no standardized outcome measures or the lack of employing general and specific measures of psychological constructs. The proportion of clients who showed improvement in the presenting problem ranged from 64% to 94% across studies (Hymmen et al., 2013): the greatest change was most evident for depressive symptoms and the least for self-harm, indicating that SST could be more useful for certain types of clients.

Clients' perceived ability to cope with their problems also improved from pre-session to post-session. They also reported feeling less stressed immediately after treatment. In particular, confidence in coping, in the form of self-efficacy, is a potential mechanism of change in therapy, as clients are more likely to participate in activities that will improve their mental health if they feel capable of doing so (Fentz, Arendt, O'Toole, Hoffart, & Hougaard, 2014; Pietrabissa, Manzoni, Rossi, & Castelnuovo, 2017; Rossi, Panzeri, Pietrabissa, Manzoni, & Castelnuovo, 2020).

3.   For Which Types of Client Does Single Session Therapy Work Best?

Following Talmon (1990), attempts have been made to identify for whom and for what types of problem SST may be useful (Cameron, 2007; Ewen et al., 2018; Hymmen et al., 2013). Cameron (2007) provided an overview that SST is mainly suitable for clients who come to therapy with some identifiable and solvable problem they are actively seeking to change (Cameron, 2007). In the review conducted by Hymmen et al. (2013), two variables were seen to most determine the response of an individual or family to SST, namely, the severity of the problem and client motivation or readiness of the client to change. In fact, the findings of most studies have revealed that individuals with more severe symptoms did not experience the same level of improvement as those with less severe symptoms. Specifically, there is an agreement that SST is not likely to be sufficient for symptom resolution for clients with a significant biological or neurological basis for their problems (including clients with major mental illness, dementia, etc.), suicidal or homicidal tendencies, major personality dysfunction (such as borderline personality disorder), psychotic problems (Campbell, 1999), or when the client is asking for longer-term ("traditional") psychotherapy (Cameron, 2007; Hymmen et al., 2013). These results mirror what is commonly observed in traditional therapy, where clients with more severe symptoms typically exhibit less favorable treatment outcomes (Lindhiem, Kolko, & Cheng, 2012).

Consistent with these findings, other investigations have shown that SST can be most effective with highly motivated, higher functioning, and less distressed clients (Hampson, O'Hanlon, Franklin, Pentony, & Fridgant, 1999; Mireau & Inch, 2009), but research on the association between initial symptom severity and SST results is still yielding mixed results (Hymmen et al., 2013). Indeed, in situations with limited resources, SST was shown to be an effective way to address a diverse range of client issues (Cameron, 2007). However, those with more severe mental problems might need additional sessions or services to achieve comparable improvements, although they might still derive benefits from a single therapeutic encounter (Hymmen et al., 2013; Miller & Slive, 2004).

In support of this, Bloom (1981) analyzed 50 years of literature on unplanned single-session encounters, suggesting that SST could potentially become the primary method for publicly-funded mental health agencies to cope with increasing service demands and long waitlists (Bloom, 1981). Twenty years later, Bloom (2001) revisited this topic, providing a summary of studies that evaluated the effectiveness of SST (Bloom, 2001). However, while uncontrolled studies indicated promising results with a "success" rate of 70–80%, there was a shortage of controlled studies and the need for more rigorous research to determine the optimal conditions for single session interventions.

Accordingly, Hurn (2005) stated that, despite the considerable potential of SST, there was a shortage of scientific evidence due to methodological weaknesses in existing outcome studies. He cautioned against viewing SST as a cure-all for every client, especially in complex cases, but supported the utility of SST in outpatient mental health settings, recognizing that it could serve as a beneficial triage system (Hurn, 2005). Another, more recent systematic review of randomized controlled studies conducted by Bertuzzi et al. (2021) reported that SST is more effective than no treatment or multi-session treatments in reducing anxiety among youth and adults (Bertuzzi et al., 2021). However, the methodological quality of the included studies was generally found to be skewed. Schleider and Weisz (2017) also conducted a meta-analysis of randomized controlled trials (RCT) of studies investigating the impact of single session interventions (SSIs)[1] on youth mental health problems and concluded that SSI has a significant positive impact with an overall small to medium effect size (Schleider & Weisz, 2017).

Although the findings of the current review suggest promise for SST, the available literature mainly consists of descriptions of services using SST as a primary approach. Research in SST continues to be affected by methodologically limited quantitative studies and bias resulting from the method of collecting outcome data (Hymmen et al., 2013).

Likewise, while the term "SST" unquestionably designates a scenario where a therapist assists a client within a single session while acknowledging the availability of additional sessions, scholars have contended that this term alone may inadvertently foster misconceptions about the nature of single-session work (Young, 2018). As such, they have introduced alternative terminology to more accurately capture the essence of this intervention method. For instance, terms like *brief intervention, single-session intervention*, or *one-at-a-time* have been proposed to better reflect the focused and time-limited nature of the therapeutic interaction (see Hoyt, Young, & Rycroft, 2021, pp. 11–15). However, a consensus within the field regarding how to refer to this approach should be formed in order to foster a more nuanced understanding of both its potential benefits and limitations. The choice of terminology should convey the targeted and time-limited nature of the intervention while also focusing on the availability of follow-up or additional sessions as needed. It should also be clear that SST is not a therapeutic approach per se, but a method for providing this service. This would help prevent misunderstandings among clients, therapists, researchers, and other stakeholders, and ensure that expectations regarding the scope and outcomes of single-session work are appropriately aligned.

Future Directions in Single Session Therapy Research

Although significant progress has been made in SST research, additional high-quality research is needed to support its evidence.

First, given the variability of the quality of the study and the preponderance of pilot/feasibility studies, additional well-designed randomized controlled trials (RCTs) are needed to fully examine the efficacy of SST. Such studies should include prespecified hypotheses and outcomes, a priori power calculations, adequate sample size, and the use of outcome measures to produce reliable, valid, and clinically meaningful data that can inform practice and policy in the field of mental health.

Another area of improvement is the exploration of the long-term effects of SST. Understanding the sustained benefits of single-session interventions over time (ideally up to one year) using multiple follow-up assessments will contribute to a more comprehensive evaluation of SST's long-term efficacy.

Further research efforts must be particularly directed toward a systematic evaluation of the cost effectiveness of SST compared to traditional long-term therapy to better guide its application and facilitate its regulation by government agencies. Indeed, "even if a psychological treatment could show strong efficacy and/or effectiveness, due to the high costs, it could never be assimilated in real clinical practice" (Castelnuovo, Pietrabissa, Cattivelli, Manzoni, & Molinari, 2016; Emmelkamp, David, Beckers, Muris, & Cuijpers, 2014). To help reach this goal, more clinics could offer SST by appointment or by walk-in, and their relative cost-effectiveness could be systematically evaluated. Comparing SST with traditional longer-term therapies or other short-intervention models or comparing single-session intervention across *different* therapeutic modalities will also provide valuable insights and guide clinical decision-making.

SST research should also focus on analyzing the therapeutic process and identifying effective techniques—particularly those that emphasize client strengths and competencies (Hoyt, 2025)—within a limited time frame. Understanding how therapists establish rapport, identify goals, and facilitate change becomes imperative for a deeper understanding of the most effective therapeutic mechanisms. Micro-analysis of sessions, including language patterns, nonverbal cues, and the timing of interventions, might contribute to this aim. Furthermore, since research findings reveal that not all clients may be equally suited for single-session interventions, it is essential to uncover the mechanisms of change and identify active ingredients that contribute to positive outcomes (Campbell, 2012). This involves continuing to explore client characteristics that can predict success in SST, such as motivation, cognitive flexibility, and the presenting issue.

Given the recognized importance of cultural considerations in therapy, further research should also delve deeper into the adaptation of SST techniques to diverse cultural contexts. As a result, within standardized training protocols personalized interventions could be developed for maximum impact. Risk management strategies and tools for ensuring the responsible and ethical practice of SSIs could also be established.

Future studies incorporating the previous recommendations could answer important questions about for whom SST may be efficacious, the optimal delivery method and intervention design for specific populations, and the possible role of single-session ideally as a "first-line" treatment within a stepped-care model.

Emerging Trends in SST Research

The landscape of SST research is dynamic and continuously evolving with emerging areas that warrant further investigation. With the rise of telehealth and digital interventions, technological advances have certainly influenced practice and research. More studies are needed to investigate the feasibility and effectiveness of providing SST through virtual platforms (Singla et al., 2023). Virtual delivery of SST may further increase willingness and ability to participate due to increased accessibility (especially among underserved populations), convenience, flexibility, and may be less distressing for some individuals.

Researchers may also begin exploring the integration of technology, including artificial intelligence and machine learning, into SST processes. The use of chatbots, virtual reality, and machine learning algorithms might potentially enhance the efficiency and effectiveness of single-session interventions.

The increasing attention to SST in publications, conferences, and training sessions will help to recognize its potential value in providing accessible, efficient, and client-centered mental health care.

Conclusions

SST has developed over the years, finding spaces of application in different contexts (public and private), with different therapeutic approaches, and in multiple areas of intervention (mental health, families, emergency, work).

Unquestionably, the interest of clinicians and researchers in studying the feasibility and clinical efficacy of SST has been due to its ecological function in providing efficient and effective services while responding to community needs. By its nature, SST can indeed improve accessibility by offering quicker access to mental health services, particularly for people otherwise facing long waitlists or who may not have the ability to commit to long-term therapy due to various constraints (Slive, McElheran, & Lawson, 2008). In addition to these practical and logistical considerations, SST can also be seen in the ethical light of respectfully empowering clients as soon as possible to achieve their self-defined treatment goals (Hoyt, 2025).

As SST gains traction, it is not without critics and controversies. Skeptics question the depth of change that can be achieved in a single session, emphasizing the importance of continued research in the field. Concerns, such as the potential for over-simplification of complex issues and inadequate assessment, are also subjects of debate. As the body of evidence supporting SST grows, so does our understanding of its potential applications, limitations, and implications for the future of mental health care. Continuous and systematic research on the usefulness and cost effectiveness of SST is vital to create effective stepped-care delivery services and reduce overall treatment costs for both clients and healthcare systems (Hymmen et al., 2013; Slive et al., 2008). Training and implementation are important and benefit from a clear, evidenced-based authorizing environment.

The mental health profession is at a crossroads and faces unprecedented challenges alongside unparalleled opportunities for growth and innovation. Embracing technology and investigating how brief interventions can be delivered efficiently in various settings, including community centers, schools, and online platforms, may open new avenues for accessible mental health care.

Note

1 *Editors' note:* see Chapter 10 (Schleider) in this volume.

References

Andreasson, S., Hansagi, H., & Osterlund, B. (2002). Short-term treatment for alcohol-related problems: Four-session guided self-change versus one session of advice—A randomized, controlled trial [Clinical Trial Comparative Study Randomized Controlled Trial]. *Alcohol, 28*(1), 57–62. https://doi.org/10.1016/s0741-8329(02)00231-8

Barwick, M., Urajnik, D., Sumner, L., Cohen, S., Reid, G., Engel, K., & Moore, J.E. (2013). Profiles and service utilization for children accessing a mental health walk-in clinic versus usual care. *Journal of Evidence-Based Social Work, 10*(4), 338–352. https://doi.org/10.1080/15433714.2012.663676

Basoglu, M., Salcioglu, E., & Livanou, M. (2007). A randomized controlled study of single-session behavioural treatment of earthquake-related post-traumatic stress disorder using an earthquake simulator. *Psychological Medicine, 37*(2), 203–213. https://doi.org/10.1017/S0033291706009123

Berman, A.H., Forsberg, L., Durbeej, N., Kallmen, H., & Hermansson, U. (2010). Single-session motivational interviewing for drug detoxification inpatients: Effects on self-efficacy, stages of change and substance use [Randomized Controlled Trial Research Support, Non-U.S. Gov't]. *Substance Use and Misuse*, 45(3), 384–402. https://doi.org/10.3109/10826080903452488

Bertuzzi, V., Fratini, G., Tarquinio, C., Cannistrà, F., Granese, V., Giusti, E.M., Castelnuovo, G., & Pietrabissa, G. (2021). Single-session therapy by appointment for the treatment of anxiety disorders in youth and adults: A systematic review of the literature. *Frontiers in Psychology*, 12, 721382. https://doi.org/10.3389/fpsyg.2021.721382

Bloom, B.L. (1981). Focused single session therapy: Initial development and evaluation. In S.H. Budman (Ed.), *Forms of Brief Therapy* (pp. 167–216). Guilford Press.

Bloom, B.L. (2001). Focused single-session psychotherapy: A review of the clinical and research literature. *Brief Treatment and Crisis Intervention*, 1(1), 75–86. https://doi.org/10.1093/brief-treatment/1.1.75

Boman, J., Lindqvist, H., Forsberg, L., Janlert, U., Granasen, G., & Nylander, E. (2018). Brief manual-based single-session motivational interviewing for reducing high-risk sexual behaviour in women—An evaluation [Randomized Controlled Trial Research Support, Non-U.S. Gov't]. *International Journal of STD and AIDS*, 29(4), 396–403. https://doi.org/10.1177/0956462417729308

Boyhan, P.A. (1996). Clients' perceptions of single session consultations as an option to waiting for family therapy. *Australian and New Zealand Journal of Family Therapy*, 17(2), 85–96. https://doi.org/10.1002/j.1467-8438.1996.tb01078.xCitations

Brooks, A.C., Chambers, J.E., Lauby, J., Byrne, E., Carpenedo, C.M., Benishek, L.A., Medvin, R., Metzger, D.S., & Kirby, K.C. (2016). Implementation of a brief treatment counseling toolkit in federally qualified healthcare centers: Patient and clinician utilization and satisfaction [Research Support, Non-U.S. Gov't]. *Journal of Substance Abuse Treatment*, 60, 70–80. https://doi.org/10.1016/j.jsat.2015.08.005

Cameron, C. (2007). Single session and walk-in psychotherapy: A descriptive account of the literature. *Counselling and Psychotherapy Research*, 7(4), 245–249. https://doi.org/10.1080/14733140701728403

Campbell, A. (1999). Single session interventions: An example of clinical research in practice. *Australian and New Zealand Journal of Family Therapy*, 20(4), 183–194.

Campbell, A. (2012). Single-session approaches to therapy: Time to review. *Australian and New Zealand Journal of Family Therapy*, 33(1), 15–26. https://doi.org/10.1017/aft.2012.3

Cannistrà, F., Piccirilli, F., Paolo D'Alia, P., Giannetti, A., Piva, L., Gobbato, F., Guzzardi, R., Ghisoni, A., & Pietrabissa, G. (2020). Examining the incidence and clients' experiences of single session therapy in Italy: A feasibility study. *Australian and New Zealand Journal of Family Therapy*, 41(3), 271–282. https://doi.org/10.1002/anzf.1421

Castelnuovo, G., Pietrabissa, G., Cattivelli, R., Manzoni, G.M., & Molinari, E. (2016). Not only clinical efficacy in psychological treatments: Clinical psychology must promote cost-benefit, cost-effectiveness, and cost-utility analysis. *Frontiers of Psychology*, 7, 563. https://doi.org/10.3389/fpsyg.2016.00563

Church, D., Piña, O., Reategui, C., & Brooks, A. (2012). Single-session reduction of the intensity of traumatic memories in abused adolescents after EFT:

A randomized controlled pilot study. *Traumatology*, *18*(3), 73–79. https://doi.org/10.1177/1534765611426788

Ellis, J.G., Cushing, T., & Germain, A. (2015). Treating acute insomnia: A randomized controlled trial of a "single-shot" of cognitive behavioral therapy for insomnia [Pragmatic Clinical Trial Randomized Controlled Trial Research Support, Non-U.S. Gov't]. *Sleep*, *38*(6), 971–978. https://doi.org/10.5665/sleep.4752

Emmelkamp, P.M., David, D., Beckers, T.O.M., Muris, P., Cuijpers, P., Lutz, W., Andersson, G., Araya, R., Banos Rivera, R.M., Barkham, M., Berking, M., Botella, C., Carlbring, P., Colom, F., Essau, C., Hermans, D., Hofmann, S.G., Knappe, S., Ollendick, T.H., . . . Vervliet, B. (2014). Advancing psychotherapy and evidence-based psychological interventions. *International Journal of Methods in Psychiatric Research*, *23*(Suppl 1), 58–91. https://doi.org/10.1002/mpr.1411

Eom, S.Y., Kim, E.S., Kim, H.J., Bang, Y.O., & Chun, N. (2012). [Effects of a one session spouse-support enhancement childbirth education on childbirth self-efficacy and perception of childbirth experience in women and their husbands] [Controlled Clinical Trial]. *J Korean Academy of Nursing*, *42*(4), 599–607. https://doi.org/10.4040/jkan.2012.42.4.599

Ewen, V., Mushquash, A.R., Mushquash, C.J., Bailey, S.K., Haggarty, J.M., & Stones, M.J. (2018). Single-session therapy in outpatient mental health services: Examining the effect on mental health symptoms and functioning. *Social Work in Mental Health*, *16*(5), 573–589. https://doi.org/10.1080/15332985.2018.1456503

Falkenstrom, F., Ekeblad, A., & Holmqvist, R. (2016). Improvement of the working alliance in one treatment session predicts improvement of depressive symptoms by the next session [Randomized Controlled Trial]. *Journal of Consulting and Clinical Psychology*, *84*(8), 738–751. https://doi.org/10.1037/ccp0000119

Fentz, H.N., Arendt, M., O'Toole, M.S., Hoffart, A., & Hougaard, E. (2014). The mediational role of panic self-efficacy in cognitive behavioral therapy for panic disorder: A systematic review and meta-analysis. *Behavior Research and Therapy*, *60*, 23–33. https://doi.org/10.1016/j.brat.2014.06.003

Gaskell, C., Simmonds-Buckley, M., Kellett, S., Stockton, C., Somerville, E., Rogerson, E., & Delgadillo, J. (2023). The effectiveness of psychological interventions delivered in routine practice: Systematic review and meta-analysis. *Administrative Policy in Mental Health*, *50*(1), 43–57. https://doi.org/10.1007/s10488-022-01225-y

Hampson, R., O'Hanlon, J., Franklin, A., Pentony, M., Fridgant, L., & Heins, T. (1999). The place of single session family consultations: Five years' experience in Canberra. *Australian and New Zealand Journal of Family Therapy*, *20*(4), 195–200.

Hansen, N.B., Lambert, M.J., & Forman, E.M. (2002). The pychotherapy dose-response effect and its implications for treatment delivery services. *Clinical Psychology: Science and Practice*, *9*(3), 329–343. https://doi.org/10.1093/clipsy.9.3.329

Harper-Jaques, S., & Simms, J. (2015). Single session walk-in therapy. *Canadian Nurse*, *111*(1), 12–13. https://www.ncbi.nlm.nih.gov/pubmed/26387233

Haukebo, K., Skaret, E., Ost, L.G., Raadal, M., Berg, E., Sundberg, H., & Kvale, G. (2008). One- vs. five-session treatment of dental phobia: A randomized controlled study [Comparative Study Randomized Controlled Trial]. *Journal of Behavior Therapy and Experimental Psychiatry*, *39*(3), 381–390. https://doi.org/10.1016/j.jbtep.2007.09.006

Hellstrom, K., & Ost, L.G. (1995). One-session therapist directed exposure vs two forms of manual directed self-exposure in the treatment of spider phobia [Clinical Trial Comparative Study Randomized Controlled Trial Research Support, Non-U.S. Gov't]. *Behavior Research and Therapy, 33*(8), 959–965. https://doi.org/10.1016/0005-7967(95)00028-v

Holst, M., Willenheimer, R., Martensson, J., Lindholm, M., & Stromberg, A. (2007). Telephone follow-up of self-care behaviour after a single session education of patients with heart failure in primary health care. *European Journal of Cardiovascular Nursing, 6*(2), 153–159. https://doi.org/10.1016/j.ejcnurse.2006.06.006

Hoyt, M.F. (2025). *Single Session Therapy: A Clinical Introduction to Principles and Practices.* Routledge.

Hoyt, M.F., Rosenbaum, R., & Talmon, M. (1992). Planned single-session psychotherapy. In S.H. Budman, M.F. Hoyt, & S. Friedman (Eds.), *The First Session in Brief Therapy* (pp. 59–86). Guilford Press.

Hoyt, M.F., & Talmon, M. (2014). *Capturing the Moment: Single Session Therapy and Walk-In Services.* Crown House Publishing.

Hoyt, M.F., Young, J., & Rycroft, P. (2021). *Single Session Thinking and Practice in Global, Cultural, and Familial Contexts: Expanding Applications.* Routledge.

Hurn, R. (2005). Single-session therapy: Planned success or unplanned failure? *Counselling Psychology Review, 20*(4), 33–40.

Hymmen, P., Stalker, C.A., & Cait, C.A. (2013). The case for single-session therapy: Does the empirical evidence support the increased prevalence of this service delivery model? *Journal of Mental Health, 22*(1), 60–71. https://doi.org/10.3109/09638237.2012.670880

Kutz, I., Resnik, V., & Dekel, R. (2008). The effect of single-session modified EMDR on acute stress syndromes. *Journal of EMDR Practice and Research, 2*(3), 190–200. https://doi.org/10.1891/1933-3196.2.3.190

Lamprecht, H., Laydon, C., McQuillan, C., Wiseman, S., Williams, L., Gash, A., & Reilly, J. (2007). Single-session solution-focused brief therapy and self-harm: A pilot study. *Journal of Psychiatric Mental Health Nursing, 14*(6), 601–602. https://doi.org/10.1111/j.1365-2850.2007.01105.x

Lindhiem, O., Kolko, D.J., & Cheng, Y. (2012). Predicting psychotherapy benefit: A probabilistic and individualized approach. *Behavior Therapy, 43*(2), 381–392. https://doi.org/10.1016/j.beth.2011.08.004

Luutonen, S., Santalahti, A., Makinen, M., Vahlberg, T., & Rautava, P. (2019). One-session cognitive behavior treatment for long-term frequent attenders in primary care: Randomized controlled trial [Randomized Controlled Trial]. *Scandanavian Journal of Primary Health Care, 37*(1), 98–104. https://doi.org/10.1080/02813432.2019.1569371

Martin, A., Rauh, E., Fichter, M., & Rief, W. (2007). A one-session treatment for patients suffering from medically unexplained symptoms in primary care: A randomized clinical trial. *Psychosomatics, 48*(4), 294–303. https://doi.org/10.1176/appi.psy.48.4.294

Miller, J.K., & Slive, A. (2004). Breaking down the barriers to clinical service delivery: Walk-in family therapy. *Journal of Marital and Family Therapy, 30*(1), 95–103. https://doi.org/10.1111/j.1752-0606.2004.tb01225.x

Mireau, R., & Inch, R. (2009). Brief solution-focused counseling: A practical effective strategy for dealing with wait lists in community-based mental health services. *Social Work, 54*(1), 63–70. https://doi.org/10.1093/sw/54.1.63

Mongelli, F., Georgakopoulos, P., & Pato, M.T. (2020). Challenges and opportunities to meet the mental Hhalth needs of underserved and disenfranchised populations in the United States. *Focus (American Psychiatric Publications)*, *18*(1), 16–24. https://doi.org/10.1176/appi.focus.20190028

Oar, E.L., Farrell, L.J., & Ollendick, T.H. (2015). One session treatment for specific phobias: An adaptation for paediatric blood-injection-injury phobia in youth. *Clinical Child Family Psychological Review*, *18*(4), 370–394. https://doi.org/10.1007/s10567-015-0189-3

Ollendick, T.H., Halldorsdottir, T., Fraire, M.G., Austin, K.E., Noguchi, R.J., Lewis, K.M., Jarrett, M.A., Cunningham, N.R., Canavera, K., Allen, K.B., & Whitmore, M.J. (2015). Specific phobias in youth: A randomized controlled trial comparing one-session treatment to a parent-augmented one-session treatment. *Behavior Therapy*, *46*(2), 141–155. https://doi.org/10.1016/j.beth.2014.09.004

Ollendick, T.H., Ost, L.G., Reuterskiöld, L., Costa, N., Cederlund, R., Sirbu, C., Davis, T.E., III, & Jarrett, M.A. (2009). One-session treatment of specific phobias in youth: A randomized clinical trial in the United States and Sweden. *Journal of Consulting and Clinical Psychology*, *77*(3), 504–516. https://doi.org/10.1037/a0015158

O'Neill, I. (2015). What's in a name? Clients' experiences of single session therapy. *Journal of Family Therapy*, *39*(1), 63–79. https://doi.org/10.1111/1467-6427.12099

Perkins, R., & Scarlett, G. (2008). The effectiveness of single session therapy in child and adolescent mental health. Part 2: An 18-month follow-up study. *Psychology and Psychotherapy*, *81*(Pt 2), 143–156. https://doi.org/10.1348/147608308X280995

Pietrabissa, G., Manzoni, G.M., Rossi, A., & Castelnuovo, G. (2017). The MOTIV-HEART study: A prospective, randomized, single-blind pilot study of brief strategic therapy and motivational interviewing among cardiac rehabilitation patients. *Frontiers of Psychology*, *8*, 83. https://doi.org/10.3389/fpsyg.2017.00083

Rodda, S.N., Lubman, D.I., Cheetham, A., Dowling, N.A., & Jackson, A.C. (2015). Single session web-based counselling: A thematic analysis of content from the perspective of the client. *British Journal of Guidance & Counselling*, *43*(1), 117–130. https://doi.org/10.1080/03069885.2014.938609

Rossi, A., Panzeri, A., Pietrabissa, G., Manzoni, G.M., Castelnuovo, G., & Mannarini, S. (2020). The anxiety-buffer hypothesis in the time of COVID-19: When self-esteem protects from the impact of loneliness and fear on anxiety and depression. *Frontiers in Psychology*, *11*, 2177. https://doi.org/10.3389/fpsyg.2020.02177

Schleider, J.L., Dobias, M.L., Sung, J.Y., & Mullarkey, M.C. (2020). Future directions in single-session youth mental health interventions. *Journal of Clinical Child and Adolescent Psychology*, *49*(2), 264–278. https://doi.org/10.1080/15374416.2019.1683852

Schleider, J.L., & Weisz, J.R. (2017). Little treatments, promising effects? Meta-analysis of single-session interventions for youth psychiatric problems. *Journal of the American Academy of Child and Adolescent Psychiatry*, *56*(2), 107–115. https://doi.org/10.1016/j.jaac.2016.11.007

Schmulson, M.J., Ortiz-Garrido, O.M., Hinojosa, C., & Arcila, D. (2006). A single session of reassurance can acutely improve the self-perception of impairment in patients with IBS. *Journal of Psychosomatic Research*, *61*(4), 461–467. https://doi.org/10.1016/j.jpsychores.2006.02.011

Singla, D.R., Schleider, J.L., & Patel, V. (2023). Democratizing access to psychological therapies: Innovations and the role of psychologists. *Journal of Consulting and Clinical Psychology*, *91*(11), 623–625. https://doi.org/10.1037/ccp0000850

Situmorang, D.D.B. (2022). "When the first session may be the last!": A case report of the implementation of "rapid tele-psychotherapy" with single-session music therapy in the COVID-19 outbreak. *Palliative & Supportive Care, 20*(2), 290–295. https://doi.org/10.1017/S1478951521001425

Slive, A., & Bobele, M. (2013). Walk-in counselling services: Making the most of one hour. *Australian and New Zealand Journal of Family Therapy, 33*(1), 27–38. https://doi.org/10.1017/aft.2012.4

Slive, A., McElheran, N., & Lawson, A. (2008). How brief does it get? Walk-in single session therapy. *Journal of Systemic Therapies, 27*(4), 5–22. https://doi.org/10.1521/jsyt.2008.27.4.5

Söderquist, M. (2018). Coincidence favors the prepared mind: Single sessions with couples in Sweden. In M.F. Hoyt, M. Bobele, A. Slive, J. Young, & M. Talmon (Eds.), *Single-Session Therapy by Walk-In or Appointment. Administrative, Clinical, and Supervisory Aspects of One-at-a-Time Services* (pp. 270–290). Routledge.

Talmon, M. (1990). *Single-Session Therapy: Maximizing the Effect of the First (and Often Only) Therapeutic Encounter.* Jossey-Bass.

Tantirangsee, N., Assanangkornchai, S., & Marsden, J. (2015). Effects of a brief intervention for substance use on tobacco smoking and family relationship functioning in schizophrenia and related psychoses: A randomised controlled trial. *Journal of Substance Abuse Treatment, 51*, 30–37. https://doi.org/10.1016/j.jsat.2014.10.011

Thom, A., Sartory, G., & Johren, P. (2000). Comparison between one-session psychological treatment and benzodiazepine in dental phobia [Clinical Trial Controlled Clinical Trial Research Support, Non-U.S. Gov't]. *Journal of Consulting and Clinical Psychology, 68*(3), 378–387. https://doi.org/10.1037//0022-006x.68.3.378

Toneatto, T. (2016). Single-session interventions for problem gambling may be as effective as longer treatments: Results of a randomized control trial. *Addictive Behaviors, 52*, 58–65. https://doi.org/10.1016/j.addbeh.2015.08.006

Urrego, Z., Abaakouk, Z., Roman, C., & Contreras, R. (2009). *Evaluation of results from a single session psychotherapeutic intervention in population affected by the Colombian internal armed conflict.* http://hdl.handle.net/10144/223391

Weisz, J.R., Kuppens, S., Ng, M.Y., Eckshtain, D., Ugueto, A.M., Vaughn-Coaxum, R., Jensen-Doss, A., Hawley, K.M., Krumholz Marchette, L.S., Chu, B.C., Weersing, V.R., & Fordwood, S.R. (2017). What five decades of research tells us about the effects of youth psychological therapy: A multilevel meta-analysis and implications for science and practice. *American Psychologist, 72*(2), 79–117. https://doi.org/10.1037/a0040360

Whicher, E.V., Utku, F., Schirmer, G., Davis, P., & Abou-Saleh, M.T. (2012). Pilot project to evaluate the effectiveness and acceptability of single-session brief counseling for the prevention of substance misuse in pregnant adolescents. *Addictive Disorders & Their Treatment, 11*(1), 43–49. https://doi.org/10.1097/ADT.0b013e3182387029

World Health Organization. (2022). *Mental Disorders.* World Health Organization.

Young, J. (2018). SST: The misunderstood gift that keeps on giving. In M.F. Hoyt, M. Bobele, A. Slive, J. Young, & M. Talmon (Eds.), *Single-Session Therapy by*

Walk-In or Appointment: Administrative, Clinical, and Supervisory Aspects of One-at-a-Time Services (pp. 40–58). Routledge.

Young, J., & Dryden, W. (2019). Single-session therapy—Past and future: An interview. *British Journal of Guidance & Counselling, 47*(5), 1–10. https://doi.org/10.1080/03069885.2019.1581129

Young, K., & Jebreen, J. (2019). Recognizing Single-Session Therapy as psychotherapy. *Journal of Systemic Therapies, 38*(4), 31–44. https://doi.org/10.1521/jsyt.2019.38.4.31

Zehnder, D., Meuli, M., & Landolt, M.A. (2010). Effectiveness of a single-session early psychological intervention for children after road traffic accidents: A randomised controlled trial. *Child and Adolescent Psychiatry and Mental Health, 4*, 7. https://doi.org/10.1186/1753-2000-4-7

Chapter 14

Walk-In Single Sessions, Then and Now

The Eastside Community Mental Health Service in Calgary, Canada

Nancy McElheran

The original Eastside Family Centre (EFC; now called the Eastside Community Mental Health Service, ECMHS) is a community-based walk-in Single Session Therapy (SST) resource that has been previously described (Slive, MacLaurin, Oakander, & Amundson, 1995; Slive, McElheran, & Lawson, 2008; Clements, McElheran, Hackney, & Park, 2011; Stewart, McElheran, Park, Oakander, & MacLaurin, 2018). The original EFC was launched in 1990 by Wood's Homes senior management with the support of the Wood's board of directors and community and political leaders. The eastside of the city of Calgary, Alberta, Canada, was selected, as it was known for its ethnic diversity and high socioeconomic need.

The focus of the walk-in service was to offer no-cost, easily accessible therapy to people in moments of need at a location convenient to them. Clients self-referred or were referred by friends, family, and/or a community professional. Walking in for a single session of therapy at the EFC was well received. Outcome data consistently indicated 80% of clients felt heard, understood, and respected. They commented positively on the quality of the service received, with 87% noting a reduction in distress after their session. Clients who decided to return for additional sessions (43%) indicated they did so because they felt the therapy met their need(s) and they could access the service in a timely fashion. The main mental health concerns presented by individuals at that time were anxiety and depression. Families and couples who attended the service also highlighted stress, anxiety, and conflict in relationships that at times led to domestic violence as their central concerns (Stewart et al., 2018; McElheran, 2021).

The infrastructure that facilitated the EFC walk-in SST service for over 30 years was key to its success. As noted in earlier reports, therapy teams, comprised of graduate-level regulated professionals, were one component of this infrastructure. Teaching and supervision of graduate-level students and community-based therapists became an integrated component of the therapy teams. One-way mirrors supported this team approach and the training/supervision. The other core component was the session structure

DOI: 10.4324/9781032693828-17

itself, adapted from the Milan therapy group (Boscolo, Cecchin, Hoffman, & Penn, 1987). This structure consisted of:

- a pre-session consultation with the team regarding the client's presenting concern and possible questions to consider
- the therapy session itself, conducted by one of the therapists from the team
- an inter-session consultation regarding the client's concerns, with suggestions as to potential interventions
- presentation of the intervention to the client
- the post-session debriefing of client feedback regarding the intervention

Many clients indicated they felt cared for by having multiple professionals attend to their mental health needs. Some would thank the team at the end of their session (Stewart et al., 2018).

The EFC walk-in SST was the first of its kind in Canada. It became the example that others would follow (see Slive & Bobele, 2011). Adaptations to the SST approach, whether it was walk-in or single sessions by appointment, were made in accordance with the particular community need. Core SST principles, such as keeping a focus on what the client needs in the moment, the creation of a collaborative alliance between client and therapist, the utilization of client strengths and resources, and interventions in the form of ideas that fit with the client's beliefs were modeled after the EFC approach and upheld across services and the country (McElheran, Harper-Jaques, & Lawson, 2020).

The Pandemic Pivot

In March of 2020, the world had to make major adjustments in response to the COVID-19 pandemic. Public health officials in Alberta mandated an immediate suspension of all in-person contact, which required the shutting down of the walk-in service at the EFC. Wood's Homes senior management group, along with the staff at Eastside, came up with the first of many creative responses to this crisis by acquiring the online virtual infrastructure necessary to offer clients single sessions by appointment (phone or video) from their homes or other private locations. The information form, previously filled out by the client when they arrived, was replaced by an intake form that was then completed with the client over the phone by the EFC crisis team and prior to their appointment with a therapist. This change, which provided the crisis team with the client intake information, allowed the therapy staff the opportunity to have "fresh eyes" on the information when they first met clients online and in keeping with historical practice. This was a first for the staff of both the crisis and therapy teams. Both staff groups readily embraced this significant shift in process. A serendipitous benefit for the client with this shift to having the crisis team conduct the intakes was the fact that if they were in crisis when they called they would have the crisis dealt with immediately. As a result, the intake information gathered either went directly forward to the therapy team or a safety-and-risk management plan would be put in place for the client until they saw a therapist. Consistent with the former walk-in service was the fact that clients could choose their appointment time. Separate and apart from this new intake process for online SST was the addition of e-therapy. Clients could email a request for therapy that was responded to in a timely fashion by the therapy teams. E-therapy became another option for clients during the pandemic. The client would describe in writing their concerns and the team would respond accordingly.

The new intake form, completed by the crisis team staff with the client over the phone and adapted from the original, accorded well with the basic principles of SST outlined earlier, i.e., determine what the client's most pressing need/concern is, what strengths and resources are available to them in the present, and determine what they see as possible outcomes/solutions to their current dilemma. In addition to asking questions regarding what the client wants/needs from their upcoming session, is a question the crisis staff ask in relation to risk. As noted earlier, when a client indicates they are at risk, the crisis staff address this concern immediately. Adding a question as to risk, and the assessment of the same by the crisis team staff, is helpful to the therapy team. The therapist follows up with the client in their session when risk may be present but is not imminent.

The following are the questions that constitute the intake form.

Table 14.1 The Eastside Community Mental Health Service virtual intake form (abridged)

(© 2022. Used by agreement. This modified questionnaire is the sole property of Wood's Homes and as such may not be copied in part or in whole without the explicit written permission from Wood's Homes.)

Presenting Concerns:

1. Is this your first time using this service?
   ☐ Yes ☐ No

2. What is the single-most important concern that you wish to share today?

3. Has this concern ever been so bad that you have any thoughts of harming or killing yourself?
   ☐ Yes ☐ No

   Suicide Risk Assessment ☐Low ☐Medium ☐High☐NA
   Comments (i.e., Intervention, Relevant Recent History):

(Continued)

Table 14.1 (Continued)

4. We know domestic violence or interpersonal violence is a problem for people and can directly affect them. Violence and abuse can be physical, psychological or even financial.

   Will domestic violence or abuse be part of what you would like to talk about in your session?

   ☐Yes ☐No

   Comments:

5. How would you rate your level of distress regarding today's concern?

   ☐1   ☐2   ☐3   ☐4   ☐5   ☐6   ☐7   ☐8   ☐9   ☐10

   Immediate Intervention Necessary? Describe

6. In regards to your concern(s) today, what things have you tried?

7. Please describe the sources of strength in your life (e.g., sense of humour, patience, intelligence, stubbornness, religious practice, spirituality, family, friends, strong will, courage, creativity, spirituality)

8. Have you had previous therapy? ☐Yes ☐No
   Comments:
   Are you currently receiving therapeutic services? ☐Yes ☐No
   Comments:

9. Do you have present involvement with Children's Services/Child Welfare? ☐Yes ☐No
   Comments:

10. What would you most like in today's session? (e.g.: information, help in making a decision, managing a conflict between, support in, ideas about managing)

    If a couple or family session, what are the first names of the clients in the session?

11. For many people, a single session with a therapist is enough to take action or to feel better. Imagine yourself at the end of the session, what will tell you things are heading in the right direction?

    Date and time of appointment:

Therapists remained rigorous in adhering to the established single session mindset that is informed by research and is key to offering this type of service whether online, over the phone, or in-person (Bloom, 2001; Hoyt, 2009; Duncan & Miller, 2000; Talmon, 1990).

The therapy staff and consulting teams were given additional technological training as needed to enable them to conduct SST sessions by appointment online (phone and video). The actual format and process for conducting a session with a consulting team followed the Milan 5-step process referenced earlier: having an online Webex pre-session discussion regarding the client's most pressing need, observing the session via a breakout room as opposed to observing behind a one-way mirror, the inter-session team consultation in the main room, creating interventions that aligned with the client's concerns, presenting the interventions, and the post-session team debriefing with suggestions for the future should the client return. Staff and consultants made the necessary adaptations to delivering single sessions of therapy online quickly and seamlessly. The flexibility of both the staff and the organization to adapt to client and community need during the pandemic was noteworthy.

Within 72 hours of the public health requirement to discontinue face-to-face contact, the Eastside virtual service was up and running. Clients were offered single-session/one-at-a-time appointments at times and locations that fit for them. Clients were "seen" in their homes, in libraries, in their cars, or other private and convenient (for them) locations. Feedback from clients indicated that some preferred the online option, while others stated they hoped for a return to in-person sessions as soon as was feasible. Therapists made similar comments, with some stating they preferred the online format because it was easily accessible from multiple locations, while others awaited a return to in-person contact.

In-person contact resumed July 2021 when the EFC team determined it would be safe to commence in-person single sessions by appointment with COVID screening protocols in place. Open-access walk-in SST resumed May 3, 2022. The decision to continue offering online single sessions was in keeping with client feedback that indicated some preferred to be seen from the comfort of their homes or other private locations.

Outcomes for the pandemic period were consistent with those seen pre-pandemic with one exception: client reports of greater subjective distress, which seemed to be directly attributable to the pandemic and its restrictions on their lives.

Case Illustration

An example of the online SST approach during the pandemic is a video session conducted with a couple who were experiencing considerable conflict in their relationship. They contacted the crisis team by phone, having heard of the service from a friend. They asked to be "seen" for a session of therapy as soon as possible. They were provided with information as to how the new online SST system worked, including the fact that they could have one session with a therapist and team and/or could book another session(s) as they needed. The crisis team staff who conducted the intake over the phone asked the couple what their most pressing concern was. As stated by the wife, Anna, her husband, John, was "harsh" in the language he was using about her parenting of their first child. She indicated that she felt intimidated by John much of the time and was now considering leaving the relationship, even though she professed her love for him. When John was asked by the same staff what was concerning him most, he stated that while he was initially "caught off guard" by Anna's concerns and her comment that she felt intimidated by him, he did concede he could be harsh in his language at times, which he attributed to his own upbringing and the strict parenting style of his parents. The couple also agreed their parenting practices could be different based on their different cultural backgrounds (Anna was from South Africa; John grew up in Canada).

The first online video session with this couple, conducted from a breakout room via Webex, found them in separate locations. Anna was in their home, while John was in their car. Both stated they felt comfortable in their respective private locations. The therapist informed them that the EFC offered a single session or one-at-a-time approach and that while they could return as often as they wished, the session that day would be complete in and of itself. Confidentiality of information was also reviewed. The therapist advised that a team of professional therapists would be available to be a part of their session online, in a breakout room, where they and the therapist would talk and would also participate in the inter-session consultation. The couple each indicated they understood and agreed.

The session started with the therapist elaborating upon the aforementioned concern. The couple was asked what each wanted from this session. Attention was paid to addressing any potential risk issues given Anna's comment that she felt intimidated at times. At the end of the 45-minute session, before taking the inter-session consultation break and after determining that neither was at risk, the therapist re-inquired as to what they would most like today. The couple indicated they needed to find new ways of talking with one another so they could move forward. Anna stated she wanted to feel more comfortable with John when they disagreed; John stated he wanted to feel that Anna was hearing his concerns, and he also wanted her to feel comfortable telling him when she felt intimidated and/or overwhelmed by his approach. The team members who attended this session in the breakout room sent possible suggestions of questions to the therapist via a "chat" message.

Following the five-step Milan model, and in keeping with the original walk-in process, the inter-session consultation with the therapist and team, conducted in the main online room, led to the following ideas for the couple to consider as an experiment: both Anna and John were commended for their ability to be open with each other and the team regarding their concerns as to how best manage the conflict that arose from their different perspectives. Their love and concern for each other's welfare was noted and commended. The couple was offered a structured way of having a conversation. They were invited to come up with a set time to sit down at a table across from each other. Each person could talk for five to ten minutes while the other person listened. The content of the conversation could be a focus on what each person wanted the other to understand about their thoughts and feelings about parenting their child and/or any other important relationship issue. At the end of that time, the partner could give feedback as to what he/she heard and understood, which could then be validated and/or modified by the person speaking, based on what they were wanting their partner to understand. After completing as many of these structured conversations as they wished, they could explore what they had learned about each other and how that might make a difference in their communication habits. They were invited to return if they wished.

The couple did return for several additional sessions, booked on their initiative through the crisis team. Each session was conducted online, via video, with different therapists and teams, depending on the day. The focus continued to be on ways to improve talking with each other in order to feel heard and understood (Söderquist, 2023). After six single sessions, booked by them and at convenient times for them, with a consistent focus on ways they could talk respectfully with each other and in ways they could hear what the other person had to say, the couple indicated they were at a point where they could have a disagreement with one another without returning to former habits of intimidation and/or withdrawal from conversations. They were commended for the work done and invited to return at any point if they needed. They commented that they found the team involvement very helpful and appreciated having both the safety and the capability of meeting the therapist and team online from their home.

The New Eastside Community Mental Health Service (ECMHS)

Coincidental with the pandemic, Wood's Homes senior executive group and the managers of the then-EFC were re-conceptualizing the services offered at the center based on changes in local community thinking and funder requirements (Beere, Page, Diminic, & Harris, 2018; CMHA, 2018; Valaitis, Carter, Lam, Nicholl, Feather, & Cleghorn, 2018; GermAnn, MacKean, & Butler, 2020). Clients were stating that community-based services had become very complex and difficult to navigate, which was reportedly very stressful. Examples offered had to do with navigating the health care system and finding a family physician. Housing was another example cited in that a housing shortage was creating both financial and living constraints for many. Funders were requiring more efficient and effective service delivery models. This information was similar to what was heard in the early 1990s that prompted the opening of the original EFC. The notion of a "hub" where multiple services could be offered on the same site and in a seamless manner (Bostock & Britt, 2014) was proposed and accepted by Wood's Homes in keeping with its mandate to adapt services to meet the needs of both clients and communities.

In September 2020 staff of the EFC and Community Resource Team (CRT) merged to become the Eastside Community Mental Health Service (ECMHS), adding new options to fit community request (Janet Stewart, personal communication, September 15, 2023). A first step was to formalize the relationship between CRT (now called the Community Counselling Team, CCT) and the EFC therapists (now called the Therapy Team). As noted, the two services worked interdependently during the pandemic to create the virtual service delivery approach. The management decision to continue offering the single session online therapy service (video and phone) while bringing back the walk-in service and continuing with the in-person by appointment service was a first step in this new integrated hub model.

A new service, called Systems Navigation, was introduced to assist clients with larger systems issues noted earlier. This approach was first introduced in primary care settings in the early 1990s (Dahlgren & Whitehead, 2021). Typically, clients come from the therapy teams, with the need for systems navigation emerging from the therapy session. The therapy team takes the first step by connecting the client with the service navigator at the end of their single session. The ECMHS staff, designated as system navigators (SNs), link clients with wellness resources, employment centers, financial supports, housing, and any other need that arises. The System Navigator establishes a relationship with clients and then connects them with the identified professional by making the first contact and introduction. This first contact is called a "warm transfer" (Jack & Wathen, 2021). This process has made a significant difference to the client experience. Client feedback indicates that in 2023, 89% of clients reported they had a clear next step; 90% reported receiving the service they needed.

Integrated Ethno-Cultural Teams are another new component in the development of the ECMHS hub. From the outset, the east side of Calgary was regarded as a multicultural sector of the city. Historically, EFC walk-in clients and callers to the crisis team were offered their session primarily in English or, as required, with the assistance of interpreters from other city resources and/or family and friends. When possible, and primarily through the community volunteer therapist group of the time, clients could receive a single session of therapy in the language of their choice. Accordingly, in developing the new ECMHS, specific attention was paid to offering single sessions in the language of the client's choice by hiring staff with language and cultural proficiency. At present, 40% of clients requesting a service have a diverse (i.e., non-Canadian) cultural background, have a preferred language other than English, and have newcomer or immigrant experience. While not all languages are available, in 2023 ten languages other than English were available to clients who requested the same (Janet Stewart, personal communication, September 15, 2023). This is a developing strength of this new hub model of service delivery.

A concept called "Caring Contacts" has also been introduced to the SST approach at the ECMHS. Previously the assessment and management of risk with clients was sufficiently important that the EFC created a risk matrix to aid therapists in identifying risk as low, medium, or high. High-risk clients were (and are) typically referred to hospital emergency rooms with a safety plan, while low- and medium-risk clients were supported to gather their personal resources around them and also create a safety plan they or their support group could implement.

In 2019, an article appeared by Links et al. in the *Canadian Journal of Psychiatry* that outlined specific steps that could be taken to intervene with risk at all levels. One of the therapy team's consulting psychiatrists brought the article forward for consideration. The ECMHS group embraced this caring contact approach. Caring contacts consist of telephone calls to at-risk clients subsequent to their single session to support them and ensure their current safety as follow up to the safety plan made as part of their session. A caring contact call is typically offered within one to two days of their session, depending on what the client prefers. It can be made by the therapist of record but can also be made by a member of the CCT. The caring contact call is made over and above other intervention(s) that emerged in their session. On occasion, and after discussion with other team members and managers, additional external resources such as police may be involved if there are urgent concerns for the client's safety and if the client is unresponsive when concern for their safety remains. Feedback from clients has been very positive to date. Clients feel cared for and have expressed gratitude for the attention received (J. Stewart, personal communication, September 15, 2023). On occasion clients will state they don't need additional support. This is respected by the team when the clients are clear with regard to their safety plan and the resources at their disposal.

The final addition to the hub service model development was the implementation of the classification system for identifying mental health concerns used by other programs at Wood's Homes starting in 2023. This change has added congruency of information with other programs at Wood's and added depth to the previous system utilized. This change has also assisted the research department of Wood's Homes in both defining and refining organizational as well as program outcomes.

One-at-a-Time Brief Therapy Case Example Illustrating the Hub Model That Includes System Navigation and the Caring Contact Approach at the ECMHS

Liz, a 70-year-old Caucasian woman, phoned the ECMHS in early March 2023 at the suggestion of a city crisis line and in response to her request for a therapy referral. All therapeutic contacts were via telephone. As stated by her, Liz was relatively new to her rural community outside of Calgary and was reporting that she felt isolated, lost, and lonely. These feelings had exacerbated longstanding mental health issues for which she had been hospitalized on numerous occasions in the past.

On first contact, Liz was crying profusely, stating she was afraid of her impulse control and thought she could do harm to herself. Initial exploration of safety resources revealed she had a daughter living in the same community who could come to her home, although Liz said she would be reluctant to call her daughter because she did not wish to be seen as vulnerable. Given the initial risk at hand, the therapy team offered a caring contact instead of a single session of therapy and focused on assisting Liz establishing her web of safety resources. Caring contacts continued over the next couple of weeks at her request and until Liz stated she no longer had thoughts of self-harm/suicide. These contacts were conducted by members of both the crisis and therapy team staff.

Once Liz re-established her sense of safety, she requested a therapy session for assistance in managing the thoughts that were "bogging" her down and creating considerable anxiety on a daily basis. As initially presented, current thoughts causing her distress were related to trauma from the treatment she received in past hospitalizations. Her descriptions of what she felt at that time were persistent and personal violations by hospital staff. These thoughts were very vivid for her in the present. She also described profound feelings of loss in relation to the recent death of a son. This more recent loss had triggered the thoughts and anxiety from the past. A contract for five to six sessions of one-at-a-time therapy was established. Liz was informed that each session would be complete in and of itself, might not be with the same therapist, and that she could determine when or if she would have a subsequent session(s). Liz responded well to both the notion of being in charge of her own therapy and her ability to choose when the sessions occurred. At the beginning of each session Liz was asked what her most pressing concern was and what she most wanted from her session. Liz consistently focused on addressing the loss of her son, as his loss was profound and painful for her on a daily basis. She felt close to him and he reminded her of his father, who is also gone from her life. These losses were among the overwhelming memories that led to her being hospitalized for lengthy periods. The therapy team found that Liz responded well to the intervention of imagining seeing her son in a warm and safe place as a way of creating boundaries for herself in addressing past suffering and loss alongside present possibilities. She was also offered tools for managing her anxiety that included some mindfulness meditation on a daily basis. By the end of the fourth session Liz was stating she felt less anxious and more at peace with herself and in her new community. She also stated she was able to think of her son at times that fit for her versus having his image present all the time. She also stated she had come to terms with the loss of her son's father. She commented that she had recently invited her daughter to her house and found it a happy experience. She requested to put remaining sessions on hold, stating she would initiate a call back if and when she needed it.

The therapist and team supported Liz's decision. At the same time, they offered her the service of the system navigator so she could become more familiar with the resources in her new community. Initially a bit reluctant, Liz did accept this assistance when she was assured there would be a person-to-person "warm transfer" between her and the community person(s). A nurse practitioner became Liz's medical back-up for her considerable medical problems. Coincidentally, Liz met a woman who lived close to her, was also alone, and who befriended her.

In summary, the current open-access hub model of service delivery was developed in order to continue offering online (video and phone) therapy services in addition to the return to in-person by walk-in and/or appointment. The ECMHS hub model of service delivery, which also includes system navigation, warm transfers, and caring contacts, has been well received by the community, which appears to value having a single point of access to a range of services. The ECMHS currently offers one-at-a-time SST in the following ways:

- Two days per week: Online (video or phone) single sessions by appointment.
- Two days per week: Both online and in-person single sessions by appointment.
- Two days per week: Open-access walk-in SST.

An Example of a Walk-In Session That Includes an Ethno-Cultural Approach

Randy, a 45-year-old man who immigrated to Canada from Mexico approximately ten years ago walked into the ECMHS on a recent Saturday. His stated concern was the loss of a relationship of several years. Randy was offered his session in Spanish by a Mexican-Canadian therapist, which he accepted, stating that while he could speak English well, he felt that in his current emotional state he would prefer speaking in Spanish. He also stated he appreciated the therapist would perhaps better understand some of his feelings, as the therapist might share similar values as he. When the therapist asked what he would like from his session he stated that he needed to find ways to manage his thoughts and feelings about his lost relationship. He said that he found that he was unable to focus on his work as an engineer, which was concerning for both himself and his employer. Randy informed the therapist that his girlfriend of four years had recently told him she wanted to pursue other relationships and had moved from the apartment where they had lived together. He was completely shocked by her decision, as they had been talking about getting married. Randy stated he was unable to sleep, was having difficulty concentrating, was not eating, and had withdrawn from all social contact since he found it too painful to be reminded of his loss when around friends. He denied any thoughts of self-harm or risk, stating he would not want to create that kind of upset for his family or friends.

After approximately 45 minutes, the team met for an inter-session consultation with the therapist. Together they created the following intervention: Randy was validated in his shock over the abrupt loss of the person he had anticipated would be his life partner. He was commended for his capacity to think of his supportive family and friends and how they were receiving his news. The team commented that Randy's surprise and shock over the sudden departure of his partner could leave him with many unanswered questions. He was offered two ideas to consider. One was to set fixed times of the day when he would think of his partner and what she meant to him. At the end of that time he would shift focus to other things, such as his work, or perhaps call a friend or engage in any other activity he enjoyed that did not involve thinking of his partner. At the same time, he was invited to write down the questions he had with regard to her leaving so that they were not circling around in his head and heart. The team also suggested he consult with his family doctor if the sleep disturbance continued. Randy was invited to return at any point to talk about what he learned from this intervention and/or if he had another issue he wished to address. Randy thanked the team, commenting that the bracketing exercise, scheduling specific times to think about the lost partner, sounded very useful.

Outcomes for this new hub service for 2023 indicate that 1,512 clients were seen. In-person sessions accounted for 969 clients (individuals, couples, and families), while 543 clients were seen either online or by phone. In-person data indicates 89% of clients experienced a reduction in distress, while 89% were satisfied with both the intake process and team approach. Online service reports indicate a 90% decrease in distress, 79% satisfaction with the intake process, and 85% satisfaction with the team.

All clients reported feeling heard, understood, and respected (94% in person, 98% online) by their respective teams.

The Wood's Homes classification system for mental health concerns, noted earlier, was launched in 2023, alongside the development of the other hub services that now constitute the hub model for the ECMHS. Anxiety and depression (now referred to as "emotional dysregulation") continue to be among the top ten most pressing issues for clients. The "emotional dysregulation" category of concerns separates suicidal ideation/intent from other emotional content, which is a helpful distinction. This classification system also offers discreet ways of understanding concerns. For example, grief and loss are a category separate from others, as are life stressors, relational difficulties (individual, couple, family), and identified mental health problems. When mental health problems such as depression and anxiety are evident but not confirmed by a diagnosis from a medical professional they are noted as "suspected." System navigation issues are classified as life stressors.

Using the Wood's Homes classification system, the top ten presenting concerns for ECMHS therapy clients in 2023 were as follows:

Evaluation of this new hub service is in its early stages. To date, client and staff feedback is positive in that they like the flexibility with which the services are currently offered. Therapy clients can phone on a day when they have booked an in-person session and change to an online session as needed. By appointment in-person sessions are valued by clients for their predictability. At the same time, the teams have commented that the walk-in days are equally interesting and satisfying, particularly as clients are coming at moments of most pressing need. The capacity to assess and manage risk is enhanced by the new caring contact approach, which has assisted the therapy teams over time. The system navigation service is an added benefit for those clients who need this service.

Table 14.2 Top 10 presenting concerns

Emotional Dysregulation: Anxiety (Suspected)
Identified Mental Health Concern
Life Stressor: Situational Crisis, Traumatic Event
Emotional Dysregulation: Depression (Suspected)
Relational: Couple/Relationship Struggles
Relational: Family Conflict
Grief or Loss: Life Transitions
Life Stressor: Larger Systems Navigation Concerns
Emotional Dysregulation: Suicidal Ideation/Intent
Life Stressor: Physical Health/Illness Concerns

The current therapy teams operate both online and in person as per the hybrid model noted earlier. Walk-in days have all team members in person. The days when clients are only online and/or online and by booked in-person appointments, therapists and consultants do the same; that is, therapists can be in person at the center while a consultant can be online and still participate as a team member. The flexibility offered by this new system has facilitated increased accessibility of psychiatric consultants in particular, as they are able to come online from their hospital or home work space. It also supports therapists and other professional consultants contributing to the team and, at the same time, practice safe health habits, which is a more sensitive issue in our current times of continuing COVID concerns.

In Summary

The new ECMHS and its hub model of service delivery continues to meet community need. At the same time, the work of the therapy team has remained consistent with the themes that underlie single session thinking and practice (Hoyt, Young, & Rycroft, 2021). The mindset and attitude that a single session of therapy may be all that is needed supports therapists in joining with their client to create an alliance for a collaborative therapy session. A one-at-a-time mindset is key to the continued successful delivery of this service. Having both an accessible and timely service to meet client need in whatever format they choose remains central to the work and assists the clients in achieving their goals. Evaluation of this new service is currently a work in progress.

Acknowledgments: My thanks to my team: the ECMHS staff: Dan Neuls, clinical coordinator; therapists Eileah Trotter, Lindsey McCallum, and Fintry Mooken; and consulting psychiatrist Dr. Maureen Pennington for their thoughtful ideas and comments. Thanks also to supervisor Laura Camacho for providing the outcome data. I am most grateful to my good colleagues and friends, Sandy Harper-Jaques and Ann Lawson, for their clarity in their suggestions for adding depth to this paper and to Dr. Bill McElheran for his editing skills.

References

Beere, D., Page, I.S., Diminic, S., & Harris, M. (2018). *Floresco Service Model Evaluation: Final Report 2018.* The University of Queensland, Queensland Centre for Mental Health Research. https://espace.library.uq.edu.au/view/UQ:168e28e
Bloom, B.L. (2001). Focused single-session psychotherapy: A review of the clinical and research literature. *Brief Treatment and Crisis Intervention, 1*(1), 75–86.

Boscolo, L., Cecchin, G., Hoffman, L., & Penn, P. (1987). *Milan Systemic Family Therapy: Conversations in Theory and Practice*. Basic Books.

Bostock, L., & Britt, R. (2014). *Effective Approaches to Hub and Spoke Provision: A Rapid Review of the Literature*. Social Care Research Associates. www.alexiproject.org.uk

Canadian Mental Health Association (CMHA). (2018). *Mental health in balance: Ending the health care disparity in Canada*. https://cmha.ca/wp-content/uploads/2018/09/CMHA-Parity-Paper-Full-Report-EN.pdf.

Clements, R., McElheran, N., Hackney, L., & Park, H., (2011). The Eastside Family Centre: 20 years of single session walk-in therapy. In A. Slive & M. Bobele (Eds.), *When One Hour is All You Have: Effective Therapy for Walk-In Clients* (pp. 109–127). Zeig, Tucker, & Theisen.

Dahlgren, G., & Whitehead, M. (2021). *The Dahlgren-Whitehead Model of Health Determinants: 30 Years On and Still Chasing Rainbows* (pp. 20–24). ScienceDirect.

Duncan, B.L., & Miller, S.D. (2000). *The Heroic Client: Doing Client-Directed Outcome-Oriented Therapy*. Jossey-Bass.

GermAnn, K., MacKean, G., & Butler, B. (2018). *Exploring Mental Health Services and Supports for Children, Youth, and Families in Calgary: A Report to the United Way of Calgary & Area*. United Way Calgary Office. Retrieved August 20, 2020, from https://www.socialimpactlab.com/wp-contect/uploads/2018/10/United-Way-Exploring-Mental-Health-Services-and-Supports.pdf

Hoyt, M.F. (2009). *Brief Psychotherapies: Principles and Practices*. Zeig, Tucker, & Theisen.

Hoyt, M.F., Young, J., & Rycroft, P. (2021). Single session thinking and practice: Going global one step at a time. In M.F. Hoyt, J. Young, & P. Rycroft (Eds.), *Single Session Thinking and Practice in Global, Cultural and Familial Contexts* (pp. 3–26). Routledge.

Jack, S., & Wathen, C. (2021). *Trauma- and Violence-Informed Care: Making Warm Referrals*. McMaster University, School of Nursing. https://phnprep.ca/resources/tvic-warm-referrals/

Links, P.S., Eynan, R., & Shah, R. (2019). Are new standards for assessing and managing suicidal patients needed in Canada? *The Canadian Journal of Psychiatry, 64*, 400–404.

McElheran, N. (2021). The story of the Eastside Family Centre: 30 years of walk-in single session therapy. In M.F. Hoyt, J. Young, & P. Rycroft (Eds.), *Single Session Thinking and Practice in Global, Cultural and Familial Contexts: Expanding Applications* (pp. 125–132). Routledge.

McElheran, N., Harper-Jaques, S., & Lawson, A. (2020). Introduction to the special section: Walk-in and single-session and booked single-session therapy in Canada. *Journal of Systemic Therapies, 39*, 15–20.

Slive, A., & Bobele, M. (Eds.). (2011). *When One Hour Is All You Have: Effective Therapy for Walk-In Clients*. Zeig, Tucker, & Theisen.

Slive, A., MacLaurin, B., Oakander, M., & Amundson, J. (1995). Walk-in single sessions: A new paradigm in clinical service delivery. *Journal of Systemic Therapies, 14*, 3–11.

Slive, A., McElheran, N., & Lawson, A. (2008). How brief does it get? Walk-in single session therapy. *Journal of Systemic Therapies, 27*, 5–22.

Söderquist, M. (2023). *Single Session One at a Time Counselling With Couples*. Routledge.

Stewart, J., McElheran, N., Park, H., Oakander, M., MacLaurin, B., Jing Fang, C., & Robinson, A. (2018). Twenty-five years of walk-in single sessions at the Eastside Family Centre: Clinical and research dimensions. In M.F. Hoyt, M. Bobele, A. Slive, J. Young, & M. Talmon (Eds.), *Single-Session Therapy by Walk-In or Appointment: Administrative, Clinical and Supervisory Aspects of One-At-A-Time Services* (pp. 72–90). Routledge.

Talmon, M. (1990). *Single Session Therapy: Maximizing the Effect of the First (and Often Only) Therapeutic Encounter.* Jossey-Bass.

Valaitis, R., Carter, N., Lam, A., Nicholl, J., Feather, J., & Cleghorn, L. (2018). *Implementation and Maintenance of Patient Navigation Programs Linking Primary Care with Community-Based Health and Social Services: A Scoping Literature Review.* BMC Health Services Research. https://bmchealthservres. biomedcentral.com/track/pdf/10.1186/s12913-017-2046-1

Chapter 15

Invitations, Embedded Hopes, and Creative Collaboration in Sweden

To Follow the Couple's Lead in One-at-a-Time (OAAT) Sessions

Martin Söderquist

Single-session/one-at-a-time (OAAT) thinking and practice challenge therapists and counsellors[1] in many ways. Listening to what the clients hope for and want, being flexible and open for the unexpected, and being concentrated and fully present in the session are some of the challenges. Truly believing in the couples' competencies and giving up the idea of the therapist being the true expert are also very important in single session. What most of all challenges therapists and counsellors seems to be the question of how to be effective with restricted time.

Searching for the best and most effective therapy model has not proved to be the answer. It has instead probably contributed to fights and conflicts among therapists, counsellors, and researchers. Common factor research, on the other hand, has shown the similarities of different therapy models and that these similarities are more important than the models in explaining positive results in therapy (Wampold, 2001; Wampold and Imel, 2015).

Miller and Bertolino (2012) reported that 13–20% of positive results from therapy can be explained by treatment and that 80–87% of the difference between clients in treatment and clients with no treatment can be explained by client and non-therapeutic factors. This implies the need for paying close attention to the couples' own competencies and resources, including their supporting network. It also raises the question for therapists and counsellors: "How can we make our contribution to a therapy/counselling session as effective and useful as possible for the couple?"

One guiding principle follows naturally: *Follow the couple's lead.*

Background

It is necessary that the single session service offered to couples is compatible with the organization and the practices of the teams working with Single Session Therapy (SST), walk-in, and OAAT. There are many different ways to do this (Slive and Bobele, 2011; Cannistrà and Piccirilli, 2021; McElheran, Stewart, Soenen, Newman, & MacLaurin, 2014; Hoyt & Talmon,

DOI: 10.4324/9781032693828-18

2014; Hoyt, Slive, Bobele, Young, & Talmon, 2018; Hoyt, Young, & Talmon, 2021).

As presented in Söderquist (2018, 2023a, 2023b) and Söderquist, Cronholm-Nouicer, Dannerup, and Wulff (2021), the Couple Counselling Team in Malmö, Sweden, has found that offering single session by appointment fits best. Since 2011 the team has offered couples the possibility of choosing OAAT counselling sessions (in person and online). The couples have the option to schedule more OAAT sessions (no guarantee to see the same counsellor next session) or making the choice of what the team calls Traditional Couple Counselling (waiting list, several sessions with the same counsellor over time an option).

We have found that couples have very different reasons for scheduling OAAT, a wide range of presented problems, and a broad palette of hopes for the session. Also important in OAAT is the couple's own choices to decide how to go on with their lives and their way forward. This can be summarized in Figure 15.1.

Different Reasons

Couples have different reasons for scheduling therapy and counselling, and often their reasons have little or nothing to do with therapy. The reasons can be: a brief kick-off to what the couple already are planning, the possibility of getting an appointment quickly due to the short waiting list or needed because of an acute relational crisis, their idea of "one session is

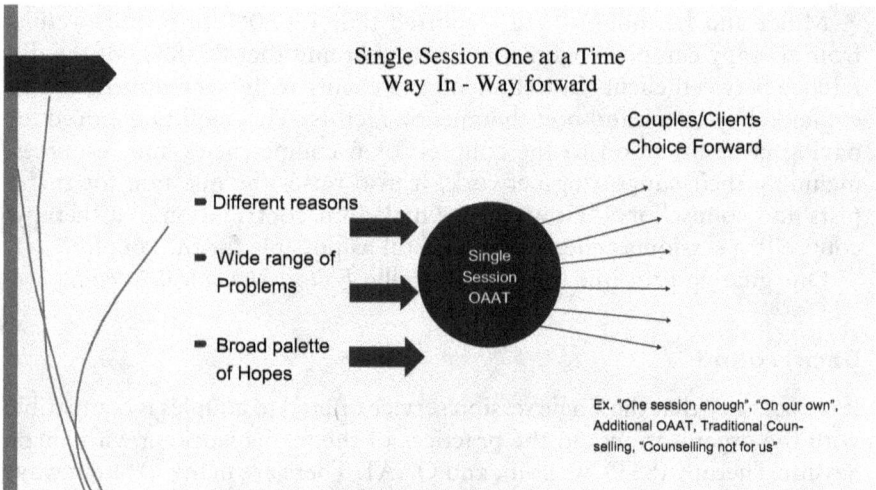

Figure 15.1 Single session one-at-a-time Way In—Way Forward.

enough," wanting to try OAAT (recommended by a relative or friend), or one partner convincing or persuading a reluctant partner to attend one session. The session can go quite wrong if the counsellor assumes the couple wants therapy.

Wide Range of Presented Problems

Couples most often mention "communication problem" (60% of the couples we have interviewed over the years), and this can be anything from minor misunderstandings, "we can't talk to each other," "he/she doesn't understand me at all," "we just quarrel," to heated discussions turning into intimate partner violence. Of course there are many other problems reported by the couples, such as infidelity, separation issues, parenting disagreements, et cetera. Every couple has their own version of what they see as the problem and the difficulties they have.

Broad Palette of Hopes

Most couples attending OAAT counselling want to solve a problem, and preferably in as short a time as possible. They schedule OAAT with hopes of developing their relationship or coming to a decision, and their problem is blocking their way forward. All couples have their own ideas of what they want, what they long for, and what they hope for. These hopes are sometimes forgotten, hidden, or embedded in the problem descriptions.

There are several hundreds of combinations of reasons, problem descriptions, and expressed hopes couples can present. You never know what you will get, and what the counsellor can do is to be open and prepared for anything by having an open mind and a flexible thinking/practice of therapeutic theories and models. Cecchin (1993) suggested that therapists be irreverent to their preferred therapy models and not be in love with their favorite models.

Couples' Own Choice Forward: An important principle in OAAT is that the couples are fully capable of deciding what they want to do after the OAAT session. There are many options for the couple: coming back for another OAAT session later, being on the waiting list for traditional counselling, deciding "one session was enough," continuing their lives on their own without counselling, or deciding that counselling "is not for us."

Follow the Couple's Lead

This means that the couples are in the driver's seat, the counsellor/therapist is a *sensei* leading from behind (Insoo Kim Berg; presentation at Salamanca EBTA conference, 1998; Berg & Dolan, 2001); or the couples are the golf players and the therapists/counsellors are the caddies (Hoyt, 2000) The couples define their problems, their tried solutions, and express their hopes, and the counsellor helps them detail these descriptions with questions, reflections, and comments.

Following the couple's lead doesn't mean accepting and following everything the couple may express. It is the responses from the counsellor to what seems to be most important and useful for the couple and non-responses for other things mentioned by the couple that create the session.

OAAT sessions are one-off experiences, focused on here and now and nearest future, focused on solvable problems and reachable hopes and goals. It is not intended to be the first session of several to be continued. Said in other words: *OAAT is keeping it simple to make the most of the session.*

This takes a lot to manage, and there are many challenges for couple therapists and counsellors, such as being dragged into long and/or endless problem descriptions and problem talk or being forced by one or both partners to take sides in their conflict. To counter these challenges and increase the possibility to make the OAAT session effective, ideas of invitations and responses, embedded hopes, and creative collaboration seem to be helpful for therapists, counsellors, and couples.

Beginning—Invitation and Responses

All therapy and counselling sessions—whatever model the therapist/counsellor prefers—begin with some kind of context marking. The client(s) and the therapist/counsellor collaboratively need to figure out important questions like: Who am I? Who are you? What do we do here? and What is the meaning of this meeting/session? Included in the context marking is also the necessity of informing the clients about confidentiality, obligation to report to Child Protection, duration and costs of the session, if a team of colleagues are present, etc. depending on the context of the session.

All social interaction can be described as taking turns by questions and answers, initiatives and responses (Aarts, 1995), or invitations and responses. These invitations and responses are both verbal and nonverbal (eye contact, tone of voice, turning away or towards, and other ways of showing interest or non-interest). Every invitation from one partner gets a response from the other partner that simultaneously is an invitation. By taking turns the couple and the counsellor co-construct and develop a dialogue and a relationship. In this way the counselling/therapy session is co-constructed by the couple and the counsellor.

In OAAT with couples, the counsellors' important and crucial part of the context marking is the invitation to the session today emphasizing what is important to the couple and what they hope for. The counsellor welcomes/

invites the couple to OAAT, and the couple invites the counsellor to their world by telling their reasons for scheduling the session, describing their problems, and expressing their hopes for the session today.

The start of the OAAT session is crucial to avoid misunderstandings and find a common project for the OAAT session. The first utterance/invitation from the couple can be crucial, like the husband saying: "My wife said to me I need to change in some ways in my behavior—she can't stand me at the moment." The counsellor can respond in many ways, of course, but very quickly needs to figure out and invite what might be most important for the couple to focus on in the session. Is it asking questions to the husband about what the wife needs to see him do after the session or next week? Is it asking the wife to clarify what she said to her husband? Or is it more effective to introduce the idea that these changes will be made in the session and asking the couple to describe how their children will notice the parents' different behaviors? This last example is what Karl Tomm and his Danish colleagues (Hornstrup, Tomm, & Johansen, 2009—in Danish; Söderquist, 2023a, pp. 31–34) call *perspective and possibility questions*.

There are always many alternative ways for the counsellor to respond and invite the couple.

Sometimes the couples introduce more or less impossible (no chance for agreement) topics, like one of the partners has decided to separate and the other partner doesn't understand or can't accept this, or a situation where one partner wants a child and the other doesn't.

How the counsellor responds to these utterances and at the same time invites the couple is crucial for the rest of the session. What seems to be most important or possible for the partners—to come to a mutual understanding, to decide they can't live together, or take a break from their discussions for a while?

All OAAT sessions are unique and there are some guidelines for counsellors to follow to make the process of invitations and responses as useful and beneficial as possible for the couples.

- Keep focus on the present/the session today and the nearest future. This is complicated enough, and one session can't solve all problems and focus on all difficulties. It is possible, though, to help the couples find out what to do and how to go on with their lives in one session or at least find a starting point. Sometimes this requires that the counsellor is benevolently stubborn to help the couple remain focused. Possibility and initiative questions are especially useful to achieve this (Hornstrup et al., 2009—in Danish; Söderquist, 2023a, pp. 31–34).
- Genuinely listen to what the couple expresses as most important to them. When couples are desperate, they present a lot of problems and difficulties and the counsellor can't respond to it all. Some of the things the couples say can be "red herrings" (distractions and dead-end streets

where the energies and ideas in the session are lost) and must simply be ignored or not even heard by the counsellor—use selective listening. Other topics or themes the counsellor responds to and at the same time invites the couple to talk about in more detail. In the end the clients' invitations and responses are more important than the counsellor's ideas and therapeutic models.

- Balance information overload and realistic hopes and goals. Not everything can be talked about or solved in an hour, and the counsellor doesn't need all information about the couple.

Embedded Hopes

In many or most therapy models HOPE is emphasized as an important goal and what the sessions aim to achieve for the clients. When the clients leave the therapy or a session with increased hope of being able to go on with their lives the therapy or counselling has been successful.

It is important to distinguish between realistic hope and hope in vain. The goal for an OAAT session must be realistic and achievable—not too big or impossible for the couple to reach. It can't be built on totally unreachable wishful thinking. Dreams are important and crucial and can be what the couple needs to handle family problems but can also stop couples from acting in the present and just waiting for the dream to come true without doing anything.

Couples schedule OAAT, counselling, or therapy for different reasons and present a wide range of problems, and this can be seen as the entrance ticket to OAAT, therapy, or counselling. They also schedule the sessions because they want and aim for something, not always directly expressed; for example, to make a decision, to come to an agreement, or to find a new way to behave together. This is probably more important than focusing on problems and difficulties in the sessions. Some couples are very clear and direct in telling what they want and hope for, but many other couples are more vague and indirect. Their hopes are forgotten, hidden, or not talked about. The story of a couple that were vague in their descriptions of why they were in OAAT and what they wanted is an example of this. What they hoped for wasn't clear to the counsellor and it wasn't until an NLP (Neurolinguistic Programming) exercise was introduced (Bandler, Grinder, & Satir, 1976) that they could turn towards each other and with great smiles on their faces simultaneously say, "Separation!" The counsellor's immediate response was "Are we done?" and the couple said "Yes—we are!" The session ended by discussing their plans for the future.

Hopes are embedded in problem descriptions, and in all problems and difficulties there are possibilities. This is the philosophy of Erickson's utilization principle—use what the client brings you. Problem descriptions can be used in brief therapy to design solutions and to be a leverage to the future for the clients (Zeig, 1980; Zeig & Gilligan, 1990; Haley, 1973; Hoyt & Cannistrà, 2023).

In OAAT it is necessary to collaboratively find the embedded hope fairly quickly. A direct way is to ask what the couple hopes for in the session so that the focus is there from the start. Questions like these can be very helpful:

- "When you leave the session today, what do you hope for us to have achieved?"
- "When you come home and see your children, what will they notice is positively different with their parents?"
- "What are your best hopes for the session today?"

There are couples that are more direct and act before the counsellor has said anything. They start the session by saying, "We want you to solve our problem!" What they hope for is clear, but the expectation is probably unrealistic. The counsellor can humorously respond by saying: "Give me a day or two (or a session or two)," "What do we start with?" or by being more future-oriented and not going into the details of the problems: "When your problems are solved—what will be the main advantages for you?" or "After the Miracle has happened, when you were asleep, and your problems are gone or solved, what do you notice and experience as different when you wake up?" (de Shazer, 1991; de Shazer, Dolan, Korman, Trepper, McCollum, & Berg, 2007).

Some couples challenge the OAAT counsellor by saying: "We want to tell our story!" or "We need to tell you about our problems" (this can take some time, the counsellor thinks). There are several options for the counsellor to respond to this and simultaneously invite the couples to describe their hopes and come to an agreement of a common project for the OAAT session:

- "When you have told your story—we have about an hour and a half, and I want to have some time close to the end of the session to share my reflections with you—what are your best hopes for the session?"
- "What do you want me to pay most attention to when you tell your story so I can give you some feedback that can be useful to you?"
- "We have this session today, and I think you need to concentrate your story to what is most important to you at the moment."

Of course, there are many more options for responses, questions, and invitations the counsellor can present to respond to the couple and simultaneously ask for their hopes.

Focusing on what the couple wants and hopes for is effective and useful for the couple. It points forward and gives a direction for the couple's future work on their own. They can't change what has been, but they can influence, modify, or change their relationship in the coming weeks or months. Sessions in which describing hopes and goals are important parts are often more filled with humour and joy. Talking about hopes, plans, and possibilities opens up clients for new possibilities.

Creative Collaboration

Is creativity inherited, or is creativity developed in interactions with others? This is a question that can be discussed forever. Steve Harvey (1990) suggests that all people have the ability to be creative, and the context/circumstances and the people they interact with help them express and develop this.

In the context of therapy or counselling sessions, creative collaboration or collaborative creativity can be a main road to help the clients to see their problems differently, to go "outside the box" and to find a new perspective, which often is a common goal for therapy and counselling. "The moments of creativity are collaboratively created in social interaction" (Söderquist, 2023a, p. 79), and these moments, even small, can be of utmost importance and sometimes a pivotal moment (Rosenbaum, Hoyt, & Talmon, 1990). In therapy and counselling pivotal moments can be described as: "A precise point in time when something appears obvious, suddenly changed and absolutely crucial" (Söderquist, 2023a, p. 17). Moments like these are not possible to plan in advance or deliberately produce but can be detected and noticed by counsellors and couples afterwards.

What Is Creative Collaboration?

There is a flow in the session when couple and counsellor take turns, invite each other, and respond to meaningful themes/focus to the couple. This flow can be experienced as an "attuned relationship" (Harvey, 1990) or described as a working alliance (Wampold, 2001; Wampold & Imel, 2015). When this process of taking turns also involves "expressive momentum"[2] (Harvey, 1990)—couple and counsellor ideas building and feeding on each other over time and creating new perspectives—the session develops further and the possibilities for new ideas are at hand. Creative collaboration can be described as playful seriousness or serious playfulness. Couple and counsellor talk about serious matters and problems but do it in playful and slightly distanced ways.

Why Is Creative Collaboration Important?

It opens up, creates alternatives/wider pictures, helps the couple see the light at the end of the tunnel, and gives the couple new experiences. The concentration and focus in OAAT of today/nearest future and what the couple is doing and planning to do requires an active and direct collaboration. This can create space for the couple and give them ideas of tools (often asked for by couples) to move forward in their relationship.

How Can Creative Collaboration Be Reached?

When the counsellor uses his/her ability to do the unexpected and improvise and uses humor (Hoyt & Andreas, 2015; Cade, 2014; Schulem, 1988) together with the couple, the chance for a constructive, collaborative, helpful, and effective session is great. The counsellor needs to be open minded and able to improvise and be playful in a respectful way and at the same time be serious. Jim Wilson (2018) has elegantly described the importance of creativity and improvising in helping families. He strongly emphasizes an open mind and a flexible and playful stance of the therapist/counsellor in therapeutic sessions.

This inviting of the couple can be achieved by introducing, for example, helicopter views, metaphors, dreams, and future discussions.

- The counsellor invites the couple to a future question, playing with time and a chance to get a new perspective to their problem by saying— "I don't have a magic stick, but let us suppose I have one and I touch you with that stick. What you want for your relationship is coming true next week—how will you notice the difference in your relationship, and how will important persons in your life notice this?" Another idea is suggesting the helicopter view: "Let us say we are sitting in a helicopter and looking at your relationship from above when you have solved your problem—what do we see?"
- Very often couples have tried to solve their problems in different ways but haven't succeeded or have ideas of how to do that but haven't gotten started yet. One of the partners may mention something like, "I need a pause button when we are in a heated discussion—I need to think," and the counsellor can give the couple the idea of creating a symbol of this pause button to use next time they are in a discussion like that (Söderquist, 2023a, Ch. 18). Another example is the couple who always start a discussion and very quickly end up in a fight. After discussions in the session (the couple really wanted to do something different) of what could be a concrete symbol and a way of halting the fight and breaking their pattern of violent behaviour, the counsellor suggests the idea that a STOP sign could be used. The couple laughed and told the counsellor, "We need to find another kind of symbol—we are police officers." Building upon ideas and suggestions from the couples is probably most effective (follow their lead)—it is their ideas and probably what they are intending to do something about. The couple's own metaphors are important to follow—the counsellor can add something (in the session

or as a suggestion the couple can do at home) that affirms the couple and simultaneously helps the couple get further in solving their problem and reaching their goals.

- Doing something unexpected and improvising respectfully is often surprising, evoking astonishment and maybe laughter. This can lead to a very positive and helpful session for the couple. The counsellor can invite the couple by saying, "You know what you need to know about me to be able to trust me and the chance to get help here. Feel free to ask me what you want!" or "I suppose you have a lot of experiences and a lot of questions about relationships. I suggest you interview me about this. Is that OK for you?" Probably these invitations from the counsellor aren't expected by the couple and they might respond positively. As always, the clients'/couple's responses are more important than the invitation from the counsellor. If they hesitate or say no the counsellor can leave the suggestion or apologize and listen to what the couple suggest instead.

Endings and Summary

In OAAT, beginnings and endings are especially important to make a complete whole with distinct starting and ending points. The context marking, invitations to the session today, and focusing the couple's hopes are important when beginning the session. Both directly and indirectly this also includes invitations to make the best of the session and aiming for ideas and plans the couple can bring home to continue their work on their own. It is optimal when the couple during the session or in the end of the session have created ideas and plans to do this. Many couples ask for ideas and suggestions from the counsellor and, of course, the counsellor can give them this during the session or at the end of the session as a reflection and summary. This ending and summary can be done in many ways:

- The couple and therapist summarize the session collaboratively.
- Counsellor takes some minutes on his/her own (individual reflection time) and ends the session with her/his reflections and suggestions to the couple.
- Writing a letter to the couple with these reflections and sending the letter after the session.
- If the counsellor has a team, the whole team can share their reflections and ideas with the couple.

There are couples asking for more sessions, and they can, of course, return for another OAAT session or be put on the waiting list for traditional counselling. If the couple raises this question, they have these options, but immediately scheduling a new session can dilute the effect of the collaborative work being done in the OAAT session. It is probably a better idea to tell the couple: "Of course you can, but I suggest you think this session today through and maybe try some of the things we have talked about and/or do something I have suggested. My idea is that you start with this for a few weeks and after that you decide how to go on. My door is always open."

Paying close attention to follow the couple's lead, inviting the couples to describe their hopes and inviting them to creative collaboration by using humor and improvisation seem to be effective and helpful for couples. For counsellors and couples this thinking and practice is a vaccination to avoid burnout and feelings of hopelessness. Most important is the possibility for everyone to enjoy the counselling sessions.

Notes

1 *Therapist/counsellor* and *therapy/counselling* are used in the text when ideas are presented in general terms. *OAAT* refers specifically to single session/one-at-a-time counselling with couples.
2 Harvey uses these terms when describing parent-child relationships when playing in dynamic play therapy. Even though parent-child and couple-counsellor relationships aren't the same, I use his terms in describing the couple-counsellor relationship in serious and playful sessions.

References

Aarts, M. (1995). *Marte Meo Guide*. M.H Aarts.
Bandler, R., Grinder, J., & Satir, V. (1976). *Changing With Families: A Book About Further Education for Being Human*. Science and Behavior Books.
Berg, I.K., & Dolan, Y. (2001). *Tales of Solutions: A Collection of Hope-Inspiring Stories*. Norton.
Cade, B. (2014). An interactional look at humour in therapy. *Australian Association of Family Therapy, 36*(3).
Cannistrà, F., & Piccirilli, F. (2021). *Single-Session Therapy: Principles and Practice*. Giunti. (Published 2018 in Italian.)
Cecchin, G. (1993). *Irreverence: A Strategy for Therapists' Survival*. Karnac.
de Shazer, S. (1991). *Putting Difference to Work*. Norton.
de Shazer, S., Dolan, Y., Korman, H., Trepper, T., McCollum, E., & Berg, I.K. (2007). *More Than Miracles: The State of the Art of Solution-Focused Brief Therapy*. Haworth Press.
Haley, J. (1973). *Uncommon Therapy: The Psychiatric Techniques of Milton H. Erickson, M.D.* Norton.
Harvey, S. (1990). Dynamic play therapy: An integrative expressive arts approach to family therapy of young children. *The Arts in Psychotherapy, 17*(3), 239–246.
Hornstrup, C., Tomm, K., & Johansen, T. (2009). Sporgsmal—der gor en forskel (Questions that make a difference). *I: Erhvervspsykologi Business Psychology, 7*(3), 2–16. (in Danish)
Hoyt, M.F. (2000). A golfer's guide to brief therapy (with footnotes for baseball fans). In M.F. Hoyt, *Some Stories Are Better Than Others* (pp. 5–15). Brunner/Mazel.

Hoyt, M.F., & Andreas, S. (2015). Humor in brief therapy: A dialogue (Part I). *Journal of Systemic Therapies, 34*(3), 13–24.

Hoyt, M.F., & Cannistrà, F. (2023). *Brief Therapy Conversations: Exploring Efficient Intervention in Psychotherapy*. Routledge.

Hoyt, M.F., Slive, A., Bobele, M., Young, J., & Talmon, M. (Eds.). (2018). *Single Session Therapy by Walk-In or Appointment: Administrative, Clinical, and Supervisory Aspects of One-at-a-Time Services*. Routledge.

Hoyt, M.F., & Talmon, M. (Eds.). (2014). *Capturing the Moment: Single-Session Therapy and Walk-In Services*. Crown House Publishing.

Hoyt, M.F., Young, J., & Rycroft, P. (Eds.). (2021). *Single Session Thinking and Practice in Global, Cultural and Familial Contexts: Expanding Applications*. Routledge.

McElheran, N., Stewart, J., Soenen, D., Newman, J., & MacLaurin, B. (2014). Walk-in single-session therapy at the Eastside Family Centre. In M.F. Hoyt & M. Talmon (Eds.), *Capturing the Moment: Single-Session Therapy and Walk-In Services* (pp. 177–194). Crown House Publishing.

Miller, S.D., & Bertolino, B. (2012). *The ICCE Manuals on Feedback-Informed Treatment (FIT)*. International Centre for Clinical Excellence.

Rosenbaum, R., Hoyt, M.F., & Talmon, M. (1990). The challenge of single-session therapies: Creating pivotal moments. In R.A. Wells & V.J. Gianetti (Eds.), *Handbook of the Brief Psychotherapies* (pp. 165–189). Plenum Press. (Reprinted in Hoyt, M.F. (1995). *Brief Therapy and Managed Care* (pp. 105–140). Jossey-Bass.

Schulem, B. (1988). The introduction of humor in supervision and therapy—Work is depressing enough without being too serious. *Journal of Strategic and Systemic Therapies, 7*(2).

Slive, A., & Bobele, M. (2011). *When One Hour is All You Have: Effective Therapy for Walk-In Clients*. Zeig, Tucker, & Theisen.

Söderquist, M. (2018). Coincidence favors the prepared mind: Single Sessions with couples in Sweden. In M.F. Hoyt, A. Slive, M. Bobele, J. Young, & M. Talmon (Eds.), *Single Session Therapy by Walk-In or Appointment: Administrative, Clinical, and Supervisory Aspects of One-at-a-Time Services* (pp. 270–290). Routledge.

Söderquist, M. (2023a). *Single Session One at a Time Counselling with Couples: Challenge and Possibility*. Routledge.

Söderquist, M. (2023b). *Single Session One at a Time. Kertaterapeuttinen työskentely parien kanssa*. Lyhytterapiainstituutti. (in Finnish)

Söderquist, M., Cronholm-Nouicer, M., Dannerup, L., & Wulff, K. (2021). Making the leap with couples in Sweden: One-at-a-time mindset in action. In M.F. Hoyt, J. Young, & P. Rycroft (Eds.), *Single Session Thinking and Practice in Global, Cultural and Familial Contexts: Expanding Applications* (pp. 163–172). Routledge.

Wampold, B.E. (2001). *The Great Psychotherapy Debate: Models, Methods, and Findings*. Lawrence Erlbaum Associates.

Wampold, B.E., & Imel, Z.E. (2015). *The Great Psychotherapy Debate: The Research Evidence for What Works in Psychotherapy* (2nd ed.). Routledge.

Wilson, J. (2018). *Creativity in Times of Constraint: A Practitioner's Companion in Mental Health and Social Care*. Routledge.

Zeig, J.K. (Ed.). (1980). *A Teaching Seminar with Milton H. Erikson, M.D.* Brunner/Mazel.

Zeig, J.K., & Gilligan, S.G. (Eds.). (1990). *Brief Therapy: Myths, Methods and Metaphors*. Brunner/Mazel.

Chapter 16

Normal Magic
Whole System Mindset in Devon, UK

Sarah Lewis

Normal Magic is a child and young person's mental health service in Devon, UK, with a collective ambition to change the way routine mental health care is provided and accessed. Our ambition is quickly coming to life.

We are a team of registered mental health professionals and practitioners with an abundance of training in traditional mental health care. We also understand and appreciate the core principles of Single Session Therapy (SST) as described by many brilliant and influential experts.[1] We ourselves are highly experienced as single session therapists, trainers, and supervisors.

I could use this space to highlight and detail the research and evidence within the SST literature. However, the mandate for this chapter is to describe our lived experience driving system change in Devon, a county in southwest England about 180 miles from London. Please be assured, the well-documented works of many leaders inform, inspire, and underpin our single session delivery model and training programs.

I presented the progress of Normal Magic at the 4th International Single Session Symposium in Rome in November 2023. That event was a three-day feast of inspiration and fuel for my personal and professional soul. When Flavio Cannistrà and Michael Hoyt asked me to write a chapter for this book, with a focus on the whole system mindset journey of Normal Magic, I was more than delighted. Here is our story so far.

Normal Magic Motivation

Our collective history working within Child and Young Person Mental Health Services brought us true insight into the challenges for children and young people accessing mental health care. NHS (National Health Service) services are often commissioned and designed with high thresholds, long referral processes, and a menu of care that does not always fit the needs

DOI: 10.4324/9781032693828-19

of those seeking help. Alongside this, there are often demand and capacity issues affecting the way help-seeking families receive timely support.

Influenced by our collective professional experiences of service design and delivery, our personal stories, and stories from people we care about, we knew something had to change with the way mental health care was provided. Our motivation was ignited.

We examined the current routine health care system in the UK. We posed ourselves two key questions:

- How can we improve access to routine child and young person mental health care, at point of need?
- Could we provide and access effective, efficient mental health care in the same way we provide and access physical health care in the UK?

Brief summary of that examination: To access NHS health care in the UK, residents register with a general practitioner (GP) at the local health center, thereafter accessing their GP through an appointment system for any health problem. Physical health problems are usually attended to with a focus on the ailment, which can often be satisfied with single appointment treatment, self-care advice, intervention, monitoring, or, when needed, onward referral to specialist health services. Once established with a GP, the person can return on an as-needed basis.

By contrast, the issues we found in accessing routine mental health care were extensive and worrisome. Local GPs let us know they routinely do have time-limited appointments (usually only 10–20 minutes long), but they are rarely specialists in child and young people mental health, and often their only option is to advise that patients be referred to child and young people mental health services or voluntary sector counseling services.

We consider this is a strangely accepted inequality to accessing routine mental health care at "point of availability" (rather than at a "point of need"—see Dryden, 2019). We decided to do something about it. Our aim is to bring parity to accessing, *at point of need*, both mental and physical health care.

The Start of Something New in Devon

Normal Magic has now worked for over a year with West Devon Primary Care Network (WDPCN), a collaboration of three GP health centers to provide 0–19-year-olds mental health care, with a difference.

When Dr. Sarah Payne from WDPCN and Normal Magic explored the possibilities of a partnership, there was an infectious energy to pilot a new method of providing child and young people mental health care. The GPs' lived intelligence of demand from their patients, their experience of barriers to accessing mental health care, alongside unanimous creative and open minds, allowed a fresh approach to be considered. Together, we designed a model of care that replicated patients' typical access to routine physical health care.

Our collaboration resulted in Normal Magic providing child and young people mental health care directly in the health centers. No referral or intake, no threshold, and no closing discharges. This means that children and young people, their parent or carer, are able to book an appointment with a registered mental health clinician in the same way they would book an appointment with their local GP. No matter how big or small the mental health concern, no matter how clear or complex the situation might be. Services are covered by the Primary Care Network (PCN) fund and are free to families. We do not tend emergencies; the NHS emergency care services attend emergencies or any hospital admission needs. Our service is for routine mental health care. However, we do at times facilitate emergency access should someone disclose suicidal activity in our sessions.

A year on and we have sustained capacity and demand. Help seekers are seen quickly and efficiently; approximately 60% are seen for a single session. Feedback from families and the GPs across WDPCN has been consistently positive and energizing. These are some typical comments from young people and parents via post-session surveys:

- "We have a clear way forward for _____ and our family and some good tips to try. We also feel confident that if needed, we could get back in touch with Normal Magic."
- "It was great from the moment we walked into the room—a great supportive environment."
- "I felt heard, understood and believed and given positive strategies to work on and build strengths."
- "I left feeling good, and know that I can contact again if I need to."
- "It's a very good system!"

Normal Magic is now commissioned to deliver child and young person mental health care, with a focus on SST, in GP health centers within Mewstone, Beacon, and Nexus PCNs. No threshold, no referral, no discharges, and closed care. This model of care is funded by PCN's Additional Roles Reimbursement Scheme, which is part of our governmental tax-supported healthcare system. This funding allows NHS health centers flexibility to recruit additional specialist roles.

Overcoming Clinical Delivery Barriers: Clinician and System Mindset

Single Session Therapy is a key aspect of our ability to provide accessible and effective care, at point of need. Delivering SST is not as easy as it sounds, yet it really is not complicated either, revolving around the mindset of the clinician, the mindset of the family, and the mindset of the system that commissions our work.

Our growing clinical team comes with a rich background of lived experiences within traditional child and young person mental health services. The WDPCN team—which by November 2023 comprised three mental health nurses and two support staff (averaging three whole time–equivalent posts—have valued specialist training and unique experiences delivering a variety of roles in complex health and education care systems. Normal Magic is more than just our name. It is a detailed, finely tuned, therapeutic engagement model designed to nurture an open growth mindset in both the clinician and the system as well as the family.

Myths and Fears

SST can hold many myths and fears, although the literature around SST is quite clear. SST does not mean help seekers can only have one session. It is also not just an initiative to attend a lengthy waiting list: its intention is efficient, high-quality care.

Consider the physical health care equivalent. We do not expect only one opportunity to access physical health care. Most physical health care appointments are delivered in a single session manner. Whether that is health care seeking for a physical ailment, for dentistry, for ophthalmology, we are often familiar with health care providers focusing on the area of concern. So why would we not create the same approach for mental health care?

Transferring Single Session Thinking Across Help-Seeking Services

We began to think about other help-giving services in Devon and became curious. Was single session thinking a transferrable model to help-giving services who were not registered mental health professionals? We began to appreciate a difference between SST and single session thinking. According to Hoyt, Young, and Rycroft (2021, p. 3):

> The essence of Single Session Thinking is to approach the first session as if it will be the only session, while creating opportunities for further work if it is requested by the client. What emerges is a collaborative,

direct, and transparent approach to providing services that puts the clint in a very active role in determining the focus and length of the work.

As Talmon (1993, p. 73) put it: "These concepts represent an alternative to the traditional model in psychiatry and psychotherapy: psychohealth replacing psychopathology, solutions replacing problems, and partnership replacing patronization, domination, and hierarchy."

We use Single Session Therapy as a descriptor of care from registered mental health professionals whose expertise is required to consider in one meeting specific mental health concerns and recovery interventions. We use single session thinking as a descriptor of care from services designed to respond to help-seeking families relating to a variety of developmental or functional concerns.

Action for Children: Devon's Children Centres

A year ago, we were fortunate to meet the senior leadership team[2] for Action for Children in Devon. Their service provides a range of child development care and parent support within local Children Centres. Their energy to improve their delivery model, encourage parents and carers in the community to ask for help, reduce barriers, and improve community engagement culminated in a scrutiny of their system mindset. This led to an opening of minds, refreshingly creative discussions, and single session thinking solutions.

We embarked on a journey of system change with them. We provided a comprehensive training package including senior leadership, consultation, all staff training, live practice in Children Centres, and ongoing single session supervision for all staff and feedback evaluation. The collaboration with Devon's Action for Children has become more than a positive partnership. It became a strategic alliance toward whole-system change, improving access at point of need. For Devon's Action for Children, single session thinking has become a focused, proportionate response to help seeking, alongside their existing menu of ongoing interventions and care. Some of the challenges with the whole-system mindset lay with concerns from staff that one session would not be enough, that safeguarding practice would be compromised, and that without the whole family assessment (which took over four weeks to complete) staff would be unable to safely advise the family regarding a solution to their problem. Trusting the families to lead their own next steps had been affected by anxiety and fear of missing something. Yet since the data showed a significant number of families dropping out of assessment processes or lingering on lengthy waiting lists, we questioned the safeguarding sense of this. Prior to the training, we spent a whole day with the county leadership team, asking, "Why are we doing it this way?" and "Are processes and referral routes inviting families in or keeping them out?" A critical turning point came when we reviewed the amount of service hours going into processing referrals. Together we reviewed a system-led process that created hours of work prior to the family being seen. We wondered about streamlining those processes and using the newfound hours to deliver single session thinking sessions.

The result of implementing single session thinking within Devon's Action for Children has been transformative, described by the leadership team as "game changing." Staff morale has improved. Access times have reduced from an average of six months to an average of three weeks. Family feedback is crucial, ensuring help giving is continually designed around community need and experience of service.

These are some of the comments parents and carers have fed back through post-session surveys:

- "You can go with any concerns and they have the best person centered approach with resources to help with lots of situations."
- "I felt empowered, encouraged and that help and support was available for area's [sic] that perhaps I wasn't overly confident with."
- "Empowered to make own decisions and choices in a non-judgmental way."
- "I felt alone with this problem before not really sure what I was doing or how to help my baby and whether or not I'm doing enough. I feel reassured that I am doing the best I can and that there is further support I can get if needed."
- "I feel receiving support as a parent isn't widely available, these sessions could really benefit parents."

Our collaboration with WDPCN and Action for Children in Devon has fueled our ambition. We are passionate advocates for whole-system mindset change. Training, in our opinion, is not enough. As we learned, implementation of the whole-system mindset is an essential ingredient to SST and single session thinking being an effective and efficient model. We are energized as we expand our comprehensive implementation and training package to other mental health specialists and community help-giving services. To date we have embarked on delivering the Normal Magic single session therapy/thinking whole-system mindset model to mental health professionals, public health nurses, an academy of providers of alternative education to students unable to access mainstream education due to medical conditions, the local education authority well-being service, and schools across West Devon.

Case Examples

The following three case examples only happened because we were seeking a new approach to child and young person mental health care. Gone were thresholds and referrals, open and closed care, replaced by a SST service where help seekers lead the way, at point of need, and are responded to and empowered.

Case 1

"Jack" (a pseudonym) was a 10-year-old boy who came into the GP health center with his mum. They had booked directly through the reception team and were seen within two weeks. No threshold and no referral or intake process.

Jack had his hood up, zipped around his face, and stated he did not want to look at me, although he did agree that he wanted to be at the appointment. I could see instantly that Jack had a restless energy and was unlikely to settle into the appointment on the traditional four-legged chair. I offered him my swivel desk chair and suggested he could use this to turn away from me or toward me, whatever he felt comfortable doing. He accepted and proceeded to swivel side to side in the chair facing away from me. I asked, "What are your hopes for meeting today?" and let them know I was all theirs for the next 60 minutes, but they could leave before then if they chose to.

Jack stated he was happy with his mum sharing their story. Mum shared that Jack was diagnosed with autism and ADHD and was having outbursts after school and into the evening. She hoped for some understanding about why this was happening and what she could do to manage the outbursts. Jack listened.

Jack was also described as a loving, happy boy who had lots of occupation that settled him through the weekends and school holidays. As Mum talked, I heard about their strong, caring relationship alongside the stress and distress after school. I asked Jack throughout if he agreed with what his mum was describing or whether he wanted to add anything. Jack shook his head no each time.

After about 15 minutes, Mum remarked that Jack was sitting still in the chair and that this was unusual. Jack said that he felt his body calm and that was why he sat still.

As Mum talked about the things Jack loved doing, I thought his activities were likely influenced by his sensory processing needs, as well as his loves and passions. I asked Mum what she noticed about this. Mum stated she did not have an awareness of sensory processing needs. I asked Mum if it would be helpful for me to share some of this knowledge and see if that was relatable to the situation in any way. She expressed interest, so I gave a brief description of sensory processing, explaining it in a way that both mother and son could understand.

By the mid-point in our appointment, Mum began sharing her own observations of Jack's sensory regulation behaviors and sensory overwhelm situations, checking with me to confirm if that was what she was observing. At times Jack added different things. Importantly for this session, he stated that the swivel chair was having an influence on his body feeling calm. We established that Jack had a variety of sensory overwhelm situations at school and they likely built up throughout the day, leading to an eruption of accumulated stress and energy after school.

I usually have paper and pens and draw in my sessions to help me create a visual of the discussion. In this case, I drew an arc to represent how we gain stressors from our daily story and how we soothe using our unique transferable Methods. Mum "got" this immediately and began to involve Jack in reflecting with her what he naturally did to self soothe; although these self-soothing methods had been seen as disruptive and boisterous.

Mum's penny drop moments[3] were seeming to happen with speed.

This led to them generating their "What next?"—their plan to start noticing Jack's Methods, for Jack to communicate his Methods when he noticed them, and together create a project that focused on mapping the Method and not simply the Story.

They asked to come back for a follow-up, which we agreed together would be in four weeks. Mum stated this would give them time to properly notice. In addition, Jack had stated that he expected I would be like everyone else and not want him back. I assured him I was always at the health center and he was welcome back whenever he wanted and needed.

Follow-Up and Comment

Four weeks later, Jack returned with his mum. He had his hood down and was carrying a large bag. He grinned and promptly sat on the floor, revealing a range of objects and a laminated sheet with various pictures on it. Mum was smiling and relaxed. Jack proceeded to inform me about their noticing and what they had learned and, more importantly, what they had changed in their life together.

Jack showed me a range of objects from the bag and in picture form that responded to senses such as proprioception, touch, and sight. Mum stated that they now had implemented a transition phase before and after school designed around sensory regulation. This was leading them to understand the story that led to sensory overwhelm, and this had also informed a plan of care at school to regulate during transitions and following demanding lessons and environment. Outbursts at home after school were no longer causing unmanageable stress and distress to Jack or Mum. Mum shared that she had also bought a swivel chair for Jack's bedroom and one was also now used at school.

There was an extraordinary amount of positive family-led changes that had taken place. Changes that were supporting understanding, communication, and acceptance. Impacts were described as important turning points in both home and school life.

Before they left, Jack asked, "if something else goes wrong, can I come back?" I said most definitely, Yes. He grinned as he held eye contact with me.

Case 2

"Layla" was 16 and attended the appointment at the GP health center alone within one week of booking the appointment. When asked what she hoped for from this session, she said she wanted help to understand her spiraling mood state and to explore ways she could stabilize her mood and feel happier again.

Layla explained that she was feeling depressed and anxious and had been feeling increasingly worse over the past six months. She revealed a year-long, "on-off" relationship with her 16-year-old boyfriend. She described a relationship where her love for the boyfriend dominated her behaviors in the relationship, regardless of how he treated her. The boyfriend was described as someone who behaved in an inconsistent manner toward her. This ranged from being loving and attentive alongside being critical and dismissive. It was Layla's first experience of loving someone.

We explored the context of "stacking"[4] to identify if there were other contributors to her feelings of depression and anxiety. Layla described a stable family life, an ability and love of learning and socializing, and no significant experience that might add a relevant layer of unhappiness to her thoughts, feelings, or behaviors.

My asking Layla for permission to share and explore together perspectives of mentally healthy loving took us further into session content. We explored love. We considered how hearts can often hold intense feelings for another, without conscious choice. Our hearts, we established, can overpower the mind, sometimes leaving us in a state of confusion between feeling and thought impacting behavior and mood. The aim of this content was to help Layla begin to identify the difference between her thoughts, feelings, and behavior. The aim was also to normalize the human instinct to love and the complexities of this. What she was feeling could be considered normal in the context of her story.[5]

To understand love, the heart, and mind, we explored the theories of healthy love, limerance, and obsessive love. I embedded a checking process throughout the session, giving space to check if each element of exploration was helpful, asking specifically why this was being received as helpful or not helpful.

The next step was to help Layla identify if her spiraling mood was connected with her experience of the described cycle of attention, criticism, and rejection. At this point in our session Layla was tearful as she spoke of realizing that her anxiety and depressed feelings were heavily influenced by this cycle.

It felt important to step back from the Story and consider what was important to Layla in terms of everyday relationships. This not only allowed me to appreciate Methods in her everyday relationships but aimed to help Layla begin to recognize her normal social standards. She spoke of a consistent group of friends and their characteristics that she felt sustained her relationships with them.

As mentioned earlier, I find it helpful to draw as I deliver a session; this allows a visual reminder of our conversation that can be built on as the session proceeds. In this part of our session I drew a basic diagram indicating Standards. This spanned Layla's Baseline of Bare Minimum; above Bare Minimum we plotted positive indicators of relationships, below Bare Minimum we plotted negative indicators of relationships.

Together we drew where her experience of her parents and closest friends were. They all plotted consistently above Baseline. I asked Layla if she felt up for plotting where her boyfriend might sit on this drawing. She immediately drew her interpretation of his effort to their relationship; this sat 80% below Bare Minimum with the occasional Bare Minimum.

I then asked Layla what she thought about what she saw in her drawing. She spoke of feeling clearer about her spiraling mood and how exhausted she felt from this. She looked at the drawing for a long time quietly, then she said, "I wish he would be up here" (indicating above Bare Minimum).

I gently reflected on the session thus far, noting that we were now 40 minutes in. I summarized her hope for the session, summarized my understanding about her description of her story, summarized my understanding of her transferable Method of sustaining healthy relationships, and summarized the abundance of Diamonds in her character strengths—Diamonds that included her noticing, tuning in to her well-being, her desire to improve how she felt, her help-seeking behavior, and her openness to explore. I reassured her that she did not need to make any big decisions, gently moving the session to the "What next?"

We spoke about the different listeners she had in her herd (her family and friends) and whether there was anyone in it that might help her reflect on our session. She laughed and stated all her friends were getting to hear about Standards. I reminded her that we come from a place of Love and Peace and not War, reminding her of her strengths of forgiveness and acceptance as well as noting her motivation to employ her agency of change. We spoke of the infancy in learning about committed relationships for both her and her boyfriend, about being transparent, communicating differently, understanding each other's expectations and standards, ultimately giving change a chance, whatever that might look like for her once she had time to digest our conversation.

Layla shared that she felt clearer about her anxiety and depressed feelings. She thanked me for my time and, as always, I asked what specifically from the session was helpful. Layla stated that she felt valued talking through how she felt, without being judged, gaining insight into her mood, thoughts, and feelings. She said she felt like a weight had been lifted from her shoulders, that she could see herself clearly again.

Follow-Up and Comment

This was the one session Layla attended. She is welcome to return whenever she wants, and she said that she would.

Case 3

The following example only happened because the whole system agreed to change. Gone was the mandatory initial comprehensive assessment; in its place, a single session where help-seekers lead the way, empowered and responded to proportionately.

Mum had arrived at the Children Centre for a planned single session appointment. (Referred by a health worker, she had received a letter inviting them to book a single session or full assessment—she chose single session.) Mum spoke of her hopes at gaining strategies to deal with the sleep issues of her two-year-old daughter "Diana."

As the story unfolded, the center staff "sat on their hands" and actively listened. Mum described a routine health care appointment had picked up on how Diana was now sleeping in a bed, having transitioned from a cot; however, she was sleeping with a side light on. The health worker had informed Mum that this was not acceptable and needed to be turned off. Mum's story revealed her own feeling of inadequacy and getting it wrong, and she had immediately followed the health worker's advice to turn the light off. The story described Diana experiencing significant distress at bedtime, not settling, and waking distressed at night. Mum shared experiencing her own increasing anxieties as bedtime arrived, struggling with feelings of guilt associated with her daughter's distress, and feeling exhausted from interrupted sleep.

As she spoke, FIDOS (an assessment tool measuring Frequency, Intensity, Duration, Onset, and Strengths) was used to ascertain any wider context of when issues had begun. The story of calm settling and all-night sleeping with a side light on were consistent. Mum stated that sometimes she fell asleep herself and the light was not turned off. Asking what happened on those nights for Diana, Mum shared that both Diana and Mum slept through the night.

The story had been happening for two months since the health worker first directed the light off.

Yet the Method of settled sleep was clear. As the practitioner reflected back the story and the previous light-on method, Mum began to experience her own empowering penny drop moments. She suddenly said, "Why am I turning the light off?"

Her disempowerment was explored, and she spoke of feeling submissive to health professionals and being someone who strived to be a great mum. The conversation turned to her own Diamonds as a mum, asking for help, knowing her own vulnerabilities, and for realizing that she knew exactly how to create happy and peaceful sleep for her daughter and herself. Mum appeared to get lost in the story, so the Method to resolution was therefore potentially blocked with spiraling consequences.

Mum thanked the Action for Children staff for helping her see what was right for her and her daughter. Her plan? The side light stays on, because bedtimes are times for stories, cuddles, peace, and sleep.

Follow-Up and Comment

Mum was spared being put through an extensive evaluation that might have further disempowered her and left her feeling inadequate. This one session was all that she needed; and she knows where to return if/when she wants.

Some Lessons Learned

Our experience using Single Session Therapy matches the evidence and reinforces our belief that SST can transform the way we provide, and access, mental health care. Since implementing SST, our specific mental health care model with PCNs has consistently shown improved access, a reduction in GP-led mental health appointments, a reduction in mental health GP duty [emergency] calls, and a reduction in onward referral to specialist services.

Normal Magic's journey is not just a story of innovation, it is a narrative of collaboration, partnership, energy, passion, and whole-system empowerment. Our journey leads us to champion Single Session Therapy as an efficient, effective delivery model in mental health care. We further champion single session thinking in any help-giving service. Having a whole-system mindset, in our experience, is an integral part of success and should not be overlooked. As Normal Magic continues to evolve and expand its reach, we believe the lessons learned from our journey will serve as a blueprint for transforming mental health care, and family care, on a broader scale.

Notes

1 For example, see Talmon (1990), Hoyt (2017), Dryden (2019), Slive and Bobele (2011), Schleider (2023), Rycroft and Young (2021), and Cannistrà and Piccirilli (2018/2021). In addition, we are inspired and influenced by the work of Carl Rogers, Aaron Beck, Insoo Kim Berg, Steve de Shazer, and John Bowlby, to name just a few.
2 Christine Cottle, Calendula Pears, and Rob Wyatt.
3 *Editors' note:* British idiom for "moments of sudden awareness or recognition."
4 "Stacking" is a term we use to consider our resilience and tipping points. For example, the straw that broke the camel's back was due to there being a whole stack of straw beneath the final straw.
5 We refer to the word "Story" to begin to introduce the idea that there is often a story occurring in our life, a narrative, a context of emotion, of thought, of behavior. We begin to introduce the idea that our unique Methods of seeking stability during hard times, the Story, are often enough to help us recover.

References

Cannistrà, F., & Piccirilli, F. (2021). *Single-Session Therapy: Principles and Practices*. Giunti. (Published in Italian in 2018.)

Dryden, W. (2019). *Single-Session 'One-at-a-Time' Therapy: A Rational-Emotive Behavior Therapy Approach*. Routledge.

Hoyt, M.F. (2017). *Brief Therapy and Beyond: Stories, Language, Love, Hope, and Time*. Routledge.

Hoyt, M.F., Young, J., & Rycroft, P. (2021). Single session thinking and practice going global one step at a time. In M.F. Hoyt, J. Young, & P. Rycroft (Eds.), *Single Session Thinking and Practice in Global, Cultural, and Familial Contexts: Expanding Applications* (pp. 3–26). Routledge.

Rycroft, P., & Young, J. (2021). Translating single session thinking into practice. In M.F. Hoyt, J. Young, & P. Rycroft (Eds.), *Single Session Thinking and Practice in Global, Cultural, and Familial Contexts: Expanding Applications* (pp. 42–53). Routledge.

Schleider, J.L. (2023). *Little Treatments, Big Effects: How to Build Meaningful Moments That Can Transform Your Mental Health*. Robinson.

Slive, A., & Bobele, M. (Eds.). (2011). *When One Hour is All You Have: Effective Therapy for Walk-In Clients*. Zeig, Tucker, & Theisen.

Talmon, M. (1990). *Single-Session Therapy: Maximizing the Effect of the First (and Often Only) Therapeutic Encounter*. Jossey-Bass.

Talmon, M. (1993). *Single Session Solutions: A Guide to Practical, Affordable, and Effective Therapy*. Addison-Wesley.

Chapter 17

Exploring SST/Drop-Ins Around the World to Increase Access to Timely Mental Health Services and Improve Outcomes for Young Australians[1]

Suzanne Fuzzard

Single Session Therapy (SST), where young people receive intervention at their first presentation, has been shown to improve outcomes. Supported generously with a Churchill Fellowship, I traveled to a number of countries to explore how the SST model developed, including the service provision, governance structures, staff recruitment, training, and supervision. This is important because currently in Australia long wait times without intervention risk young people moving away from seeking help with worsening of mental health outcomes, hopelessness, self-harming, and suicide. As a rural manager and practitioner, I was particularly interested in how staffing models could be adapted to sustain SST in regional and rural areas. It is my hope that local and national youth mental health services will consider some of the recommendations from this report and that funders, policy-makers, and government agencies will be equally interested in this and its application to service design and delivery to enhance our mental health system for young people.

Brief Highlights and General Observations

My study started with a particular focus on exploring service delivery models that enable timely access to youth mental health services and how SST and drop-in (walk-in) services might support this. However, it became so much more: conversation around access to mental health services raised topics with many I visited about social justice and equity of service delivery. It also raised discussion around a need to review how we are responding to the distress expressed by young people and whether we are over-pathologizing young people to the detriment of growing young people's hope, agency, and resilience. Many of the services and people I visited around the world spoke of a system of care that did not seem just. The less resourced you were, and if you lived in less affluent and/or low populated areas, the less access to mental health services you had. It also appears to me that the more complex your problems were deemed, the longer you

DOI: 10.4324/9781032693828-20

tended to wait for specialist services. Often young people were excluded from other services, as they had been considered "too complex." It is cruelly ironic that the more in need you are, the more often you sit on waiting lists. Challenging the status quo, reviewing current evidence, remaining curious and listening to lived experience feedback were common shared values of the services I visited. They saw neither SST or drop-in programs as the panacea for all mental health concerns, but rather saw the valuable contribution this professional work could offer to many people in distress that was timely and focused on intervention. For many young people it could be enough and has the capacity of reducing pressure on more intensive mental health services. For those needing more, they also gain more timely support. Here I will first share some general observations; then describe some encounters with particular SST leaders and programs; and then conclude with some recommendations.

General Observations

- SST and drop-in services, through their nature of being timely and engaged in exploring a client's strengths and skills, alongside understanding the challenges, offer hope and increase personal agency. These two key factors are central in reducing suicidality and distress. I have reflected that in this context "timeliness" may be just as important as the amount of time offered to a client. Our current systems and ways of responding to mental health needs and distress through extensive triage/assessment processes is creating barriers to access—SST and drop-in services open up access. These models need to be designed to suit the local community and this also has implications for staffing.
- When you offer a drop-in service, you have a nil Did Not Attend (DNA) rate!
- Clinical services are found to be the hardest to access yet are focused on our highest-need client group. Many non-clinical services see this high-need client group while they await access to clinical services, as they appear to have fewer barriers. They seem less constrained to just "get on with seeing people," while clinical services spend significant time and resources triaging and privileging assessment prior to providing treatment. Consider the notion of "No more, no less than is needed" (Duvall, Young, & Kayes-Burden, 2012). This policy paper from Canada provides useful insights relevant to Australia.
- It is important to see drop-in/SST options as part of an integrated range of stepped-care options and I would argue should be the front of service delivery for young people seeking mental health care.
- Service design elements need to be considered, such as who can refer and book appointments. Client-directed booking systems and privileging

client/family-initiated referrals have a positive impact on the level of motivation at first appointments.

- Practice considerations also need attention and should be in line with single session thinking: privileging this one session as a possible only session/opportunity. Note-taking systems are transparent, with a focus on being useful to the client and accessible to them prior to leaving.
- Another key observation was around how to use your most experienced clinicians' wisdom, especially when you have early career staff. Investment in supervision is essential. A variety of supervision models were observed to make SST work across a broad range of staff skills. Some services provided in-session live supervision of the entire consultation. Others met before, during, and after the session. Some used the break in the session to meet with a colleague/supervisor. It is important that services have sufficient funding for adequate supervision for drop-in and SST programs. Staff need to feel supported in providing treatment with "just enough" assessment questions and know when a client requires a different service response.
- Another observation involved the possibility of single session thinking (versus therapy) being taught across a range of roles and different scope of practice. I saw some wonderful examples of how peer workers for clients and families were utilized in a drop-in model. Also of note were the important role that digital mental health services can play as a part of comprehensive service offerings, again shaped by single session thinking.
- Organizational and manager support is crucial to enact change and to step away from traditional systems of risk management/triage, and there is a need for government to engage in a policy shift to enable this to occur more commonly across our service system.

The age at which young people can provide their own consent to accessing health and mental health care is a consideration needing further discussion. This can be a barrier to access, especially if you are to offer a drop-in program to young people. This consideration also needs to account for the impact of family inclusion in youth care and raises the question of services having a workforce able to engage effectively with families.

- Another highlight were conversations I had with several people I visited around "questioning our questions." How might we challenge ourselves and systems to look at the questions we ask clients and the consequences of these to clients' view of themselves? Perhaps service delivery and design could be judged on the extent to which they help promote a sense of agency, avoid blame, or encourage hope?

- I also believe services could consider their partner organizations and how to extend their drop-in workforce through shared staffing and joint practice, training, and values around SST. This would ensure a more extensive roster for drop-in services to your local community.

There are many extraordinary services and evidence around the world using single session thinking in practice. Many do not know of each other, and many organizations and governments do not know of the huge body of practice and research evidence for this field.

- Supervision is essential to the implementation and sustainability of drop-in and SST models and is crucial in enabling barrier-free and safe access to young people. As such, this needs to be incorporated into funding to implement drop-in and SST models.
- Growing an international community of practice for SST, single session thinking, and single session interventions (SSIs) is important for dissemination of research in the mental health field.
- SST and SSIs share the following fundamental core ideas and values (see Hoyt, Young, & Rycroft, 2021, p. 5):

  1. Attitude—treating the session "as if" it might be the only one and hence making the most of every encounter, underpinned by the paramount acceptance that one session could be (and often is!) enough
  2. Accessibility—responding in a timely manner without any unnecessary barriers to clients receiving help when they are most ready
  3. Acting Now—accepting that the best opportunity to address change is NOW, no matter the diagnosis, severity, or complexity of the problem, and
  4. Alliance—asking what clients want to achieve by the end of the session so that the therapist and client can work collaboratively, in the here and now, toward that goal.

Encounters Along the Way

My Churchill Fellowship took me around the world, visiting both services and programs working with young people and families and also to conferences and meetings with leaders in the field of SST, SSIs, and drop-in programs. The following reflections from these conversations and presentations are my own and may not necessarily reflect the leaders/presenters or organizations.

Here I will first describe some of my encounters, then offer some observations and recommendations.

1. Michael F. Hoyt—San Francisco

What a privilege on my travels that my first stop should be with Michael Hoyt, a psychologist in independent practice and extensive author/editor of multiple publications on SST (see Hoyt, 2025). Michael is one of the originators, along with Moshe Talmon and Robert Rosenbaum, of the SST approach. In 1990 Moshe Talmon began publishing findings from practice and defining the art of SST, with Bob and Michael joining this important development at the Kaiser Permanente Medical Center. This work developed from an observation that more than half of the patients attended only one session, even when more was available and that when follow-up occurred the majority reported significant improvement in their original concern and noted positive ripple impacts on functioning in other areas of life.

The team then considered, what if we had planned for these single sessions; both the therapist and the client knowing this one session may be enough? What more could be done, and what change in focus and energy might occur?

In conversation with Michael I see the importance in understanding and appreciating the history of the development of SST. I also saw the ongoing passion to teach new generations of therapists. I talked with Michael about how to maintain this passion, despite a system of care that continues to focus on lengthy assessment and treatment planning and a growing inequality of access to mental health care based on income and geography. It highlighted to me the importance of a community of skilled SST professionals across the world coming together. This is both for the sustainability of individual therapists but also for growth of the field. The important publications in this area from these professionals bring together growing areas of SST across the world and has seen this community of practice grow. I was looking forward to attending the 4th International Symposium, hearing from many of the originators alongside those developing this work over the last 35 years. A workshop with Michael[2] in Rome, Italy, was fittingly to be my last appointment on my Churchill Fellowship.

2. Bob Rosenbaum—Sacramento, California

Michael introduced me to Bob Rosenbaum. Conversation with Bob (and Michael) had me further thinking about "the culture of time": that more than thinking of just making the most of this moment in time we need to be in the moment with our clients. SST is often questioned as to be devaluing of a client's history (especially around a client with significant trauma) and not able to create sufficient relationships in such a brief encounter. In talking with Bob I was left to reflect on the effect of multiple sessions on a client's sense of hope and dependency on a system (often ill equipped to maintain this care). It also assumes that assessment for the sake of diagnosing someone into a particular category is useful and Bob asks: "When is the way services are delivered just wasteful?" They highlight that one size doesn't fit all and providing SST is a skilled practice requiring not only training and supervision but ongoing challenge to a mindset that sees assessment, triage, and long-term therapy as the only/best way.

I have observed that these leaders in SST have, for over 35 years, been agitating for system change and questioning the constructs from which we operate. I also got to meet newer therapists in the field of SST who are continuing to advocate for change and grow the evidence base for this work. At the Family Therapy Conference I attended in Calgary (discussed later) the same question was being asked of therapists: to consider their role in social activism. Challenging the status quo in a system and asking: Is it equitable? Is it accessible? Is it helping?

3. *Bridget Beachy and David Bauman—Yakima County, State of Washington, USA*

Bob Rosenbaum introduced me to Bridget Beachy and David Bauman, an amazing duo leading a dynamic service in primary health, alongside GPs/physicians in Yakima, 2.5 hours outside of Seattle. This visit and opportunity to consult with Bridget and David was "SST on Steroids"! This service saw clients of all ages present to a GP (general practitioner). GPs saw the client and if identified at this appointment by the client and/or GP that a psychological/behavioral health session might be helpful it would be offered. GPs would message behavioral health consultants requesting this, and the available behavioral health consultant would accept, generally within minutes of the request. The client would receive a warm handover from the GP and the GP would leave the room. Clients were informed that sessions were approximately 30 minutes long but could be shorter or longer depending on need. Understanding and accepting the context of someone's life is central in considering what change and new perspectives might be possible or acceptable to the client (see Cahill, Martin, Beachy, Bauman, & Howard-Young, 2024). Acceptance and Commitment Therapy is a central therapeutic modality to this service delivery model. Being assertive and directive around the process are also important skills.

Notes are created during the session into a notes template, they are further developed in a short break prior to the client leaving, with this being printed out for them to take away.

In order for this service to flourish, in a challenging funding environment in the USA, master's level and post-doctoral psychology students apply to complete placements with them, and this both enhances the workforce as well as contributes to the growth of skilled psychologists able to work with a single session mindset offering drop-in appointments. They are selective around those they accept, both as students and staff, and interview around mindset and fitting with the values and culture of this service. They also undertake an up to eight-week intensive training/on-boarding program into their model/way of working and the skill set required. New staff and students also work in co-therapy with experienced staff and receive supervision.

Importantly they also collect feedback and outcome data that they publish within their service that builds support for the value of the program offered in a health community that frequently questions the credibility of brief work. They collect satisfaction data from not only the client, but also the GPs and employees—who are some of the most satisfied staff groups within their agency. Some recent data they shared with me from January 2024, in which they had 1,219 visits that had 80% being less than 37 minutes. They also shared that from client satisfaction feedback they ranked in the 100th percentile around provider time spent when compared to other community health centers in the state (doing traditional mental health service delivery). Their data demonstrates that clients are getting what they need and want in timely, shorter SST consults.

This visit has me thinking further about how we might enhance our general practice model to ensure timely and brief access to psychological care that is in line with holistic health care. It also highlighted to me the importance of building a workforce with a shared vision and skill set around brief interventions/therapy and the orientation programs you provide to new staff.

4. Karen Young—Alberta, Canada

Karen has been for many years both a practitioner and trainer in brief therapies working from a narrative theoretical perspective (see Young, 2018). She has been involved in an important policy shift in mental health reform in 2012 in Ontario. The policy paper commissioned by the government reviewed current mental health service delivery at that time and called for a shift in funding to privilege mental health services offering drop-in SST-oriented services. The values and evidence explored in that policy document, titled "No More, No Less" (Duvall et al., 2012), is a must-read for our own Australian policymakers and funders, as many parallels exist within our health system and population. Further, Karen went on to work with the colleagues that credential health professionals to increase the understanding of the high level of skill required to practice in this area of psychotherapy (see Young & Jebreen, 2020).

In discussion with Karen, I was interested to explore how training in single session thinking and work might be useful across many professionals and service delivery options, such as peer workforce, vocational workers, and drug and alcohol programs. Identifying the scope of practice for these roles was something Karen raised; being clear about what staff with these work roles were expected to provide within this framework, what was single session mindset and informed work versus Single Session Therapy. We discussed how shared values and mindset of a multidisciplinary workforce might provide holistic service that is "No more, no less" than a client needs. This idea was further evidenced in my visit to services across Canada and the UK and later explored by various presentations at the SST symposium in Rome. Providing wrap-around services with a shared value of single session thinking has the potential to ensure clients are not unnecessarily directed into therapy-based services when a more functional, practical service delivery model is called for or an intervention that is much more client-directed online. I reflected on an interesting point Karen raised around funders seeming to be excited to provide significant resources to developing new assessment tools, especially around triaging and streaming clients into service pathways. She posed the question: "What is it that has funders so excited about this area of work, and how could we see this excitement (and funding) turned into accessible treatment models?"

The training Karen offers in narrative therapy, within a single session framework, had me consider the role of specific models of therapy and suitability to the SST framework. On my journey I met services that required their staff to be trained in a particular therapeutic model that shaped the delivery of the session and supervision. Some were Narrative Therapy, Solution-Focused Therapy, Acceptance and Commitment Therapy, and Contextual Interviewing. Many staff I spoke with talked of the value of being trained not only in Single Session Therapy/thinking but also a particular evidence-based therapeutic model that shaped the questions they asked. Early career staff spoke of the increased confidence and competence they felt with a clear model. They spoke of the importance of sharing this theoretical skill set with colleagues and supervision being shaped by these models. Supervisors and leaders spoke of the importance to their services having a shared skill set and training, as it ensured greater consistency in service delivery, no matter the practitioner. It also helped shape the supervision questions asked and service processes such as note templates and the way other service pathways were described.

For some services and more experienced clinicians a greater range of therapeutic tools were often drawn upon within their work, such as Systems Theory and Family Therapy, Dialectical Behavior Therapy (DBT), and Cognitive Behavioral Therapy (CBT). This pointed to the importance of experienced staff providing supervision to help further expand the thinking of clinicians as their skills developed. It also ensured clients were directed to suitable alternative pathways/clinicians should this be required.

Consideration of suitable models of therapy and training programs that both emphasize SST training and evidence-based models of therapy, alongside protocols, note-taking templates, and supervision, especially for a less experienced and early career clinician, is something I would like to explore further for my services. I am interested in this for a rural location, as obtaining an experienced mental health workforce is an ongoing challenge.

5. The Foundry—British Columbia, Canada

This program, an integrated youth service that commenced in 2015, offers multiple streams of service delivery, similar to and influenced by the headspace model. Of interest to my visit is the inclusion in their model of drop-in services. Young people enter their programs via drop-in/SST appointments, it is the core business of their programs. This model relies on stepped-care opportunities for those needing other parts of the service internally or externally. Other services are available, including assessment as needed. The drop-in staff are supported through training in Solution Focused Brief Therapy (SFBT) and generally an in-session supervision break. SFBT is based on solution building rather than problem solving. Use of "the break" varied at sites, but I noticed it was very much appreciated by new career professionals. For many the break was seen as essential, given that if you were working in longer-term therapy with a client you would have time to reflect and supervision between sessions. In SST the session break is your chance to reflect, as you may not see the client again. Many spoke of the importance of this supervision to the retention of staff and the incredible learning opportunities for workers this provided. It also gave clients a session with multiple perspectives, maximizing their single session experience. The structure of the supervision break varied but generally checked in around the survey the young person completed and their goals, alongside checking in around any safety concerns. Primarily the supervision aligned with SFBT and so encouraged a focus on "Solution Talk" rather than slipping back into "Problem Talk."

A peer workforce for young people is also an integral part of the Foundry model, and in some centers a peer family worker was employed. Also of interest was a peer-led coordinator/supervisor model to prevent worker drift. I was told how this can occur when supervision to peer workers occurs by clinicians, having peer workers' role becoming confused with a clinical role. Having experienced peer workers coordinate and supervise a peer workforce was found to prevent this.

I visited four different Foundry Centres. The implementation of the model varied depending on the workforce and age of the service establishment and client group attending. Like Australia, Canada has a publicly-funded health system. Like Australia, Canada has a colonial history that has seen significant impacts on First Nations communities.

A highlight was the many collegial conversations I had with leaders and staff in the centers sharing experiences and a common passion for working with young people. I also got to join supervisors in observing the journey for a young person through their drop-in. Another highlight was seeing the integration of a peer workforce into a drop-in service, with Port Hardy (who had only just opened their doors), for example, having a client able to connect with a peer worker in the session break. This seemed to me a wonderful opportunity for young people to debrief their session, should they wish to, while the worker debriefed with a supervisor. It had young people meet other workers/parts of the service, maximizing their experience of the service. In the true mindset of a single session, in which we consider a young person may only attend once, it maximized the range of programs they are exposed to.

At another Foundry site I saw the wonderful work of peer workers connecting with young people in the waiting area, especially if they needed to wait until a clinician became available through drop-in. Peer workers engaged through activities such as a jigsaw in the waiting area, providing welcome packs, and cooking biscuits to share. All helped to enhance a client's experience of the service and offered a lived experience perspective. Caregivers may also be referred to a family peer supporter or navigator.

The drop-in services were generally on a first-come, first-serve basis with no pre-booking and, for some teams, was at scheduled times of the week, not every day. Generally, if they could be pre-booked it was only via client/family referral. It became evident that drop-in in British Columbia did not have the barrier of underage consent, as young people over 12 years of age were able to access services without parental/caregiver consent. This was an interesting consideration I had not really thought about in relation to the challenge for our Australian program in offering a true drop-in (versus via appointment) program.

Generally, for our service we will seek parental consent if under 16 years of age. Only under particular circumstances would it proceed to a mature minor consideration. How this creates barriers for young people in accessing services needs to be considered. However, this raised interesting reflections around constraints to family inclusion and how this might be managed to encourage family-inclusive practice where possible.

The importance of family/caregiver input is recognized across the world in working effectively with young people and skills for staff to navigate this work are also important. Finding a way in which we might offer a drop-in program to all young people 12–25 years of age, without the barrier of seeking consent deserves further exploration, whilst still working with young people to retain family inclusion where feasible and helpful.

Single Session Family Consultation, a model of family inclusion adopted by headspace through collaboration with The Bouverie Centre, La Trobe University in Melbourne was something I was able to share in my visits to centers across the world (see Fuzzard, 2021; O'Hanlon & Rottem, 2021).

The other interesting way the Foundry staffed their drop-in was in partnership with consortium partners and lead agency staff who were provided the same training as the in-house staff to deliver the SST using SFBT. Consortium helped make up the roster to ensure sufficient staffing of the drop-in by qualified staff. All model fidelity and core training around the single session drop-in model and SFBT model was delivered by the national organization, Foundry Central Office Team.

6. Wood's Homes, Eastside Community Mental Health Services—Calgary, Alberta, Canada

Eastside CMHS offers a drop-in program at no cost from a mental health team that started in 1990 as Eastside Family Centre. This was led at the time by Arnold Slive (see Slive, MacLaurin, Oaklander, & Amundson, 1995), a psychologist and clinical director for Wood's Homes. This drop-in without appointment is currently available two times a week; at other times the client can book for this single session. It was wonderful to meet many of the therapists involved from inception to now, working to maintain a model that works.

This service works entirely from a team-based model with the drop-in a core program offering immediate service to anyone presenting on a first-come, first-serve basis (see McElheran, 2021; and Chapter 14 this volume). The team is made up of a variety of mental health professionals, including family therapists and students. The hub of staff includes other programs such as System Navigators, who generally review the intake form completed by the client(s) and clarify any information prior to presenting to the mental health team. Crisis workers are another internal referral point. It was clear this team worked collaboratively with clients to ensure the best fit if follow-up was offered, using a stepped-care approach.

The System Navigator presents the intake form to the team, and a pre-session conversation occurs to develop helpful questions for the therapist going into the room. All sessions are watched live via the team. The team is supported by a supervisor called a Shift Coordinator, who is a highly skilled SST clinician, notably able to create a nurturing, collaborative, and safe team environment. All sessions have a break, in which the team provides input/support to the therapist. A post-session review also occurs. The client is asked if they have any questions for the team. Clients know they are getting the input of a team, and the therapist knows they are supported. Interventions are ensured to fit with the goal of the client.

The client can consider a range of services they might choose from such as crisis support, system navigation, therapy, or ongoing access via the drop-in. They may also be referred to external agencies. The team also offered a check-in phone call that was scheduled if it was felt this might be helpful. This was called a "Caring Contact," a beautiful description from a truly caring system/team.

This is a rich therapy service for the client (that may be enough) and an incredible training opportunity for students and new graduates in the field. I also noticed this was a service that attracts and maintains its staff, with people seeking to volunteer to work in this team to gain experience.

A question I found interesting that they ask in their feedback form is: "If you didn't have this appointment, where would you have gone?" Their research has shown, many clients chose this program over attending a hospital emergency department.

I also had the opportunity to visit a youth-based program offered by Wood's Homes in Calgary called the Opportunity Hub. This service provided day programs, including groups and a cooking training opportunity in a commercial standard kitchen, alongside a shop that sold things made within the program. Upstairs was a live-in drug rehabilitation/housing program. They were considering including an SST option and increasing a family support option, perhaps through single sessions for families. This certainly had me consider our weekly drop-in psycho-social program for young people and how we might begin to offer SSTs via drop-in at the same time.

7.   Calgary Family Therapy Conference—Alberta, Canada

The theme of the Family Therapy Conference was Generativities and Disquiet. The presentations at this conference had me reflect on individuals, services, and systems attempting to respond to the disquiet of seeing behaviors of individuals, organizations, and systems that do not match your values. Many of the presenters also called for therapists to show courage in responding to this noticed disquiet at a social activism level. However, it was also noted that to be generative and come up with new ways of responding, safety is needed. This is evident as a therapist when working with clients and families looking to move toward change in their lives. It is also true of leaders of change and organizations seeking to make change to a system they don't see working. There was a call to therapists and leaders to think global and act locally.

8.   *Child and Youth Mental Health Service (REACH)—Townsend, Ontario, Canada*

Scot J. Cooper (2024; also see Chapter 24 this volume) is a Narrative psychotherapist, having trained with Karen Young. Karen, in fact, put me in touch with Scot, who manages a service called REACH in Townsend, Ontario. This is a Child and Youth Mental Health Service. I had the pleasure of meeting with both Scot and Constance Harvey over two days. I was able to join a clinician in a family session and talk to the staff there.

This service offers a drop-in service a couple of times a week, alongside other parts of the service that include Discovery Sessions (collaborative assessment meeting), ongoing services and group programs, family-based support both in and out of home, and a crisis stabilization program. Again, drop-in models were optimized by ensuring clients got "No more or no less" than they needed and that stepped-care programs were available and offered with careful consideration prior to the end of the session. From the initial form completed by the family/client the team meets to explore useful questions and allocate the clinician(s) who will provide the session.

Speaking with Scot and the team, I found the conversation around the impact of our assessment and triage questions and how they orient people to a way of thinking about themselves and acting so helpful. No question (or program) is neutral, they have the opportunity of influencing the identity of self. This might both be toward hope and personal agency or against this. Language matters, and this service gave considerable thought to their processes, questions, program names, documentation, group programs, and hence training to staff through a lens that fit with their core values. It had me consider how our services could be shaped, developed, and evaluated further through our values and those clear evidence-based factors that improve mental health. Factors such as hope-giving and strength-based principles. Supporting growth of an identity that is rooted in a sense of personal agency, resilience, and being able to contribute to others. Also focusing on opportunities within services for young people creating connection and supporting functional goals.

A collaborative document is created in the session (using a template) with an emphasis on being hope-friendly in the retelling of the client story. Clients/families have the chance to correct it before leaving. The break provides a chance for the clinician to finalize this before checking back in with the client and printing off. The worker meets with a supervisor, and questions are shaped by the Narrative SST conversation map (see Cooper, 2024). Co-working is encouraged in this service, especially supporting new staff into the service. "Double listening" is a core skill that has staff listening for both the problem and stories of difference—an excellent skill for not only therapists in sessions but for leaders and organizations/systems.

How can we listen for what is both the problem and what has, and is, making a difference to providing timely, accessible, and evidence-based mental health care to reduce distress and loss of life?

9. David Humphreys and Bishop's Stortford Primary Care Service—Hertfordshire, UK

While in the UK I was able to meet up with David Humphreys, a Churchill Fellow (2016) and consultant systemic psychotherapist from the UK. We met at the Calgary Family Therapy Conference. I visited the service he works for that demonstrates how small pockets of funding, shaped by dynamic thinkers, can be offering equitable, accessible mental health services to young people. David works within a medical clinic in Hertfordshire. This small team of a GP, health coach, occupational therapist, care coordinator, and social prescriber and psychotherapist/family therapist work to keep access and navigating their program simple, while providing wrap-around holistic care. This program demonstrated the benefits of social care in reducing the need for clinical services or reducing suffering for many whilst awaiting a specialist program. A GP leads this program, and the client is seen first by the GP.

10. Camden Walk-in Service—London

I literally walked into this service, having seen them advertised online. They operated in the evenings and on weekends, providing a drop-in opportunity for people over 18 years of age with mental health concerns and homelessness. When I dropped in, they had a few clients already arriving. It was explained to me that this service was not a clinical service but could offer up to three sessions of counseling, social connection, and social activities such as board games and art. This all occurred alongside a friendly, welcoming team that provided refreshments, warmth, and conversation. Staff explained that many people who attended had significant mental health concerns, but it was unlikely they would obtain tertiary-level mental health services due to long wait times and they would only attempt access in an emergency. Staff would support a client to the emergency department to await review of their mental state. This service highlighted many comments I had heard around the world; specialist mental health services were the hardest to access, yet many high-need clients readily access services from non-clinical services with ease. Many described significant barriers for a client in accessing mental health services and had given up on these programs unless in crisis. How we might embed mental health clinicians within these easy-to-access settings, such as homelessness services, to offer SST I think should be considered.

11. Child and Adolescent Mental Health Services (CAMHS)— Cambridgeshire and Dorset, UK

Katy Stephenson (2023; also see Chapter 11 this volume), a British family and systemic psychotherapist, introduced me to CAMHS services in the UK, at which she had been bringing SST prior to moving to Australia. I was able to visit with Cambridgeshire services who were working with local partner organizations to explore opportunities for embedding SST with a stepped-care model. They had a project position in the region from an organization whose role was looking at building connections between services to explore the possibility of innovations via collaboration within the local area. This made me think about the importance of roles that perhaps sit across services in a local region to explore possibilities for innovation that build on each organization's resources and skill set with shared values. I also reflect on the challenges of this, especially for clinical services, when health is funded by various levels of government and tendered out to non-government agencies (see Cottam, 2018).

When I met with other CAMHS services in Dorset that worked as specialist programs in the areas of intellectual disability and eating disorders it was interesting to hear how they were considering innovative practices. This included the use of single sessions or Single Session Family Consultations to enable greater access to these client groups who often received highly skilled and wonderful services, but all too often left many languishing on waiting lists for up to two years. Conversations reminded me of how hard it can be to sustain practice change in large systems but how one leader, with one more staff member (and one more staff member . . .) can make a difference and create change.

It was wonderful to share ideas with therapists on creative therapeutic ideas, which also could be used in service planning workshops. I was reminded of the great value of cross-fertilization of ideas with services locally, nationally, and internationally. The International SST Symposia (discussed later) that have occurred now four times has been an amazing opportunity for this connection. It is now being further enhanced, with new initiatives offering online SSIs (Schleider, 2023). Thank you to Katy for getting an SST network up and running across the world and inviting me into this and to Helen van Empel (see next) for inviting me to co-facilitate a LinkedIn group that we hope can be an easy space to share thoughts, research, literature, programs, and support for the single session community.

12. Helen van Empel—Amsterdam, The Netherlands

I was able to meet with Helen van Empel in Amsterdam. She is a psychologist and Director of her One Session Employee Empowerment Service (see van Empel, 2023; also Chapter 12 this volume). This service demonstrates how therapists can provide SST within a corporate setting. Primarily this program offers employee assistance programs (EAPs) funded by the employer. It is entirely via video call, and the client can book in directly via a menu of service offerings. Working with an IT specialist, Helen has designed a platform that clients can navigate (Yet.nl) to help orient them to what service they might most want/need at that time. This may include an SST appointment with a psychologist but may also include a life coach, career coach, or leadership coach, ensuring the best specialist is available and decision-making is led by the client. The inclusion of online booking for clients and the ability to choose what they most need at the time from a menu of services is something I think we ought to consider for our public service design, putting the client in the driver's seat for access and agency. It may also reduce demand on therapy services as young people navigate what service most fits for them at this time, such as vocational, drug and alcohol, group programs, and so on. These programs should be well integrated to enable smooth transition between programs as needed, using a stepped-care model and enable good clinical governance.

13. *International Single Session Symposium—Rome, Italy*

The SST symposium held in Rome November 10–12, 2023, was the fourth such International Symposium ever held. What a wonderful place to have the great "thinkers and doers" of single session work in one place from across the globe! Rome is a place of history and invention, and the SST4 International Symposium invited an opportunity to hear from those involved as the pioneers of SST. This was alongside newer innovations and ways in which single session thinking is transforming care in other spaces, such as in peer support, digital platforms, and the corporate sector. It was also an opportunity to create international networks and gather support and possibilities for research across the world in this growing field.

The Italian Center for Single Session Therapy, with Flavio Cannistrà as co-founder and co-director, hosted the symposium and demonstrated how a team of passionate and like-minded colleagues can work to create an international conference.[3]

Recommendations and Conclusion

There is no doubt young people and their families, in Australia and internationally, are coping with unprecedented levels of stress in a world that is uncertain environmentally, politically, economically, and socially.

Single session and drop-in-oriented services that provide timely access fit with the natural help-seeking behaviors of human beings. When we have a problem or crisis, we are more likely to be motivated to consider change. I wonder if the way we design our systems, however, has influenced help-seeking patterns and expectations such that we now expect long-term therapy (and indeed, "therapy") to solve problems. Many young people attend expecting to be "fixed" by a therapist. I have noticed that when young people don't continue with therapy or planned appointments they can report feeling they are therapy "failures" or are labeled by the system and workers as "avoidant" or "resistant." Systems decide how complex a client's problems are and what programs are needed, and often clients are told that only specialists can help with certain problems. What I also observe is that these specialists' programs often have the longest wait times for access or do not exist for rural and regional clients.

Around the world research demonstrates the most common number of sessions a client attends psychotherapy is one. SST and SSIs have been developed to ensure if the client only attends one session that both the client and the therapist is of the mindset to maximize this time they have together, with knowledge that more sessions are possible—leading to greater access and improved outcomes for young people. Importantly, SST/SSIs do not suggest other therapeutic modalities and more intensive programs are not needed, but rather that clients should be receiving "No more no less" than is required. Having a single session mindset to service delivery can ensure this principle is upheld and the client's lived experience and guidance in treatment is at the forefront.

Recommendations

A review of policy and funding for mental health services ought to occur. With a strong government policy document commissioned in 2012 in Ontario, Canada (Duvall et al., 2012), there is a useful precedent to consider for Australia.

- All stakeholders, including clients, families, practitioners, researchers, and those commissioning services, should be encouraged to reflect on and have conversations about questions such as "How well are we responding to those seeking help?" "What is the impact on clients of our current delayed and complex system responses?" "How could we address the issue of timeliness, and what would this look like in terms of how we design service delivery systems?"
- SST and drop-in models should be part of a complete mental health service system that provides no more, no less than is required. They should be implemented at the "front door" of service systems to ensure some level of intervention/therapy is delivered at that first point of contact. Work from a "no wrong door" policy and offering different service

pathways does require cohesive service delivery across state, federal, and non-government programs to support a stepped-care approach.

- Supervision is essential to the implementation and sustainability of drop-in and SST models and is crucial in enabling barrier-free and safe access to young people. As such, this needs to be incorporated into funding to implement drop-in and SST models.

It can be easy for services and clinicians to drift back to "old ways of thinking" that see clients unnecessarily assessed and streamed into intensive service options at the insistence of the system/worker rather than responsive to the client's current help-seeking journey. Staff need to feel supported in making decisions around service pathways and any safety concerns with a client. Managing risk is a very important aspect of mental health services, and for many young people receiving timely intervention is what reduces risk. Rural areas that have limited services, often higher complexity, and limited experienced staff may need to consider online live supervision options to support drop-in services. Supervision models of a drop-in service need to consider local context.

- In establishing drop-in and SST-oriented services for young people a few practice and implementation issues ought to be considered:
  - Consent issues for under 16-year-olds to attend a drop-in program.
  - Referrer priorities and young person access to self-directed booking systems.
  - Collaborative note-taking processes that promote transparency and client-led conversations and care planning.
  - Reviewing partner relationships and opportunities to share rostering for drop-in programs.
  - Promoting feedback opportunities for young people and families that identify the importance of timeliness of access and where clients might have gone in the absence of this access.
  - Considering the role of the follow-up phone call and its purpose.
- Exploring with funders the contribution of SST alongside GP services as part of a primary care service.
- Growing an international community of practice for SST, single session thinking, and SSI is important for dissemination of research and will support policy change and practice as well as service development.

Conclusion

I had the privilege of meeting a range of workers and young people from around the world. To be able to bring together a number of these people to help contribute to our work in Australia would further enable policymakers, funders, leaders, lived-experience young people, and clinicians to join in a re-envisaging of our mental health system. The international therapeutic, academic, and research community in SST and SSI is growing from the pioneers of over 35 years ago, and I am proud to be a part of this.

Notes

1 This is a condensed version of my 2024 Churchill Fellowship Report. Please visit https://www.churchilltrust.com.au/fellow/suzanne-fuzzard-sa-2022/ for the complete report. Special thanks to the Churchill Trust and, in particular, the Elvie Munday Award, with much appreciation to the folks at The Bouverie Centre and headspace Victor Harbor and Murray Bridge and the incredible young people and families our headspace program provides services to, as well as to the various people and organizations I was privileged to visit. Indeed, Churchill often spoke of the importance of taking risks and to be brave.
2 *Editors' note*: See Chapter 5 of this volume.
3 *Editors' note*: Many of the chapters in this book are based on those presentations.

References

Cahill, A., Martin, M., Beachy, B., Bauman, D., & Howard-Young, J. (2024). The contextual interview: A cross-cutting patient-interviewing approach for social context. *Medical Education Online, 29*.

Cooper, S.J. (2024). *Brief Narrative Practice in Single-Session Therapy*. Routledge.

Cottam, H. (2018). *Radical Help*. Hatchette UK.

Duvall, J., Young, K., & Kayes-Burden, A. (2012). *No more, no less: Brief mental health services for children and youth*. www.excellenceforchildenandyouth.com

Fuzzard, S. (2021). Embedding single session family consultation in a national youth mental-health service: Headspace. In M.F. Hoyt, J. Young, & P. Rycroft (Eds.), *Single Session Thinking and Practice in Global, Cultural, and Familial Contexts: Expanding Applications* (pp. 133–139). Routledge.

Hoyt, M.F. (2025). *Single Session Therapy: A Clinical Introduction to Principles and Practices*. Routledge.

Hoyt, M.F., Young, J., & Rycroft, P. (2021). Single Session Thinking and Practice going global one step at a time. In M.F. Hoyt, J. Young, & P. Rycroft (Eds.), *Single Session Thinking and Practice in Global, Cultural, and Familial Contexts: Expanding Applications* (pp. 3–26). Routledge.

McElheran, N. (2021). The story of the Eastside Family Centre: 30 years of walk-in Single Session Therapy. In M.F. Hoyt, J. Young, & P. Rycroft (Eds.), *Single Session Thinking and Practice in Global, Cultural, and Familial Contexts: Expanding Applications* (pp. 125–132). Routledge.

O'Hanlon, B., & Rottem, N. (2021). Single Session Family Consultation (SSFC). In M.F. Hoyt, J. Young, & P. Rycroft (Eds.), *Single Session Thinking and Practice in Global, Cultural, and Familial Contexts: Expanding Applications* (pp. 66–76). Routledge.

Schleider, J.L. (2023). *Little Treatments, Big Effects: How to Build Meaningful Moments That Can Transform Your Mental Health*. Robinson.

Slive, A., MacLaurin, B., Oaklander, M., & Amundson, J. (1995). Walk-in single sessions: A new paradigm in clinical service delivery. *Journal of Systemic Therapies*, *14*, 3–11.

Stephenson, K. (2023, December). Single session thinking: Its global impact and role in therapeutic services. *Context*, *190*, 29–31.

Talmon, M. (1990). *Single Session Therapy: Maximizing the Effect of the First (and Often Only) Therapeutic Encounter*. Jossey-Bass.

van Empel, H. (2023). *Single Session Therapy: Help je Cliënt Korte en Krachtig Voorut*. Boom Publisher. [In Dutch: Translates as *Single Session Therapy: Help Your Client Move Forward Briefly and Powerfully*.]

Young, K. (2018). Change in the winds: The growth of walk-in therapy clinics in Ontario, Canada. In M.F. Hoyt, M. Bobele, A. Slive, J. Young, & M. Talmon (Eds.), *Single-Session Therapy by Walk-In or Appointment* (pp. 59–71). Routledge.

Young, K., & Jebreen, J. (2020). Recognizing single-session therapy as psychotherapy. *Journal of Systemic Therapies*, *38*(4), 31–44.

Part IV

SST Techniques and Practices

Chapter 18

Strategic Dialogue and Hypnotherapy Without Trance

Giorgio Nardone

As science has shown us through the centuries: The best way to introduce a method is by using a real example of it:

"My Father Wants to Poison Me"

They arrived in distress from a little town from the south, sent by their family doctor, after a forced hospitalization in a psychiatric ward that had not come to any therapeutic effect. To the contrary: it had made the situation worse. The parents and their 17-year-old son sat down, the son in the middle, very thin, emaciated, and pale, staring at his mother. The latter, in a state of turmoil, began to speak while her husband seemed clearly annoyed.

> Professor, we are desperate, my son has not had any food or water for weeks. We give him I.V. solutions to keep him alive. . . He refuses all food because he thinks that his father wants to poison him and that I am unable to protect him from him . . . The doctors have already given him many drugs for months but nothing has changed, but thanks to them we got him to take the food.

While the woman, full of anguish, explained the situation, the father snorted and the son remained unperturbed, stiff in his posture, leaning toward his mother, with his back to his father. I interrupted the explanation with a hand signal, and turning to the young one I said: "Excuse me, I have a question . . . If your father wants to poison you it means that he wants to kill you, so if you don't have any food or water until you are dead you are playing his game." The boy made a leap on his chair and exclaimed: "That I had not considered . . . How do I find a way around him putting the poison in the food or drinks, though?" "OK," I answered, "You should know that, in history, the fear of being poisoned by the food that the nobility ate was solved using tasters who would try the meals to test if they were poisoned before the prince would try them." The boy

DOI: 10.4324/9781032693828-22

quickly replied: "But I don't have tasters . . . The only one that could do it is my mother, but I don't want her to die in my place." "You're right, I appreciate your noble spirit, but I have to say that you didn't consider that we could make your father the one who tastes your food before you eat it . . . so we put the poisoner in the position of being poisoned." "Brilliant!" exclaimed the boy with a satisfied smile. "So we put him with his back against the wall. . . But who can convince my father, who hates me, to do all this?" To which I responded: "Given that he is here, I can try."

Then, turning to the father, who had watched our dialogue astonished and stupefied, probably thinking that I needed perhaps as much care as his son, "Would you be willing to do this for your son?" "I would do anything for him. . . Of course I could do it if it would help him!" We agreed on all the details and the procedure to be carried out, and as we arranged everything father and son looked at each other and talked with apparent hostility.

A few days later I received a phone call from their doctor, who informed me that a miracle seemed to have occurred: the young man had resumed eating and no longer saw his father as his poisoner. I told him that nothing miraculous had been done except the application of a specific therapeutic technique, namely, putting oneself in the perspective of the phobic delirium by finding its logic and, thanks to that, redirecting the phenomenon with its "reasonableness" toward an evolution that would make it no longer maladaptive but effective and functional. "A technology that is sufficiently evolved in its effects is indistinguishable from magic" (Clarke, 1968). It is good to consider that, as is well known to experienced clinicians, in cases of adolescent "psychotic episodes," if one succeeds in dismantling the phobic delusion it rapidly decays, even in one single session, like a building undermined at its base, and most of the time it does not recur. If, on the other hand, one fails in this arduous task, the delirium tends to radicalize, becoming a true psychotic disorder.

This is a concrete example of a *hypnotherapy without trance* (Nardone, 1996; Nardone & Watzlawick, 1993) session: tuning in (Loriedo, Zeig, & Nardone, 2011) with the patient's perception of reality even when it could appear as bizarre or "crazy" and thus driving him to grasp a new and affirmative perspective of reality. The therapist should not enter in contradiction or conflict with the patient's previous narrative ("Please, correct me if I'm wrong"—Nardone & Salvini, 2007/2018, p. 19), but he must be capable to redirect the patient's perception toward a therapeutic change.

All this can be achieved by applying in our modern context ideas already known by—for example—the Hellenic sophists, who indicated the same techniques in their *art of persuasion*; or philosopher and mathematician Blaise Pascal, who prescribed what to do when you desire to induce a change in man's mind and behavior by using the same principles of persuasion. As Santayana said: "There is nothing new under the sun, just what has been forgotten." However, readapting wisdom and *techne* to the contemporary scientific theory and practice, it is certainly something relevant and advanced.

All that has to be considered when thinking about a particular way to act in a single session context, and it also elucidates very well a required mindset for the psychotherapist to have if he or she is to be both effective and quick in his or her performance: Flexibility, great wisdom, the capacity to assume non-ordinary points of view, and being a great performer while using performative communication (Austin, 1962). This appears as one of the most fascinating images of a brief strategic therapist, who is capable of pushing the specific trigger points in a pathological homeostasis, starting an immediate process of therapeutic change. This is the other—and not less important—face of the coin when conducting a single-session therapy: rigor and systematicity.

As stated, this type of treatment is precisely tailored to the needs of the problem and to the specific features of the person in treatment by differentiating the techniques based on the specific pathological variant. Even when these techniques are rigorously replicated, they will differ in the language and type of therapeutic relationship, always adapting to the unique characteristics of each patient and family system. Indeed, a fundamental aspect of the strategic approach to psychotherapy is the coexistence of *regularity* and *originality* in the therapeutic intervention (Nardone & Balbi, 2015; Nardone & Portelli, 2005; Nardone & Valteroni, 2020).

To elucidate the process, let me refer to the evidence-based strategy for conducting the first session with juvenile anorexia cases seen at the Centro di Terapia Strategica (Nardone & Valteroni, 2020; Jackson, Pietrabissa, Rossi, Manzoni, & Castelnuovo, 2018). The session starts with the investigation of the disorder. This is carried out firstly through a series of strategic questions, which accurately identify the type of anorexic eating disorder, and confirm the fact-finding and diagnostic observations through paraphrasing. The paraphrasing technique is based on providing a summary and evaluation of the answers given by the patient, thereby seeking agreement between patient and therapist. Thus, it is a method for creating an effective therapeutic relationship.

Once the type of problem has been identified, the next therapeutic maneuver is a reframing[1] of the responsibility of the parents with respect to the health of their daughter and the potential deterioration of her condition, including the most unfortunate possible outcome. In such cases, the girl may hold her parents "hostage" through emotional blackmail, ensuring that they acquiesce to her demands. Through the therapeutic maneuver, parents are made guardians of the well-being of their underage daughter with regard to her anorexia; they are held accountable to concrete responsibilities. In this way, they coalesce and regain their parental authority over their daughter and can avoid the guilt of being complicit in her dangerous pathology. After having redefined the family dynamics, we agree with the parents that, if their daughter's weight loss reaches a particular threshold of risk, which can vary from person to person, they must take her immediately to a hospital for forced feeding. In doing this, we also talk directly to the patient and explain what would happen in this scenario, using a strongly evocative image: "They will insert a tube through your nose and blow you up like a balloon." This suggestive technique is repeated several times to obtain an overload effect. It is a bit like predicting what the young anorexic patient would like to avoid—that is, to be forced to regain weight quickly.

In just one session a new climate has emerged, both for the parents and for the daughter, who now becomes, in turn, a hostage to her own actions and to the inevitable reaction of her parents, who are now bound to their medical responsibilities. At this point we proceed by proposing a sort of *illusion of alternative* (Watzlawick, 1978).

> You can avoid all this if you agree to gradually regain half a kilogram per week, no more than this. . . Otherwise there will be a tube that will blow you up like a balloon and you will regain several kilograms all at once. Of course, you might be thinking that after that you could start losing weight again, but then there will be the tube again and it will blow you up like a balloon . . . If you agree to gradually and slowly regain half a kilogram per week, we can plan together how to achieve this and help you reach your target weight without making you gain a single gram more.

Technically, this is called a *therapeutic double bind* (Watzlawick, 1978), and it is a powerful technique to make the unacceptable acceptable. Once this crucial step is achieved, the attitude of the girl is usually resigned and accepting. At this point, we completely change our communicative and relational register. We propose directly to her a suggestive dialogue about what she would really like to eat, as if the desired food would not make her gain weight.

> As we have agreed to fight our enemy, we must now agree on how to deal with food. At this point, let me ask you another question: If you could eat without fear, what would you like to eat more than anything? Let's make a ranked list of the tastiest foods for you.

There is an evident dilation of pupils, the sign of her pleasure mechanisms activating, and she says: "Pizza!" I reply: "Soft crust or thin?" She: "Thin and very crunchy so that it crackles between your teeth." And I carry on: "With hot, stringy mozzarella cheese or with a lot of overflowing tomato sauce?" The tip of her tongue touches her lip. "With hot, stringy mozzarella cheese!"

The evocation of images of her favorite food triggers genuine pleasure in the patient. Research shows (Doige, 2016) that guided imagery produces sensory effects that are not unlike the real ones. This is a powerful vehicle for change, especially when it is adopted with people who no longer allow themselves pleasure because of fear.

Together, we draw up a ranked list of her favorite foods, and together we decide what to start with when she resumes eating, so as to avoid regaining more than half a kilogram each week.

The parents are briefed thus: "You have the important task of arranging the agreed foods, making them available on the table and staying with her until the end of the meal, without talking about her problem and without insisting that she eats." I then repeat that they will have to stay there until she has finished and for some time after. "Then, at least one of you will have to stay with her for the next two hours to talk or to do some activities, such as clearing the table." This maneuver represents an evolution in comparison to our previous interventions with anorexic patients (Nardone, Milanese, & Verbitz, 2005) that shows how the model is capable of adapting its application to the always changing evolution of the disorders.

In more than 80% of the studied cases, young anorexic patients follow the initial agreement and start to gain weight gradually. Of course, this is only the initial phase of the whole therapy, but, considering the usually huge resistance of these patients, we could use a paraphrased quote from the Pythagoreans and Aristotelians: "A good start is half the work done."

The strategic dialogue used in the first session with anorexia patients is both an original ad hoc calibrated therapeutic maneuver tailored to the particular patient and her singular psychological disorder, and also—when applied to a great number of patients producing the same effects—it becomes an effective, repeatable, predictive, and transmissible therapeutic strategy.

It is also the most specific component of a successful Single Session Therapy, which enlightens us about the need for the therapist to have a mindset based on rigor and systematicity. In other words: to be an artist as well as a scientist.

Further Illustrations of How Art and Science Are the Two Sides of the Same Coin When We Perform a Single Session Therapy

A few more examples:

Little Dirt Protects From Big Dirt

This complex reframing was developed in the early nineties to deal with cases of obsessive-compulsive disorder involving preventive sanitation measures, which are particularly resistant to change:

> And so, you have your whole house sanitized, making it the temple of cleanliness. You have sanitized yourself, making yourself completely sterilized and you demand that your family members do the same . . . and here it is where the problems actually emerge . . . because you have to defend the clean you have achieved! . . . And this is what makes you terrified by any possible intrusion of dirt into your Big Clean . . . that is to say that it is the Big Clean you made that induces the fear of the Big Dirt that will ruin it . . . the Big Clean creates the Big Dirt, of which you are terrified . . . therefore, the more you create the Big Clean, the more you create the Big Dirt. [. . .] If you want to reduce up to eliminating your crippling phobia, you should contemplate the idea that the best way to defend yourself from the Big Dirt is creating a Little Dirt, which defends you from the Big Clean that creates the Big Dirt. [. . .] If you create a Little Dirt, cleaning everything, but leaving a small part of your house not perfectly clean . . . if you sanitize yourself, but leaving, for example, a finger that is not perfectly sanitized according to your standard . . . thanks to this Little Dirt you would avoid creating the idea of the Big Clean that creates the idea of the Big Dirt.

This surprising and suggestive reframing must be repeated in a redundant way, like an actual hypnotic formula, to make it acceptable to the person with obsessive-compulsive disorder that the idea of creating their daily "Little Dirt" protects from the phobia of the "Big Dirt." What seemed impossible is made possible. If the person applies the effect of the reframing, the Little Dirt represents the "therapeutic violation" to the obsessive-compulsive clean dogma, that is, the virus of change. It is a virus because change expands in an exponential way and creates an avalanche effect; the snowball thrown on the snowy slope grows larger by rolling and becomes an unstoppable avalanche.

The same type of reframing applies with great effectiveness also to the compulsive obsession of control and order, in which instead of dirt, the object of the elaborate maneuver is the small "lack of control" that protects from the phobia of the complete lack of control, or the "small disorder" that protects from the phobic "big disorder." In the latter case, we also use the analogic image of entropy, the very slow natural evolution of things, thanks to the break of an equilibrium that evolves into one of a higher type: the small disorder allows people to create a higher order.

Fear of Fasting

A second "historic" reframing has become a best practice in the treatment of binge eating (Castelnuovo, Manzoni, Villa, Cesa, & Molinari, 2011; Pietrabissa, Manzoni, Gibson, Boardman, Gori, & Castelnuovo, 2016; Jackson et al., 2018). This reframing is used to turn the tendency to reduce food intake for the fear of losing control and end up bingeing, typical of this clinical picture, into the fear of food restriction. In this way, the rigidity of the disorder is completely subverted and directed toward its extinction.

Usually, in front of these patients it is proposed:

You, like all of your "colleagues" of the disorder, think that in order to limit your colossal binge eating you should strictly control, by reducing almost up to fasting, what you allow yourself to eat . . . but, actually, it is precisely this that produces the binge eating. Fasting and restrictions, if carried out to the extreme, increase the desire of what we limit ourselves to eat, until the impulse becomes unstoppable and we end up stuffing ourselves with what we turned down . . . any prohibition increases the desire of what is forbidden to us . . . it is natural to think that it is binge eating that may cause the next and necessary fasting . . . but in fact, the mechanism works in reverse . . . it's the fast that generates the binge . . . you restrict your food intake, you fast, and in doing so you increase your desire, which becomes more and more urgent, of desired but not allowed food, until you lose control and end up binge eating a great amount of it . . . If you want to reduce binge eating and take control of food, you should be afraid of fasting and restricting your food intake, since it is this that leads you inexorably to the loss of control and binge eating . . . the more you restrict, the more you end up being overwhelmed by the frustrated desire . . . as after all it is happening . . . It's the fast that creates the binge and not the binge to create the fast.

Also in this case, the restructuring is redundantly proposed during the session and left as a topic to think about until the next appointment. As the reader can well understand, it is a subtle way to induce a change without asking for it directly. It is a way to introduce into the mind of patients, a

266   Single Session Therapies

new—for them—unambiguous vision of the functioning of their problem and creating an aversion to what, so far, they have tried to do to fight it. To summarize, it is like "leading the enemy up into the attic and then removing the ladder."

Relational Prostitution

A reframing used very often is the one oriented to change people's attitudes and relational behaviors characterized by always wanting to ingratiate themselves to others. This continuous need for confirmation is based, most of the time, on a deep sense of insecurity with respect to one's own desirability. An insecurity that induces people to constantly seek out confirmation, to avoid contrasts and conflicts, and to please others as much as possible. When, in the first session with the patient, this relational script clearly emerges, this dysfunctional interaction model is reframed as follows:

> What you have so well described to me highlights the fact that you appear incapable of activating and sustaining contrasts and that you try to constantly indulge the people around you to avoid facing their rejection. We could say, by using a provocation, that you practice relational prostitution. To please others . . . to avoid being rejected, you always agree with the other person . . . you always make them feel you are on their side . . . relational prostitution, as I understand it, is a script that has the purpose of defending yourself from the terror of not being considered enough . . . actually, from the certainty of not being able to make others like you if not by being perceived as a safe and complicit ally. All of this, reiterated in time, becomes something spontaneous . . . not something voluntary or forced . . . so much to appear as a character trait, when, instead, it is a learned behavior that has become acquisition . . . no one is born a relational prostitute . . . one becomes it for the need to defend themselves from rejection that otherwise appears to be inevitable.

If the person nods and remains, as usually happens, struck by this redefinition of their being in relation to others, we proceed:

> But I would like you to consider the fact that this is a lethal existential trap . . . what you achieve through your relational prostitution and the pleasure of receiving confirmation from others, you achieve it for what you do, not for what you are! You are convinced, if you haven't experienced it already, that if you stopped your relational prostitution and showed what you really are . . . people, accustomed to seeing you following your script, would reject you . . . or simply would be upset. . .

All of this corresponds to a kind of belief that you have built: "If I don't want to be rejected, and if I want to continue to receive confirmation about my desirability, I must continue with my relational prostitution and never expose myself for what I know I really am" . . . but by doing this you are desperately lonely! You are condemned to recite a script that, tragically, confirms that you cannot please others, except by prostituting yourself . . . what you do to avoid being lonely makes you desperately lonely.

After this reframing, strongly evocative of pain, even people who are most convinced of their own undesirability persuade themselves to change and to run the risk of being liked for what they are and not for what they do. They can then be guided to change their relational patterns and to discover that it is much more difficult not to please others completely than to please them at least enough.

All these examples of suggestive-strategic reframing require to be truly tailored to each one of the patients and to be adapted to him or her in terms of language and relational attitude, otherwise, even if the logic of the maneuver is the correct one, its power will be drastically reduced. We must never forget that the therapeutic process is the sum up of logic, language, and relation. In other words: cognition, emotion, and communication. So, to do the right thing in the wrong way can make it turn into a failure.

In a seemingly contradictory statement, the same technique changes every time because of its adaptability to the always different singularities and characteristics of each patient. However, this shouldn't surprise us, because in scientific research and application there is always requested an observation of the "regularities" in a phenomenon as well as in its "singularities." In such a way, rigorousness and creativity interact with each other, creating a new therapeutic emergent quality.

It's important to highlight that before applying one of the numerous suggestive-strategic maneuvers set up for solving specific problems, it is fundamental to have investigated thoroughly the patient's situation and condition, as well as his or her *redundant and failing attempted solutions* (Watzlawick, Weakland, & Fisch, 1974; Weakland, Fisch, Watzlawick, & Bodin, 1974).[2] Using the strategic dialogue's discriminatory questions, followed by orienting questions, and alternating them with elucidating paraphrases that build up an agreement between the patient and the therapist while evaluating the problem to be solved, appears to be very useful and capable of preventing the possibility of the therapist becoming a sort of manipulative prophet.

To conclude this exposition, I'd like to suppose that the reader has understood how complex and tiring it is to become a really smart psychotherapist, capable of inducing rapid and effective changes in a patient's mind and behavior. The paradox is that for an effective use of brief therapy an even more sophisticated and refined training is required, in comparison with the one required for the practice of long-term therapy.

It sounds like when Blaise Pascal in 1656 wrote to a friend: "My Dearest: I apologize for writing a long letter like this one, but I hadn't the time to write down a shorter one."

Notes

1 "To reframe, then, means to change the conceptual and/or emotional setting or viewpoint in relation to which a situation is experienced and to place it in another frame which fits the 'facts' of the same concrete situation equally well or even better, and thereby changes its entire meaning" (Watzlawick, Weakland, & Fisch, 1974, p. 95).
2 Thus Watzlawick (in Watzlawick & Hoyt, 1998/2001, p. 149) explained: "One of the basic principles of systems theory is that every system is its *own best* explanation. . . . What matters to me (exclusively) is the patient's specific problem; and what he has done so far to 'solve it,' i.e., the *attempted solution*, which in our perspective is the main factor that maintains and exacerbates the problem."

References

Austin, J.L. (1962). *How to Do Things with Words*. Harvard University Press.

Castelnuovo, G., Manzoni, G.M., Villa, V., Cesa, G.L., & Molinari, E. (2011). Brief strategic therapy vs. cognitive behavioral therapy for the inpatient and telephone-based outpatient treatment of binge eating disorder: The STRATOB randomized controlled clinical trial. *Clinical Practice and Epidemiology in Mental Health*, 7, 29–37.

Clark, A.C. (1968). *2001: A Space Odyssey*. New American Library.

Doige, N. (2016). *The Brain's Way of Healing: Remarkable Discoveries and Recoveries from the Frontiers of Neuroplasticity*. Penguin Books.

Jackson, J.B., Pietrabissa, G., Rossi, A., Manzoni, G.M., & Castelnuovo, G. (2018). Brief strategic therapy and cognitive behavioral therapy for women with binge eating disorder and comorbid obesity: A randomized clinical trial one-year follow-up. *Journal of Consulting and Clinical Psychology*, 86(8), 688–701.

Loriedo, C., Zeig, J.K., & Nardone, G. (2011). *Trance Forming Ericksonian Methods*. The Milton Erickson Foundation Press.

Nardone, G. (1996). *Brief Strategic Solution-Oriented Therapy of Phobic and Obsessive Disorders*. Jason Aronson.

Nardone, G., & Balbi, E. (2015). *The Logic of Therapeutic Change*. Karnac Books.

Nardone, G., Milanese, R., & Verbitz, T. (2005). *Prisoners of Food*. Karnac Books.

Nardone, G., & Portelli, C. (2005). *Knowing Through Changing: The Evolution of Brief Strategic Therapy*. Crown House Publishing.

Nardone, G., & Salvini, A. (2007). *The Strategic Dialogue: Rendering the Diagnostic Interview a Real Therapeutic Intervention*. Karnac Books. (Republished 2018 by Routledge.)

Nardone, G., & Valteroni, E. (2020). *Advanced Brief Strategic Therapy for Young People With Anorexia Nervosa: An Effective Guide for Clinicians*. Routledge.

Nardone, G., & Watzlawick, P. (1993). *The Art of Change: Strategic Therapy and Hypnotherapy Without Trance*. Jossey-Bass.

Pietrabissa, G., Manzoni, G.M., Gibson, P., Boardman, D., Gori, A., & Castelnuovo, G. (2016). Brief strategic therapy for obsessive-compulsive disorder: A clinical and research protocol of a one-group observational study. *BMJ Open*, 6(3), e009118. https://doi.org/10.1136/bmjopen-2015-009118

Watzlawick, P. (1978). *The Language of Change: Elements of Therapeutic Communication*. Norton.

Watzlawick, P., & Hoyt, M.F. (1998). Constructing therapeutic realities: A conversation with Paul Watzlawick. In M.F. Hoyt (Ed.), *The Handbook of Constructive Therapies* (pp. 183–197). Jossey-Bass. (Reprinted in Hoyt, M.F. (2011). *Interviews With Brief Therapy Experts* (pp. 144–157). Brunner-Routledge.)

Watzlawick, P., Weakland, J.H., & Fisch, R. (1974). *Change: Principles of Problem Formation and Problem Solution*. Norton.

Weakland, J.H., Fisch, R., Watzlawick, P., & Bodin, A.M. (1974). Brief therapy: Focused problem resolution. *Family Process, 13*(2), 141–168.

Chapter 19

When "How" Wins Over "Why"

The First Three Main SST Interventions According to the Method of the Italian Center for Single Session Therapy

Federico Piccirilli

Many years ago, my son approached me, his eyes sparkling with curiosity and a ready question on his lips.

"Dad, what do you do?" Instead of answering with the usual "I'm a psychologist," I decided to capture his attention with a slightly different story by replying: "I'm waiting for an hour!" Wise as only children can be, my son looked at me questioningly. His small head, full of ringlets at the time, tilted slightly, as if trying to comprehend a complex mystery.

"Dad, will you wait an hour? What does that mean?" Smiling, I leaned toward him, his wide eyes fixed on mine, and began to narrate.

"You know, my love, in an increasingly hectic world, with people seemingly running all the time, there is a special job I do. Wait an hour."

My son looked even more puzzled. "You wait an hour? But what happens in that hour?" "Well, actually, I don't wait for an hour in the common sense of the word. That hour is a special opportunity I give to myself and the people who are with me. It is an hour in which they can share their thoughts, their feelings, their fears, their dreams and everything that makes them feel good or bad. It is an hour where they can be themselves without judgment."

My son's face suddenly lit up. "So, you help people to be happy?" "Yes, in a way, I try to find the way to be serene. I try to help people find solutions to their problems and feel more peaceful. It's like helping people tidy up and find their way in this world."

My son nodded sagely. "Dad, I think your job is strange. *An hour to spend with people you don't know is really an endless time.*"

From an occasional but valuable event, having always practiced short therapies, I decided to deepen and adopt, by virtue of my son's reflection on "infinite time," a single-session mindset in my daily work. Added to this was my clinical experience, which led me to reflect on the conventionality of "prolonged" therapeutic sessions. I could see that often—dare I say, "almost always"—significant changes can take place in a surprisingly

DOI: 10.4324/9781032693828-23

short period of time. The importance of the "here and now" and the obser-vation that many people benefit immediately from a focused intervention convinced me of the value of the path I was taking.

The adoption of Single Session Therapy (SST) in my work is the result of a professional evolution, driven by the search for efficiency, listening to people's needs, and my continuous passion for innovation in the field of psychotherapy. This approach reflects my vision of a therapeutic interven-tion as a unique opportunity for change, in line with my philosophy of valuing individual resources and not labeling people, but rather treating them with a personalized approach that respects their uniqueness, doing it one hour at a time.

Creating Meaningful Change in a Single Encounter

This chapter examines the first three key interventions adopted by the Ital-ian Center for Single Session Therapy. In this perspective, the "how" of the intervention becomes more important than the "why."

To develop our SST method (Cannistrà & Piccirilli, 2018/2020) we were inspired by the structure of a brief therapy session as proposed by Michael F. Hoyt in 2009 in his work *Brief Psychotherapies: Principles and Practices*. He outlines five key phases, which we adapted and enriched by inserting specific therapeutic maneuvers. Some of these maneuvers were taken directly from Hoyt's directions (also see Hoyt, 1995, 2017, 2025), while others were developed or adapted by us.

The five stages of the method, with their respective maneuvers and tech-niques, are:

1. *Pre-treatment.* This phase focuses on gathering preliminary informa-tion and administering a questionnaire. It is based on the idea of form-ing an initial idea of the person, which is essential for orienting the session.

Techniques used:

a. Preliminary information gathering: this involves obtaining a gen-eral overview of the problem presented by the person and his or her history.
b. Questionnaire administration: this is used to disseminate the idea of change and enhance resources, thus providing a basis for the session.

2. *Initial phase.* The single session concept is introduced, and the problem presented by the person is defined. Goals are clarified and priorities

are identified, constantly soliciting feedback to establish an effective therapeutic alliance. This approach draws on the therapeutic alliance theory outlined by Bordin (1979), which emphasizes the importance of collaboration, agreement on goals and tasks, and therapeutic bonding in facilitating the change process.

Techniques used:

a. Problem definition: clear and operational identification of the problem presented by the person.
b. Clarification of goals and identification of priorities: establishing what the person expects to get out of the session.
c. Requesting constant feedback: active involvement of the person in the therapeutic process.
d. Establishing the therapeutic alliance: creating a relationship of trust and collaboration with the person.

3. *Middle phase.* The person's theory of change (Duncan & Miller, 2000), resources, and exceptions to the problem, as well as the solutions already tried and found to be dysfunctional (see Nardone & Salvini, 2004/2018), are investigated. The importance of compliments, feedback, and suggestions is emphasized, drawing on the motivational interviewing techniques of Miller and Rollnick (2002). Solutions are explored and experimented with in session, constantly making sure to be in tune with the person.

Techniques used:

a. Investigation of client's theory of change: exploring how the person views the possibility of change.
b. Exploration of resources and exceptions: identifying times when the problem does not occur or resources are not yet used.
c. Analysis of attempted dysfunctional solutions: discussing past attempts to solve the problem and why they did not work.
d. Compliments, feedback, and suggestions: acknowledging the person's progress and offering constructive suggestions.
e. Exploration and experimentation with in-session solutions: trying new strategies for dealing with the problem.

4. *Final stage.* Involves assessment of any items missed, prescription of specific tasks, an overall evaluation of the single session, and making explicit the "open door," i.e., availability for future meetings if needed. Bureaucratic issues are also addressed, and instructions are given for follow-up or (possible) next appointment.

Techniques used:

a. Evaluating missed items: making sure all important aspects have been addressed.
b. Prescribing tasks: assigning activities or reflections to carry on after the session.
c. Single session evaluation: discuss the person's impressions of the session.
d. Explication of the "open door": reassure the person about availability for future meetings if needed.
e. Instructions for follow-up/next appointment: arrange future steps and bureaucratic issues.

5. *Follow-up.* Feedback is requested after a period of time to evaluate the effectiveness of the intervention and consider the need for a new appointment, reiterating the "open door" policy.

Techniques used:

a. Requesting feedback after time: obtaining a post-session evaluation to understand the long-term impact of the intervention.
b. Assessment of need for reappointment: deciding whether additional sessions are needed based on the person's needs.
c. Explication of the "open door": maintaining a sense of continued availability and support.

Single Session Therapy represents a significant shift in the psychotherapy landscape, emphasizing the importance of a focused intervention capable of generating change in a single encounter. Each of these phases is crucial to the success of SST, ensuring that each session is able to generate a significant impact on the person's life.

The Initial Phase

The initial phase of SST is a key moment in the therapeutic process. During the first 10–20 minutes of a one-hour session, the basis for the entire encounter is established.

The introduction of the single session mindset is a process that challenges traditional notions of therapy. Inspired by Milton Erickson (1967) and others (e.g., Iveson, George, & Ratner, 2014), the therapist changes the common perception of therapy as a long-term process by introducing a different perspective from the beginning. The view that change can begin immediately in the same session, in line with G.M. Carpetto's (2008) normalization techniques, represents a significant conceptual leap and lays the foundations for purposeful development.

In this context, the role of the therapist also changes. The client is told that he/she has the freedom to assess the need for further sessions. This not only redefines the therapist from a problem solver to a facilitator of the healing process (a method expert) but also emphasizes the discovery of the person's resources (the client is the content expert), strengthening their autonomy and active involvement in the therapeutic process.

Problem definition follows a focused approach. The focus is on specific problems, defined in operational terms and articulated through the person's language and perspective. This approach, inspired by Watzlawick (1978; also see Gergen, 1999; von Glasersfeld, 1984) and the principles of radical constructivism, requires a high level of listening and adaptation on the part of the therapist, who must tune in to the person's language and provide clarification when necessary. This intervention, together with the importance of setting SMART goals as described by Doran (1981; discussed later), facilitates a clear structuring of the pathway and initiates a process of cognitive and emotional restructuring.

Another key element is the importance of ongoing feedback to ensure that therapy is tailored to the person's needs. Inspired by feedback-informed treatment (Miller & Duncan, 2004), this approach enables effective and ongoing communication between therapist and person, improving the quality of the relationship and the effectiveness of therapy.

Finally, the creation of an effective therapeutic alliance in the first moments of therapy is crucial. Curiosity and genuine interest, as emphasized by Hoyt (2009, 2017, 2025), together with the joint definition of therapeutic goals, highlighted by Norcross (2011), establish a relationship of trust and cooperation. This alliance is not only a means of achieving therapeutic goals but becomes a key element in the person's change and development.

The First Three Key Actions

The process unfolds in a symphony of harmoniously interwoven techniques and mindsets. From challenging traditional concepts to creating an effective therapeutic alliance, each step is designed to facilitate the person's evolution. The single session thus becomes a journey where change begins with the very first session and develops through a tailored therapeutic pathway, guided by the needs and resources of each individual.

1. Define the Problem in Operational Terms

At the heart of SST is the idea that a "problem" can be better understood by breaking it down into specific, operational elements. This concept has its roots in Lazarus and Folkman's (1984) theory of rational action, which emphasizes the need for a detailed understanding of the problem in order to deal with it effectively. Rational action theory suggests that emotions are the result of cognitive appraisals of situations. Therefore, defining the problem in operational terms allows therapists to identify the specific cognitive evaluations that contribute to people's unwanted emotions.

Defining the problem in operational terms means giving a detailed description, including specific relevant behaviors, feelings, thoughts, or situations.

Suppose, for example, that we have a person who reports "social anxiety." To develop an operational definition, the therapist might ask the person to describe a specific situation in which they experienced social anxiety. The person might respond by describing a recent experience during a work meeting, with follow-up questions detailing who was there, what was said, what thoughts and feelings occurred. This helps to make the problem clearer and more understandable for both parties.

Let's take a closer look at another example of how the therapeutic application of operational definition can pave the way for personal improvement.

Case Example

"Claudia" (a fictitious name), a woman in her thirties, faces recurrent and destabilizing episodes of panic attacks. These episodes occur with an almost predictable frequency of twice a week, flare up particularly in crowded places, and follow a pattern of symptoms that include heart palpitations, breathing difficulties, and dizziness, leading to an intense sense of fear and isolation.

The session with Claudia starts with a detailed analysis of the problem. The client and therapist together outline the specific contours of the panic attacks, highlighting not only their frequency and duration but also specific triggers such as closed and crowded environments. This process of definition is crucial, as it transforms the problem from a broad and elusive entity into a series of observable and manageable phenomena.

The session continues by defining behavioral patterns, in particular Claudia's tendency to avoid potentially triggering situations, a strategy that, although intended to protect her, paradoxically reinforces the cycle of panic attacks and limits her social and professional life. The session explores strategies that Claudia has already tried, such as breathing and distraction, providing an important basis for understanding what has not worked in the past and what could be improved.

In this context, it is crucial to analyze how panic attacks fit into Claudia's wider life context, affecting her social interactions and work performance. This provides insight into the function of the problem in Claudia's life, highlighting how panic attacks are not just isolated episodes, but part of a broader fabric that influences and is influenced by her lifestyle and daily interactions.

2.   Clarifying the Objective and Setting Priorities

Clear and measurable goals could be set thanks to the problem definition and the subsequent mapping of Claudia's resources and strengths. These goals, aimed at promoting concrete changes, are the culmination of the problem definition process and the basis for the personalized treatment plan. The problem becomes a set of specific, observable, and manageable phenomena, rather than something broad and undefined. This not only gives Claudia a sense of understanding and control over her challenges, but also guides the therapist in formulating a treatment plan that is rooted in the individual's reality.

Locke and Latham's (1990) SMART model emphasizes the importance of clear and measurable goals. During the session, the therapist and the person work together to formulate a specific and achievable goal. Goals must be Specific, Measurable, Achievable, Relevant, and have a defined Time frame, which helps to maintain clarity and motivation for the person during treatment. In the case of a person with social anxiety, the therapist could work with her to set a SMART goal such as "reduce anxiety in social situations within three months."

Another Example of the Therapeutic Application of SMART Objectives

"Marco," a young 28-year-old engineer, contacted me to get help managing his work-related stress and anxiety, which were negatively affecting his productivity and general well-being. The session conducted with Marco is an example of how effective goal setting can guide a journey. Marco is facing an increasing level of stress and anxiety related to his work environment, a condition that not only compromises his productivity but also affects his general well-being, causing difficulties in concentration and sleep disturbances. These symptoms become particularly acute around important work deadlines, a time when the pressure seems to become unbearable.

In working together, we focused on setting SMART goals that would provide a clear and measurable path to change. The goals were calibrated to be specific and directly linked to the problems Marco wanted to address: reducing his stress levels at work and improving his sleep quality. To ensure that these goals were realistic and measurable, I encouraged and Marco agreed to use tools that would accompany him outside the therapeutic context (beyond the single session), such as a sleep diary to monitor actual sleep hours and a daily self-rating scale for stress levels. These tools not only provided concrete feedback on progress, but also helped to keep him focused and aware of his progress.

The goals were translated into a workable action plan. Marco committed to spending time each day practicing time-management techniques such as the "tomato technique" (a time management technique developed by Francesco Cirillo, 2019) to improve his concentration at work. He also decided to establish an evening routine, including reducing his exposure to screens before going to bed, to improve the quality of his sleep at night.

In leaving the door open, I encouraged Marco to keep a diary in which he records his progress and the challenges he faces, a process that not only provides useful information for the therapist but also helps Marco actively reflect on his journey. A follow-up session was also arranged after three weeks to assess progress and make any adjustments to the action plan.

This focused approach and the formulation of SMART goals not only gives Marco a sense of direction and control over his "problems," but also a clear and measurable framework for dealing with and managing work-related stress and anxiety. Well-defined and realistic goals are key to optimizing the effectiveness of the session, allowing Marco to leave with a concrete plan of action and a clear vision of what he hopes to achieve.

3. Asking for Constant Feedback

Ongoing feedback during a session is a fundamental practice in SST. The therapist asks the person about the progress of the therapy and satisfaction with the progress, and the overall effectiveness of the therapeutic process. This allows therapists to adapt their strategies and approaches to the person's needs and preferences, helping to optimize therapeutic effectiveness. Miller and Duncan (2004; also see Lambert, 2010; Prescott, Maeschalck, & Miller, 2017) emphasize that feedback, used systematically, is essential for improving therapeutic effectiveness. This approach paves the way for a deeper understanding and serves as an essential guide for the therapist, especially in a context where time is "limited" to a single session.

By assessing step by step whether the person finds the strategies discussed useful and whether he or she feels listened to and understood enables the therapist to make timely changes in real time to improve the effectiveness of the session. Besides its function of guidance and evaluation, feedback plays an essential role in building the therapeutic relationship. Feeling heard and valued can significantly increase the person's engagement and empowerment in the process. This aspect strengthens the co-operation and trust between the person and the therapist, which is crucial for the success of the session. Feedback is therefore not just an evaluation tool, but an active mechanism that helps to make each session as fruitful and transformative as possible.

Another Example of Using Constant Feedback in a Single Encounter
Can Be Seen in the Story of "Marta"

A 35-year-old woman, "Marta" requested a consultation for a specific problem: anxiety arising from her recent job promotion. Right from the start of the session, we clarify the goals to be achieved. I listened carefully as Marta expressed her concerns, asking targeted questions to better understand her situation.

Throughout the session, I relied on constant feedback. After each significant step in the conversation, I asked Marta to share her thoughts and reactions. This kept the therapy focused on her specific needs and ensured that we proceeded in a direction that she found helpful and comforting. As the session progressed, I used Marta's feedback to calibrate the intervention. If a strategy or idea did not resonate with her, we explored alternative paths. The dynamic nature of the process ensured an intervention in line with her expectations and needs. I also encouraged her to reflect on her thought process and emotional reactions, promoting greater awareness and helping her to recognize and enhance her self-regulation and problem-solving skills.

Toward the end of the session, I synthesized Marta's feedback and integrated it into a personalized action plan. I asked for her opinion on the proposed plan, allowing for further modifications based on her input. This turned the therapy into a collaborative process, where Marta took an active role in her own evolution and growth.

As well as helping the client feel heard and understood, feedback also provides valuable information for the therapist to use in order for him or her to feel effective and satisfied in their professional activity.

A Methodical Person: Report of a Single Session Therapy

"Luca" contacted the Italian Center for Single Session Therapy with a specific request for a one-session therapy. With a history of psychotherapy courses behind him, Luca was faced with a dilemma that had been bothering him for years: his obsessive search for the perfect "study method," which paradoxically had left him in the stagnant state of an unenrolled out-of-course student.

During our one session we navigated the waters of his concerns, in accordance with the SST method. It was clear that Luca, in his zeal, had lost sight of the forest in order to focus on the trees, i.e., he had gotten bogged down in the details of study methods without making any real progress in his academic pursuits. Using constant feedback and rephrasing, we began to draw a map to guide him out of the maze of his obsessive thoughts. It

was a revelation for Luca to realize that he had already absorbed everything about study methods that he needed to learn effectively. I suggested
that he abandon the search for new methods and rely on what he had
already internalized, a kind of "non-method" that worked automatically
and effortlessly.

Luca reported in the online follow-up:

Good morning, Dr. Piccirilli. I'm writing to you 14 days after the interview. As I said in the session, I gave up all control and solutions (practicing the "no method"). The first days were emotionally difficult, but
I discovered that I was still doing what I had to do and the world did not
collapse on me. On the contrary, I started to function again, like gears
that had been stuck for years starting to turn again.

I am not sure how this is possible (because I am not as efficient as
I used to be), but I have actually been much more productive in the
last two weeks than in the previous two months. And most of all, I feel
freer. Sometimes I recognize the tendency to go back to the old script,
but I block it out, I have a kind of useful fear. I can only thank you with
all my heart.

Luca's story is a complex web of aspirations and obstacles, rooted in a
deep insecurity and an obsessive search for perfection. The central problem
presented itself as a paradox: the more Luca tried to optimize his study
method, the further he moved away from his goal of graduating. This
relentless pursuit of efficiency had turned studying into an end in itself,
rather than a means to an academic end.

Luca had developed a kind of meta-study, a continuous and manic
analysis of different learning methods. Initially intended as a way of maximizing time and effectiveness, this process had become a real obstacle.
Every day, instead of concentrating on the content of his lectures, Luca lost
himself in analyzing, testing, and modifying his study methods. The result
was an endless cycle of perfecting techniques that, paradoxically, took him
further and further away from his real goal: graduating.

The aim of the SST was therefore twofold. On the one hand, it was
necessary to help Luca recognize and dismantle this self-destructive cycle,
allowing him to see how his obsession with the perfect method had become
a brake rather than an accelerator. On the other hand, it was crucial to
guide him toward acceptance and trust in the study method he had already
internalized, and to teach him to appreciate the effectiveness of a more
spontaneous and less controlled approach. Essentially, the aim of this single
session was to help Luca realize that he already had the skills and abilities
to learn effectively. The key step was to shift his focus from the relentless

search for the perfect method to the practical application of what he had already learned. The proposed "non-method" aimed to free him from the cage of his own expectations and obsessions, allowing him to adopt a more fluid and natural approach to studying that would not only improve his productivity, but also give new space to his personal life and well-being.

Luca's story, with all its facets and complexities, effectively illustrates the potential transformative power of Single Session Therapy. SST is not only effective for specific problems but also for more complex situations, such as Luca's, where an obsessive drive for efficiency and perfectionism was a barrier to personal and academic success. His story highlights the importance of recognizing and enhancing a person's inner resources, rather than focusing excessively on external techniques and methods.

Future Perspectives

SST, as illustrated by the method of the Italian Center emphasizes the creation of significant changes in a single therapeutic encounter. The method is developed through five key phases: pre-treatment, initial phase, intermediate phase, final phase, and follow-up, each with specific objectives and techniques. These phases are based on principles such as clear and operational problem definition, setting SMART goals, and active involvement of the person through constant feedback.

These fundamental elements guide the person on a path of self-discovery and allow the therapist to establish an effective therapeutic alliance, which is crucial to the success of the intervention.

Luca's case in particular demonstrates the effectiveness of the method in tackling complex and deep-rooted problems. His story, marked by an obsessive search for the perfect study method, reflects a common dilemma in the modern world, where the quest for perfection often hinders personal and professional progress. SST, with its emphasis on the "how" rather than the "why," allowed Luca to overcome his blockage, free himself from the shackles of his own expectations, and embrace a more natural approach to learning.

The theory and practice of Single Session Therapy can be a powerful tool for change, offering people the opportunity to confront and overcome problems through a tailored method that emphasizes the importance of enhancing individual resources and treating each person as a unique entity, respecting their individuality, and promoting a sense of autonomy and resilience.

Time and I: Reflections of a Psychotherapist

Time has deep meaning in my professional life as a psychotherapist, where every day is a journey through the temporal dimensions of human existence. Time, in its inexorable march, has always had a significant effect on me. Sometimes it surprises me with its speed, while at other times it seems to slow down, almost immobilizing me in the constant ticking of the seconds.

Since the beginning of my career, I have been fascinated by the philosophical concept of time. Heraclitus, over 2000 years ago, said that you never bathe in the same river twice. The idea that each moment is unique and that we are constantly changing has always guided my approach.

In my clinical practice, every encounter is a proof of the changing nature of existence. Our bodies, for example, change from moment to moment, and we find ourselves navigating this constant diversity. Memories, thoughts, emotions: everything is transformed, constantly slipping away.

I have studied the theories of time of philosophers such as Hegel, Bergson, and Heidegger. I have always felt that time is more than just a succession of events; it is a force that shapes our lives.

Over the years I began to see the therapeutic "framework" as something flexible, malleable, according to the needs of each individual. The rigidity of the original rules was replaced by a more adaptable approach, capable of responding to the unique dynamics of each person.

Time and its interaction with the therapeutic process has always been at the center of my thinking. Why do we meet weekly, monthly, or yearly? These questions have led me to use time not only as a measure but as a therapeutic tool, adapting it to the individual stories of my patients. Over the years, my aim has been to make a positive difference to people's lives by helping them find a new, more functional, and satisfying balance. This mission to help is driven by the belief that therapy (and my work as a psychotherapist) should be about making ourselves unneeded, giving people the tools to deal with their problems themselves.

In this journey toward fulfilling my "mission," the most consistent and natural approach for me is the practice of Single Session Therapy. In this context, each one-hour session becomes a significant step toward self-efficacy and emotional independence for people.

References

Bordin, E.S. (1979). The generalizability of the psychoanalytic concept of the working alliance. *Psychotherapy: Theory, Research & Practice*, 16(3), 252–260.

Cannistrà, F., & Piccirilli, F. (2018). *Terapia a Seduta Singola: Principi e Pratiche*. Giunti. (Published in English in 2020 as *Single Session Therapy: Principles and Practices*.)

Carpetto, G.M. (2008). *Interviewing and Brief Therapy Strategies: An Integrative Approach*. Pearson.

Cirillo, F. (2019). *La tecnica del pomodoro. Il celebre metodo per gestire al meglio il proprio tempo e diventare efficienti e organizzati*. Tre60.

Doran, G.T. (1981). There's a S.M.A.R.T. way to write management's goals and objectives. *Management Review*, 70(11), 35–36.

Duncan, B.L., & Miller, S. (2000). The client's theory of change: Consulting the client in the integrative process. *Journal of Psychotherapy Integration, 10*(2), 169–187.

Erickson, M.H. (1967). *Advanced Techniques of Hypnosis and Therapy* (J. Haley, Ed.). Grune & Stratton. (Published in Italian in 1978 as *Le nuove vie dell'ipnosi*. Astrolabio-Ubaldini.)

Gergen, K.J. (1999). *An Invitation to Social Constructionism*. Sage.

Hoyt, M.F. (1995). *Brief Therapy and Managed Care*. Jossey-Bass.

Hoyt, M.F. (2009). *Brief Psychotherapies: Principles and Practices*. Zeig, Tucker, & Theisen. (Published in Italian in 2018 as *Psicoterapie brevi. Principi e pratiche*. CISU.)

Hoyt, M.F. (2017). *Brief Therapy and Beyond: Stories, Language, Love, Hope, and Time*. Routledge.

Hoyt, M.F. (2025). *Single Session Therapy: A Clinical Introduction to Principles and Practices*. Routledge.

Iveson, C., George, E., & Ratner, H. (2014). Love is all around: A solution-focused single session therapy. In M.F. Hoyt & M. Talmon (Eds.), *Capturing the Moment: Single Session Therapy and Walk-In Services* (pp. 325–348). Crown House Publishing.

Lambert, M.J. (2010). Yes, it is time for clinicians to routinely monitor treatment outcome. In B.L. Duncan, S.D. Miller, B.E. Wampold, & M.A. Hubble (Eds.), *The Heart and Soul of Change: Delivering What Works in Therapy* (2nd ed., pp. 239–266). APA Books.

Lazarus, R.S., & Folkman, S. (1984). *Stress, Appraisal, and Coping*. Springer.

Locke, E.A., & Latham, G.P. (1990). *A Theory of Goal Setting and Task Performance*. Prentice Hall.

Miller, S.D., & Duncan, B.L. (2004). *The Outcome and Session Rating Scales: Administration and Scoring Manual*. Institute for the Study of Therapeutic Change.

Miller, W.R., & Rollnick, S. (2002). *Motivational Interviewing: Preparing People for Change* (2nd ed.). Guilford Press. (Published in Italian in 2014 as *Il Colloquio Motivazionale*. Erickson.)

Nardone, G., & Salvini, A. (2004). *Il dialogo strategico*. Ponte alle Grazie. (Published in English in 2018 as *The Strategic Dialogue: Rendering the Diagnostic Interview a Real Therapeutic Intervention*. Routledge.)

Norcross, J. (Ed.). (2011). *Psychotherapy Relationship That Work: Evidence-Based Responsiveness*. Oxford University Press. (Published in Italian in 2012 as *Quando la relazione terapeutica funziona. Vol. 1 & 2*. Sovera.)

Prescott, D.S., Maeschalck, C.L., & Miller, S.D. (Eds.). (2017). *Feedback-Informed Treatment in Clinical Practice: Reaching for Excellence*. APA Books.

von Glasersfeld, E. (1984). Introduction to radical constructivism. In P. Watzlawick (Ed.), *The Invented Reality: How Do We Know What We Believe We Know? (Contributions to Constructivism)* (pp. 17–36). Norton. (Published in Italian in 1988 as *La realtà inventata*. Feltrinelli.)

Watzlawick, P. (1978). *The Language of Change: Elements of Therapeutic Communication*. Norton. (Published in Italian in 1988 as *Il linguaggio del cambiamento*. Feltrinelli.)

Chapter 20

Finding the Beauty in Every Encounter

The Aesthetics of a Single Session

Pam Rycroft

By now there has been much written about the rationale, the process, and the service provision advantages of an approach to therapy built on the finding of Moshe Talmon and his team that most clients attend therapy just once (Hoyt & Talmon, 2014; Rosenbaum, Hoyt, & Talmon, 1990; Talmon, 1990). Being aware of this finding, it simply makes sense to shift our own therapeutic frame such that the first (and possibly only) session is re-cast, not as a gentle beginning of an ongoing relationship but as a complete therapeutic enterprise in itself—albeit with an open door for further therapy.

Beauty? Seriously??

SST may not be for all practitioners. It requires a particular mindset (Cannistrà, 2021) and a particular energy. But, I believe, it also offers a particular reward. I have heard many a practitioner describe an SST approach with words such as "refreshing," "energizing," and "invigorating." I have watched colleagues moved to tears and have myself experienced a sense of wonder again and again to know that a single encounter can be a healing, change-making experience.

Michael Hoyt (2021, pp. 35–36) has written about the hope and joy of SST:

> How we therapists choose to conceive and construe our clients and our work together can help enhance a sense of what the dictionary defines as joy: a feeling of delight, happiness, and gladness, and a source of pleasure.

I'd like to springboard from this idea and consider the beauty of SST. But further—the implications of *expecting* beauty! The aesthetics. I don't just mean having thoughtfully decorated consulting rooms (though the environment of course plays an important role). I'm talking about an aesthetic attitude—a way of orienting oneself to the world—or in this case, to single session work.

DOI: 10.4324/9781032693828-24

The neuroscientists are telling us that expecting beauty in the therapeutic encounter can help therapists tolerate uncertainty and stay tuned to the process of change. Sarasso and associates (2022) from the Brain Plasticity and Behavior Changes Research Group at the University of Turin write of the human tendency to fit new experiences into existing neural templates in order to avoid the anxiety associated with the unknown. The risk then is that we shut out information that doesn't fit with our existing predictive models and miss the opportunity to learn and grow. They see an aesthetic attitude as one of being open to the beauty of an experience—and, further, of expecting beauty. They go as far as to suggest (p. 3):

> current developments in neuroaesthetics have indeed renewed the interest in the link between knowledge/meaning and beauty [. . .] perhaps supporting the hypothesis that aesthetic sensibility and competences are key factors for the success of the therapeutic encounter.

Not to pretend that the immediate outcome of every single session is beautiful, but to suggest to you that an appreciation of the process—of the form and structure, of the rhythm, the therapist's presence, the interactional dance, and the "music" in the process of a single session—can enhance the therapist's and, in turn, the client's experience of SST. As Roubal and colleagues (2017, p. 6) write:

> To be aware, awake, with senses active, and at the same time relaxed, allowing you to be touched by what happens. [. . .] To remain confident that chaos does indeed make "sense," and that with sufficient support a meaning will emerge. The therapists are not disoriented, but present. They are not idle, but are ready to join the "dance" that unfolds at the boundary where clients and therapists make contact.

But how and where do we find the beauty in a single session?

Aesthetics and Pragmatics

The common view of aesthetics is that it has to do with one's taste and appreciation of beautiful things: a fine piece of art, a sculpture, a poem, a musical composition, etc. This view can be connected back to Immanuel Kant (1790/2000), who called these "judgments of taste." Aesthetic pleasure, as he saw it, comes from the free play between imagination and understanding.

Some writers have sought to broaden this view of aesthetics. For example, Joseph Kupfer (in Zukowski, 1995, p. 45; also see Farber, 2017) sees everyday activities as infused with aesthetic qualities. He uses the example of a basketball game, being "more enjoyable when appreciated as an aesthetic whole, with its

changing rhythms, its sudden grace, and its dramatic tension, finally, deci-
sively, resolved." Seen thus, appreciation of the game is focused on its process
rather than its outcome. As Zukowski points out, Kupfer (whose own interest was in education) invites us to appreciate and create aesthetic value in the
everyday—in particular, those activities that have social significance.

Gregory Bateson (1980)—anthropologist, scientist, cybernetician, and
psychologist—was known for asking: "What is the pattern that connects?"
In his 1983 book *Aesthetics of Change*, Brad Keeney demonstrates how
cybernetics provides an aesthetic understanding of change: "a type of
respect, wonder, and appreciation of natural systems often overlooked by
the various fields of psychotherapy, in Bateson's view" (p. 8). Following
Bateson, he avoids any dichotomy between aesthetics and pragmatics (that
is, techniques/interventions/practical skills), seeing them as recursively
interconnected, with aesthetics as a contextual frame for practical action.
As Keeney points out (1983, p. 187) Bateson held that any action "if it be
planned at all, must always be planned upon an aesthetic base."

More recently, Wulff and St. George (2007) also highlight the relationship between aesthetics and pragmatics in an article intriguingly titled
"Family Therapy, You Make Me Feel Like Dancing." The authors liken
the process of family therapy to the process involved in learning ballroom
dancing. As they see it, in particular the dance moves (the pragmatics)
become dancing when they are coordinated with music, with a partner,
and with other couples on the dance floor. This coordination of the moves
with those contextual elements is the aesthetic.

Thus, the aesthetic goes beyond the basic pragmatics—BUT it can't
exist without them.

A special edition of the 2018 *Journal of Clinical Psychology* was dedicated to what therapists can learn from the arts. The editor, Jesse Geller,
writes of three basic convictions: firstly, that successful therapists work
creatively, whether or not they see therapy as art or science; secondly, cul-
tivating an aesthetic perspective can enhance a therapist's capacity to serve
creatively as an agent of change; and thirdly, that there are valuable lessons
in therapy to be learned from the arts. Within the edition, various writers
look to things learned from dance, painting, music, and the literary arts
that can be applied to therapeutic work. I will refer to a few here.

Process, Structure, and Form

Back, for a moment, to that basketball game and the idea that, when
appreciated as an aesthetic whole, what becomes apparent are its changing rhythms, its sudden grace, and its dramatic tension, followed by its
resolution—in other words, the process rather than the outcome. Does
this description find any echo in your own single session experience? It

certainly does in mine. There is a kind of therapy "dance" with a changing rhythm that occurs across the session. It may not end in resolution as such, but in so far as it is a kind of microcosm of a whole therapy, complete in itself, it offers the opportunity for a good mutually determined ending (we tend to call it *closure*) that is rare in longer-term work.[1]

Of course, in our work with clients, we all seek positive outcomes. But imagine for a moment abandoning any investment in the outcome and simply working in and with every moment. Give yourself the opportunity to imagine truly abandoning the ego involved in hoping to bring about positive change and in simply being as fully present to every moment as it is possible to be. In fact, I believe that an aesthetic attitude in single session work is about exactly this: being fully present to the moment, the here and now, while holding the gestalt, the whole process in mind. This requires an appreciation of form, of rhythm, of the interactional "dance" with its "dramatic tension" and its moments of "sudden grace."

In thinking about process, I think about the form or structure that "contains" it. This takes me to a sort of "map" that we have used at The Bouverie Centre in our teaching of SST, which came about when students asked for some broad guidelines in conducting a session. Described in more detail in Rycroft (2018) and Rycroft and Young (2021), in its essence it involves three phases: a good beginning, a good (if murky) middle section, and a good ending (see Figure 20.1).

Now we were certainly not the first to come up with this three-part idea: some would say it goes all the way back to Aristotle's *Poetics* (see Pivnick,

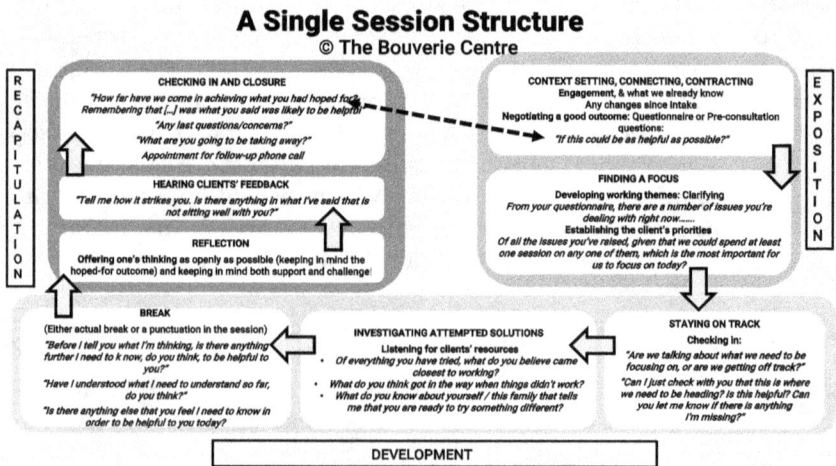

Figure 20.1 The Bouverie Centre's single session "map."

2018). In relation to single session work in particular, Keeney and Keeney (2014, p. 441; 2019) use the analogy of a three-act play for every session, with:

> The beginning act with its communications concerning problems and crisis is bridged to a middle act that enables more choices of understanding and action that, in turn, enables further movement toward a more resource-focused final act.

Personally, I love a musical analogy, in particular, the sonata form. This involves a beginning section, called the *Exposition*; a middle section (*Development*); and a final section called the *Recapitulation*. It may also have small additional parts at the beginning (an *Introduction*) and at the very end (called a *Coda*). The major themes emerge in the first section; are played with and developed in the middle section; only to return in the reflective final section, having changed through the influence of that middle section.[2]

Good beginnings in SSTs also promote the expression of our clients' major themes. As shown in Figure 20.1, this can happen through a pre-session questionnaire and/or at the beginning of the session itself, with questions such as: "If our time together today could be as helpful as possible, what is it you would walk away with?" And if there are a number of themes: "Of all the issues you've raised, what is the most important, do you think, for us to focus on today, here and now?" This helps in engaging/creating a working alliance and finding a focus (that is, establishing what is likely to be a good outcome for the session). One of my own long-held beliefs about therapy that was challenged by an SST approach was the idea that a therapeutic relationship takes time to build and that trust is often hard won. And we know that the therapeutic relationship is central to good outcomes. While our clients are the heroes of change, Duncan, Miller, Wampold, and Hubble (2010) call the alliance the "soul of change" and remind us of Bordin's (1979) three-part definition of the therapeutic alliance involving a relational bond, agreement on the goals, and also the tasks of therapy. So: in its invitation to clients to determine what is important to talk about here and now and what a good outcome looks like, as well as in staying close to the client's experience—working in a truly collaborative way—an SST approach is well placed to create a good therapeutic relationship and lead to a positive outcome.

The (often murky) middle section of a single session is the most exciting (and sometimes nerve-wracking) phase. I call it "murky" because it can feel that way. Here we are balancing a number of things: hearing the complaints or the distress story while listening for possibilities for change;

wanting to give our clients space to tell their story while being conscious of the limited time we have for intervening; allowing for the "variations" in their themes while staying on track—trying to hold a sense of what is most important here and now; etc. And, of course, the more people in the room or on the screen, the greater the balancing act! I also call it "sometimes nerve-wracking" because it can be difficult to sit with the uncertainty in this middle part of the session.

Something that helps hold both the gestalt (a sense of the session as a whole) while working within the moments (see Staemmler, 2006) is the art of moving between content and process, or "checking in," as we call it, with our clients via questions such as: "Are we talking about what we need to be focusing on, or are we getting off track?" or "Can I just check with you that this is where we need to be heading? Is this helpful, or not so much? Can you let me know if there is anything I'm missing?" And in the last part of this middle/development section, with (hopefully) an idea of what our clients are struggling with, our own thoughts about what may help in moving even a step closer to what they want, as well as an idea of our clients' resources, it can be useful to prepare for the final, more reflective section. We do this by asking questions such as: "Before I tell you what I'm thinking, is there anything further I need to know, do you think, to be helpful to you?" or "Have I understood what I need to understand so far, do you think?" Generally, if we have taken the time to understand what's important here and now, as well as having checked in with our clients along the way, it is rare that anything new comes up here. If it were to, then a decision would need to be made about whether it is connected with what we have already heard or whether it may need to be acknowledged as something that can't be dealt with today but should be followed up on.

The final (*Recapitulation*) section (where themes are brought back but changed by what has happened in the development section) is said, in sonata form, to be a reflective phase. In our single session "map," it is also a reflective phase. Some may be fortunate enough to have access to a reflective team (e.g., Young, Prentice, Macri-Riseley, Fitch, & Pati-Tasca, 1997; Harris & Crossley, 2021), but there doesn't have to be a team to use this last part of the session to "think aloud" in front of the client(s), to use one's own honest responses to their story and one's own ideas about what might help. It may vary from a suggested idea or strategy for a step forward (if ideas or strategies were asked for) to something as simple as reflecting a client's dilemma or their stuckness—but doing it with honesty and authenticity. This is a time for acknowledging what the client or clients walked in with, what might have emerged from the conversation that ensued, and a check-in about what they are taking away. In this way, the ending comes full circle, connecting back to the beginning of the session (as represented in Figure 20.1 by the broken line with double arrows).

Then there may be a sort of equivalent of the musical *Coda* in a follow-up—by phone, online, or in person. For those like me, who believe that therapy begins well before any therapy session and ends well after, a follow-up conversation provides valuable feedback about what clients took away, how it was used (or not), and what they want and need therapeutically (if anything) from that point on.

Structure and form are the container for process, and the process helps to determine the form. I am suggesting here that some version of a good beginning, a good (if murky) middle section, and a good ending provide a gestalt that allows for many different models, styles, and therapeutic "pivot chord" moments (Rosenbaum et al., 1990) as well as "moments of sudden grace."

Rhythm—and Sometimes Working "Off the Beat"!

Each person brings to therapy their own themes, their own "music," and their own rhythms that are played out in the mutual interchange between client and therapist as they speak and listen to each other (Geller, 1994). As therapists, we are (consciously or unconsciously) adapting our own rhythms and adjusting the balance between listening and speaking to meet the needs of the particular client or clients we are with at any one time. Our interactional rhythms can be containing and pleasurable or challenging, even threatening. As Geller (2018, p. 206) puts it:

A dialogue that is rhythmically synchronized with respect to the exchanging of the roles of listener and speaker has the effects of softening the bodily boundaries that separate the participants and stimulates a sense of bodily closeness.

Of course, rhythm is not limited to sound: there are rhythms in bodily movements and in eye contact also. It is possible that, if we as therapists find ways to attend to both our clients' and our own rhythms more consciously, finding a shared tempo, we may be able to generate greater choice in our responsiveness—perhaps matching some clients' rhythms in order to reduce their anxiety, or finding a contrasting rhythm when a challenge is called for.

In an article dedicated to exploring what psychotherapists might learn from jazz music, David Johnson (2018, p. 250) writes:

Jazz in particular is a relevant art form with which to compare psychotherapy, because jazz turned music into an improvisational conversation (with structure). The psychotherapeutic interaction, though certainly structured, is in its essence also an improvisational conversation between two people.

He sees a strong link between the way jazz musicians both hold a theme and improvise on that theme according to what is felt in the moment.

Johnson tells the story of Louis Armstrong deciding in 1925 to do something that hadn't been done before. He departed from the standard beat and played just a little before or a little after the beat, before finally picking up the beat again. When asked why he consciously played off the beat, reportedly Louis answered: "Because I know where the beat is!"

To play within a clear frame (in jazz, a 32-bar structure) while sometimes breaking the "rules" and playing off the beat can lead to greater vitality and dimensionality in therapy, Johnson suggests. To do this, he says (pp. 258–259), will be to embrace "a greater sense of risk, allow more moments of surprise, and tolerate greater uncertainty, not just for the client, but more critically for the therapist." However, as Johnson points out, it is always important for the therapist, like Louis Armstrong, to know where the beat is!

Mindset—Yes. But Also "Heart-Set" and "Body-Set"

Flavio Cannistrà (2021, 2022) has highlighted beautifully the fundamental role of mindset for successful Single Session Therapy work. As he writes (2022, p. 77): "How we look—which is directed by our mindset—influences what we see, and what we see influences how we proceed."

This brings us back to our own (and our clients'!) expectations. Being open to the possibility that change can happen, even in a single encounter, adds hope, commitment, and focused hard work to the enterprise.

Eighteen months after the death of her mother, a young client attended a single session at The Bouverie Centre with her father. This followed a conflict between them, which led to a Child Protection notification. In an interview about their experience of the single session, the father put it this way:

> So being the one session, you wanna get as much as you can out of it, so you put more into it . . . you sort of tend to push it a bit more.

And the fifteen-year-old, in comparing her SST experience to some weekly school-based counseling, said:

> When I first started with [individual counselor] I knew I'd be seeing her more, so it [. . .] took me longer to get out what I wanted to get out, whereas when I came here, I got it all out in one shot. I liked that better because with [individual counselor] you wouldn't really get to the inside stuff as much [. . .] whereas it was straight to the point when we were here. [. . .] And I like that better because you do get it all out, whereas if you have a few more sessions I don't think you do.

So, yes—both the therapist's and the client's mindsets play a huge role in an SST.

But what do I mean by heart- and body-set? I mean the need for us as therapists to embrace the excitement and ready ourselves for the emotional "dance" that a single encounter provides. Following Talmon (1993), working from a philosophy that holds our clients as the experts on their own lives enables us to share the responsibility for the outcome with them. But we need to be as resourced as we can be, not as "The Experts," but to use our expertise to help our clients get where they want to get. We need courage to embrace the unknown and the skill and flexibility to adapt our rhythm, our tone, our techniques, and our own "use of self." Being as open-minded and open-hearted as possible, ready with all of our senses attuned, physically and emotionally. Being prepared to face uncertainty and to learn from it through curiosity. Being prepared to hold the beat while going off the beat—if and when it's likely to be helpful.

Being fully present—which sounds easy but isn't. This takes energy and commitment. We're human, and we may need to "check in" with ourselves, physically and mentally, in order to let go of anything that might present an obstacle to our being fully available to the work. For co-therapists, too, this pre-session time can be an important prelude. Because they will need to attend to the rhythm of their own co-therapy "dance," as well as to their "dance" with the client(s). Honest discussion between therapists about any fears, concerns, or likely triggers can be helpful here. Sharing things like: "When I get anxious, I tend to . . ." and "What I'd love from you, if you notice that, is . . ." (For a delightfully honest discussion about co-working as SST therapists with different theoretical preferences, see McGrane & Findlay, 2021.)

Presence and Extraordinary Presence

In a chapter from the 2017 book titled *How and Why Are Some Therapists Better than Others?*, authors Jeffrey Hayes and Maria Vinca pose the question of how therapists overcome all the obstacles (exposure to unpleasant feelings, images, words, and behaviors) to fully engage with their clients and attune to their needs. The truth is, they suggest, therapists are not always present. We're human: we can become overwhelmed by clients' emotions, actions, or lack of progress. Or bored. Or triggered in some way to respond in unhelpful ways.

I hear too often of therapists seeing clients back-to-back, one after the other, with little or no time between to reflect on the previous session or prepare themselves to be as fully present as possible for the next. Just as pre-session questions can be so useful in preparing our client for a single session, therapists' own questions to themselves are also useful. What are we carrying? What judgments, preconceived ideas, distracting thoughts, or feelings are we holding? The more we can empty ourselves of potential distractions, the more we create room to be truly present to whomever we see next.

Hayes and Vinca (2017, p. 95) go on to consider the differences between "ordinary presence" and the rarer "extraordinary presence." Defining "presence" as being aware of and centered in oneself while maintaining attunement to and engagement with another person, "extraordinary presence" is

> a state in which one feels fully and deeply collected, relaxed, open, and watchful. [. . .] One feels energized without a sense of excitement, alert without hyperarousal, sensitive without being identified, calm without being removed.

While these authors regard this as a particularly rare quality, and while we can't all be a Milton Erickson or a Carl Rogers,[3] I want to suggest that the context of an SST has the potential to bring forth in therapists a sense of presence that goes beyond ordinary. The focused nature of a single session means we work hard, in each moment, to understand then help our clients in finding a path forward. This, I believe, leads to a high level of alertness and a seeking of attunement with an energy that is quite different from that experienced in work with ongoing clients. With any first meeting, there is a particular kind of anxiety (or excitement): an edge which primes us to pick up on all the information available to us (not just verbal, but also people's appearance, their expressions, body language, tone of voice, how they carry themselves, where they choose to sit, and so on). In the ongoing work, these things become familiar, and I believe we stop noticing the significance of them in the same way. We can forget what we learned about our clients in that first meeting from our observations as well as from our own responses to them. I can't help but wonder whether this sense of presence (that is perhaps more likely in a first or only meeting) and the connection that follows is what we all seek in the work, and whether this in fact is part answer at least to where the beauty lies.

From Anxiety to Curiosity

It is very normal for even experienced therapists to feel some anxiety prior to and/or during a single session. There are natural tensions, as mentioned, particularly in the middle phase of the session. Our desire to be helpful can lead to a focus on the outcome rather than the process—often resulting in the therapist working too hard—what Michael White (personal communication, 1989) used to call "getting ahead of the clients." According to an aesthetic view, staying with the process and holding an expectation of beauty helps us as therapists distance from our own desire to change the client and the situation, which is likely, paradoxically, to prevent full understanding and connection (Sarasso, Francesetti, Roubal, Gecele, & Ronga, 2022).

Aesthetic pleasure, these same authors tell us, can only follow a certain amount of mental work—a tolerance of uncertainty (or "defied predictability," in their terms), where the temptation to ignore what doesn't fit easily into our own existing frameworks of understanding is resisted. This is the "murky" part. Because of this, and as the ultimate opening to a new understanding, aesthetic experiences could be seen as both disruptive and transformative at the same time.

It is curiosity that is the link between aesthetics and pragmatics and that generates a shift from anxiety to a sense of awe and wonder about what is happening. This is not just about clever questions, but about a stance—a whole orientation to the work—the sort of curiosity that reflects genuine interest in the person and the drive to understand them.

In his book *The Gift of Therapy*, Irvin Yalom (2009) exhorts us to treat every therapy as a new therapy and to work with the here and now. Each client will teach us how to work with them if we are able to tune in to and resonate with their themes. There may be a mixture of harmony and discord, and if we are working with couples or families it will be a polyphony rather than a duet. But if we can find some resonance, this is also where the beauty is. It may happen in a moment, or it may take longer. There may be opportunities for pivot chord moments (Rosenbaum et al., 1990) or those "moments of sudden grace," or it may be simply a shared struggle to make sense of what is happening here and now. Using curiosity and all our senses to stay tuned to our clients in the moment-by-moment work, contained by a sense of the shape and form of the whole, is our best opportunity to find the beauty.

Coda

A coda musically is a sort of "last word." Therapeutically this may involve a final check-in that connects back with our clients' original "theme" or "themes," as well as any arrangements for following up.[4]

Here is my Coda:

SST provides the context for therapists to see a session as a coherent whole, a gestalt, to blend good pragmatic skills and techniques with an aesthetic attitude—the capacity to "hold the process" (the form, the rhythm, the timing, the flow, the pattern of connections) while attending to the moments, even when it doesn't necessarily feel anything like a Beethoven sonata—and being open to the beauty of the work regardless. In preparing ourselves well and expecting beauty, we are more likely to sit with uncertainty, to stay in the difficult moments and the "moments of grace" and to make the most of every session.

Notes

1 While the psychotherapy literature tends to cast the ending to psychotherapy (often called "termination") as a mutually determined, congratulatory, graduation and farewell, experience suggests that such happy endings are rare. Most ongoing therapy ends by default when the client decides not to attend any more. An SST, on the other hand, allows for a clear closure, creative endings (see Hoyt, 2017; Hoyt & Rosenbaum, 2018), and a mutual decision about "where from here."

2 For a great example, listen to the first movement of one of the many wonderful performances of Beethoven's "Moonlight Sonata" on YouTube.

3 Carl Rogers (in Baldwin, 2000, p. 30) himself reflected on the role of presence: "I am inclined to think that in my writing I have stressed too much the three basic conditions (congruence, unconditional positive regard, and empathic understanding). Perhaps it is something around the edges of those conditions that is really the most important element of therapy—when my self is very clearly, obviously present."

4 As Rosenbaum (in Hoyt & Rosenbaum, 2018, p. 322) has written: "We can often end therapy effectively by borrowing a musical technique. Many musical pieces end with a restatement of the beginning theme. Because there have been intervening musical developments, this is not a mere repetition but a return that provides and consolidates the different perspectives that have emerged. Often the statement is followed with a coda that gives a satisfying sense of closure."

References

Baldwin, M. (2000). Interview with Carl Rogers on the use of the self in therapy. In M. Baldwin (Ed.), *The Use of Self in Therapy* (2nd ed., pp. 29–38). Haworth Press.

Bateson, G. (1980). *Mind and Nature: A Necessary Unity*. Dutton.

Bordin, E.S. (1979). The generalizability of the psychoanalytic concept of the working alliance. *Psychotherapy: Theory, Research & Practice*, 16(3), 252–260.

Cannistrà, F. (2021). The vital role of the therapist's mindset. In M.F. Hoyt, J. Young, & P. Rycroft (Eds.), *Single Session Thinking and Practice in Global, Cultural, and Familial Contexts: Expanding Applications* (pp. 77–88). Routledge.

Cannistrà, F. (2022). The single session therapy mindset: Fourteen principles gained through an analysis of the literature. *International Journal of Brief Therapy and Family Science*, 12(1), 1–26.

Duncan, B.L., Miller, S.D., Wampold, B., & Hubble, M. (2010). *The Heart and Soul of Change: Delivering What Works in Therapy* (2nd ed.). APA Books.

Farber, B.A. (2017). Becoming a more effective psychotherapist: Gaining wisdom and skills from creative others (writers, actors, musicians, and dancers). In L.G.

Castonguay & C.E. Hill (Eds.), *How and Why Are Some Therapists Better Than Others? Understanding Therapist Effects*. APA Books.

Geller, J.D. (1994). The psychotherapist's experience of interest and boredom. *Psychotherapy: Theory, Research, Practice, and Training, 31*(1), 3–16.

Geller, J.D. (Ed.). (2018). Special issue: The transformative powers of aesthetic experiences in psychotherapy. *Journal of Clinical Psychology, 74*(2), 197–268. (whole issue.)

Harris, R., & Crossley, J. (2021). A systematic review and meta-synthesis exploring client experience of reflecting teams in clinical practice. *Journal of Family Therapy, 43*(4), 687–710.

Hayes, J.A., & Vinca, M. (2017). Therapist presence, absence, and extraordinary presence. In L.G. Gastonguay & C.E. Hill (Eds.), *How and Why Are Some Therapists Better Than Others? Understanding Therapist Effects*. APA Books.

Hoyt, M.F. (2017). The last session in brief therapy: Why and how to say "when." In M.F. Hoyt (Ed.), *Brief Therapy and Beyond: Stories, Language, Love, Hope, and Time* (pp. 153–176). Routledge.

Hoyt, M.F. (2021). The hope and joy of single session thinking and practice. In M.F. Hoyt, J. Young, & P. Rycroft (Eds.), *Single Session Thinking and Practice in Global, Cultural, and Familial Contexts: Expanding Applications* (pp. 29–41). Routledge.

Hoyt, M.F., & Rosenbaum, R. (2018). Some ways to end an SST. In M.F. Hoyt, M. Bobele, A. Slive, J. Young, & M. Talmon (Eds.), *Single-Session Therapy by Walk-In or Appointment: Administrative, Clinical, and Supervisory Aspects of One-at-a-Time Services* (pp. 318–323). Routledge.

Hoyt, M.F., & Talmon, M. (Eds.). (2014). *Capturing the Moment: Single Session Therapy and Walk-In Services*. Crown House Publishing.

Johnson, D.R. (2018). Playing off the beat: Applying the jazz paradigm to psychotherapy. *Journal of Clinical Psychology, 74*, 249–260.

Kant, I. (2000). *Critique of the Power of Judgment* (P. Guyer, Ed.; P. Guyer & E. Matthews, Trans.). Cambridge University Press. (Originally published in German in 1790.)

Keeney, B. (1983). *Aesthetics of Change*. Guilford Press.

Keeney, H., & Keeney, B. (2014). Deconstructing therapy: Case study of a single session crisis intervention. In M.F. Hoyt & M. Talmon (Eds.), *Capturing the Moment: Single Session Therapy and Walk-In Services* (pp. 441–461). Crown House Publishing.

Keeney, H., & Keeney, B. (2019). *The Creative Therapist in Practice*. Routledge.

McGrane, T., & Findlay, R. (2021). Families at first sight: Practice innovations towards making family SST more friendly and effective. In M.F. Hoyt, J. Young, & P. Rycroft (Eds.), *Single Session Thinking and Practice in Global, Cultural, and Familial Contexts: Expanding Applications* (pp. 267–277). Routledge.

Pivnick, B.A. (2018). Behind the lines: Toward an aesthetic framework for analytic psychotherapy. *Journal of Clinical Psychology, 74*, 218–232.

Rosenbaum, R., Hoyt, M.F., & Talmon, M. (1990). The challenge of single-session therapies: Creating pivotal moments. In R.A. Wells & V.J. Giannetti (Eds.), *Handbook of the Brief Psychotherapies* (pp. 165–189). Plenum Press.

Roubal, J., Francesetti, G., & Gecele, M. (2017). Aesthetic diagnosis in gestalt therapy. *Behavioral Sciences, 7*(4), 70. https://doi.org/10.3390/bs7040070

Rycroft, P. (2018). Capturing the moment in supervision. In M.F. Hoyt, M. Bobele, A. Slive, J. Young, & M. Talmon (Eds.), *Single Session Therapy by Walk-In or Appointment* (pp. 347–365). Routledge.

Rycroft, P., & Young, J. (2021). Translating single session thinking into practice. In M.F. Hoyt, J. Young, & P. Rycroft (Eds.), *Single Session Thinking and Practice in Global, Cultural and Familial Contexts: Expanding Applications* (pp. 42–53). Routledge.

Sarasso, P., Francesetti, G., Roubal, J., Gecele, M., Ronga, I., Neppi-Modona, M., & Sacco, K. (2022). Beauty and uncertainty as transformative factors: A free-energy principle account of aesthetic diagnosis and intervention in gestalt psychotherapy. *Frontiers in Human Neuroscience.* https://doi.org/10.3389/fnhum.2022.906188

Staemmler, F. (2006). The willingness to be uncertain: Preliminary thoughts about interpretation and understanding in gestalt therapy. *International Gestalt Journal, 29,* 19–42.

Talmon, M. (1990). *Single Session Therapy: Maximizing the Effect of the First (and Often Only) Therapeutic Encounter.* Jossey-Bass.

Talmon, M. (1993). *Single Session Solutions: A Guide to Practical, Effective, and Affordable Therapy.* Addison-Wesley.

Wulff, D., & St. George, S. (2007). Family therapy, you make me feel like dancing. *Contemporary Family Therapy, 29,* 87–97.

Yalom, I. (2009). *The Gift of Therapy.* HarperCollins.

Young, J., Prentice, G., Macri-Riseley, D., Fitch, R., & Pati-Tasca, C. (1997). Three journeys toward the reflecting team. *Australian and New Zealand Journal of Family Therapy, 18*(1), 27–37.

Zukowski, E.M. (1995). The aesthetic experience of the client in psychotherapy. *Journal of Humanistic Psychology, 35*(1), 42–56.

Chapter 21

Single Session Therapy in Japan

Perspectives on Past, Present, and Future Methods and Tactics

Keigo Asai

After describing the current situation and challenges of Single Session Therapy (SST) in Japan, this chapter introduces the mindset and models that could be developed as SST to fit the Japanese culture and also describes the potential for the development of SST in Japan.

The First Wave of SST in Japan[1]

The beginning of SST in Japan was first observed in the late 1990s. The first Pan-Pacific Brief Psychotherapy Conference was held in 1995 and the second in 2001, both with Michael Hoyt as a featured speaker (Japanese Association of Brief Psychotherapy, 1996, 2004). Moshe Talmon also visited Japan as a guest speaker at the Japan Telephone Consultation Conference in 2000, which led to the translation of his seminal work, *Single Session Therapy*, in 2001 (Talmon, 1990/2001). However, for about 20 years thereafter, there was no translation or publication of books on SST, and no major SST trend was seen. There are two possible reasons for this. First, in Japan, there is a strong belief that change takes time. One of the few articles in the literature on SST in Japan questions the idea that therapy can be completed in a single session (Tanji, 2007). Another reason is confusion regarding brief therapy. The postscript to the Japanese edition of *Change: Principles of Problem Formation and Problem Resolution* describes brief therapy as "the ultimate single-session therapy" (Watzlawick, Weakland, & Fisch, 1974/1992). In addition, when Talmon visited Japan in the 2000s was also the time when brief therapy was greatly expanding in Japan (Itakura, Sato, & Editorial Committee of Interactional Mind, 2011), and it is possible that SST and brief therapy were seen as the same thing. Since the translation of Talmon's book, several conference presentations, reports, and articles have used the term *SST*. They described an interview structure in which therapy is conducted only once (Nishikawa, 2007), or therapy that results in one-session termination (unplanned

DOI: 10.4324/9781032693828-25

single-session therapy), as SST (Itakura et al., 2011). Most studies have used the term SST in an undefined manner.

Second Wave of SST in Japan

However, major changes were in order in this situation. In 2021, an on-demand workshop on SST was held at the National Foundation of Brief Therapy Japan, an academic conference on brief therapy, with Flavio Cannistrà as the guest speaker (Cannistrà, 2021). The workshop included lectures on the history, mindset, approach, and demonstration of SST by Cannistrà. Many practitioners and researchers learned about SST for the first time here. Since this workshop, *Single-Session Integrated CBT* was translated in 2023 (Dryden, 2022/2023) and *Single Session Therapy: Principles and Practice* was translated in 2024 (Cannistrà & Piccirilli, 2021/2024). SST in Japan is expected to develop further from here on.

Japan's Unique Models of SST

For SST to develop in Japan, it is not sufficient to merely import foreign ideas; an approach that fits the Japanese context is required. Currently, there is no unique approach in the Japanese context, such as the Italian Center for Single Session Therapy Method (Cannistrà & Piccirilli, 2021). However, there are some potential approaches that could be uniquely developed in Japan, such as the Single Session Solution $(3S)^2$ (Wakashima & Nihonmatsu, 2022) and the Revision of the Three Steps Model, which is a brief therapy model (Wakashima, Noguchi, Kozuka, & Yoshida, 2012; Wakashima, Kamoshida, & Nihonmatsu, 2023).

The 3S conducts a multilayered assessment of the individual and the system in a single session and concludes the therapy with suggestions and interventions regarding "what can be done now." Thus, the idea is to aim for completeness of therapy in one session. Another way to describe this would be through the "vertical process," which means to consider the "vertical" work that is done during one session while it is working in the "horizontal" process of a multiple-sessions therapy (Cannistrà & Piccirilli, 2021). The attitude toward realizing this idea is the 3S approach, which is to clarify what is needed now for the client, treat the client as their own expert, and proceed with the therapy.

The Three Steps Model is a brief therapy approach developed in the course of providing psychological support following the 2011 Great East Japan Earthquake (Wakashima et al., 2012). It has recently been revised to be used in contexts other than disaster relief (Wakashima et al., 2023). The therapy proceeds in the following three steps:

Step 1: Treating symptoms, illnesses, and problems with a nonconfrontational, accepting attitude, which includes normalizing the problem, clarifying the problems that accompany it, and reframing it to find meaning in the symptoms and illness.

Step 2: After asking the client about the "worst time," their current state is investigated to identify differences from the worst times and the present. A scaling question, with "10" for the worst time and "0" for the previous period of normal life, may also be used. Reversing the general scaling question and the numerical values not only reveals the differences from bad times but also helps identify the behaviors[3] and resources that have helped to improve it. The client may be asked to continue doing what has helped him/her so far. In addition, the therapist can share with the client the perception that symptoms and problems have subsided over time. If this was the worst time for the client, the therapist could discuss how to move through this period.

Step 3: Clients are advised to "behave differently than before." This can be the severing of a vicious circle in MRI brief therapy or blocking dysfunctional behavior (Cannistrà & Piccirilli, 2021; also see de Shazer, 1991; O'Hanlon, 1999). However, this step may not necessarily be performed if the client is able to navigate Step 2 successfully on their own.

This model primarily focuses on and facilitates the client's *natural recovery* rather than the therapist's intervention. Focusing on natural recovery incorporates the ideas of Morita therapy, which was originated by Shoma Morita in Japan and is a psychotherapy that focuses on accepting suffering as it is and conceptualizing unpleasant thoughts and feelings as natural and uncontrollable phenomena (see Morita, 1998). If 3S and natural recovery are seen as a "mindset," each step of the Three Steps Model may be seen as a specific approach.

Case Examples

Three case studies on the application of the 3S and the Three Steps Model are presented here. Parts of the cases were adapted so that individuals could not be identified.

Case 1: A Child Who Changed the Way She Perceived the Problem by Looking at the Time Frame (Asai & Asai, 2024)

In this case, the author was involved as a school counselor. The client was "Kimiko" (a pseudonym), an 11-year-old sixth-grade girl attending public primary school.[4] Kimiko offered to talk to the school counselor, and counseling was conducted. The school counselor visits the school approximately once a month. Because sessions would be at least a month apart, each session was approached as a potentially complete experience.

Prior to counseling, information about Kimiko was obtained from the homeroom teacher, who clarified that when Kimiko entered grade 6, she was placed in a different class from her friends, with whom she had been in the same class for five years. Because of this change, she now had no close friends in the sixth grade.[5] In principle, elementary schools in Japan have fixed classes for one to two years, and students spend most of their time at school with classmates in the same class. Therefore, not being able to get on with friends in the same class can lead to maladjustment in school life. In the class to which Kimiko belonged, other children were concerned about Kimiko being aloof and approached Kimiko, but she did not join them and preferred being alone. In particular, Kimiko was the only child in this class planning to go to a secondary school different from the other children, and her homeroom teacher was concerned if she would adjust well in the new school. Therefore, the homeroom teacher often approached Kimiko and asked her about her story.

Kimiko told the counselor that it was a real shock for her to be separated from her good friends and that in her current class she was often left alone when making groups in classes. The counselor then asked her: "What do you hope will change here for you to be happy you came to counseling today?" Kimiko responded that she wanted to have friends in the class and be part of her peer group.

The therapist conducted therapy using the Three Steps Model with a mindset (3S) of what is needed for the client now and focusing on Kimiko's natural recovery.

Step 1: The therapist listened to Kimiko's story and normalized her current situation of being separated from her friends.

Step 2: With "natural recovery" in mind, the counselor asked her about her toughest moments (which she scored 10 on a 0–10 scale), to which Kimiko replied, "deciding on the school trip group[6] six months ago," and that she was currently "between 5 and 6." She mentioned the reason for the present score was that some of her classmates approached her and made her join their group, she had a good time on the school trip, and that it was not as bad as when she had to choose a group. However, because Kimiko was unable to recognize and articulate her own behavior regarding the reduced score, the therapist made her realize the reality that things had improved over time.

Step 3: Kimiko had also mentioned that three of her classmates were easy to talk to or she was not scared being engaged with them. The therapist then asked her to find classmates other than these three who she could befriend, without actually having to talk to them. The intention of this intervention was to have Kimiko herself find the exception, as she did when deciding on the group for the school trip. Kimiko seemed reluctant, but when the therapist emphasized that she only needed to observe them, she was open to trying it.

In a follow-up session, Kimiko reported that she was unable to find new classmates with whom she was unafraid to engage; however, since she had only a short time left to spend with her current classmates, she realized that her current situation was good enough. The counseling was terminated, as Kimiko wanted to discontinue it. In the feedback from the homeroom teacher, the counselor found that though her staying alone had not changed, Kimiko responded when other children approached her and sometimes engaged with them happily.

Case 2: An Intervention in Mother-Daughter Interaction Following the Accidental Death of a Family Member (Asai, 2023)

The client, Ms. "Tanaka," a 32-year-old office worker currently living alone, came for counseling because she was worried about her mother, who lives away from her. The counseling was, in principle, one session, but the client could continue if she wished.

Six months prior, Ms. Tanaka's father had died in a car accident, a sudden misfortune for the family. The family was devastated, especially Ms. Tanaka's mother, who still blamed herself that she did not do enough for her husband. Ms. Tanaka has been struggling to talk to her mother. Her mother is a caring person but rarely relies on other family members. It was the first time Ms. Tanaka saw her mother blaming herself, and she wanted her mother to rely more on Ms. Tanaka. Since Ms. Tanaka currently lives apart from her mother due to her work commitments, she is unable to see how her mother is doing and support her (for example, helping her with shopping), even if they do not talk. Since her communication with her mother was mostly through daily calls and messages, her limited involvement seemed to make her anxious.

The therapist discussed the session plan, and they concluded that the most difficult thing for Ms. Tanaka was not knowing what to say when her mother made blaming remarks about herself; this is what they would address. The therapist used the Three Steps Model with a mindset (3S) of what is needed for the client now, focusing on Ms. Tanaka's mother's and Ms. Tanaka's natural recovery.

Step 1: The therapist normalized the following two perspectives for Ms. Tanaka: (1) it is a natural reaction for Ms. Tanaka's mother to blame herself, as all members of their family experienced the sudden loss of a loved one; and (2) it is natural for Ms. Tanaka to not know what to say in response to her mother's comments, as she is going through a difficult time herself.

Step 2: Ms. Tanaka said that her mother's blaming herself had somewhat lessened from when it was at its worst, which was evident in the reduced number of calls and texts in which her mother blamed herself. Therefore, the therapist shared with Ms. Tanaka that her mother was calmer than before. She agreed that the frequency had decreased; however, it was still difficult for her when it happened.

Ms. Tanaka then reported that when her mother called or texted, a routine exchange took place at the start, but as it continued, the mother spoke to Ms. Tanaka in a negative, self-blaming way, for example, "It is my fault that your father died." Ms. Tanaka would say "Don't say that" in response but was unsure and unconvinced whether these words were helpful to her mother and whether she was really dealing with the situation correctly. Her mother appeared relieved, but in subsequent calls/texts she would blame herself again; it was clear that this vicious cycle was being repeated.

Step 3: It was assumed that Ms. Tanaka's mother would calm down further over time, but the therapist suggested the following intervention as a change in behavior from previous ones: Ms. Tanaka would "deliberately" rely on her mother as opposed to wanting her mother to rely more on her. Given her mother's personality, it would have been difficult for her mother to change and rely on Ms. Tanaka immediately. Therefore, it was anticipated that when Ms. Tanaka relied on her mother, the mother would feel that her daughter, Ms. Tanaka, was still a handful—and the content of communication would change from blaming herself to something about Ms. Tanaka. Specifically, Ms. Tanaka would send her mother calls and texts needing pampering with the following content: "I don't like living alone, can I come home this weekend?" The intervention was also intended to change the phone calls and text messages originating from the mother. Until now, Ms. Tanaka had always been at the receiving end of her mother's phone calls and was often not ready for the conversation. This would give her time to prepare for the conversation. Ms. Tanaka was satisfied and eager to try the intervention when the intentions behind it were explained.

Follow-up session: One-and-a-half months later, replying to the therapist's follow-up message asking if additional sessions were required, Ms. Tanaka responded with a happy message that no additional sessions were required and that her request for a transfer near her mother's home was granted. Her mother also felt reassured to have her back, which made her realize that her mother was relying on her. Through a combination of coincidental forces, the major issue of relating to her mother was resolved in one session.

Case 3: Where Attempts to Perform Eye Movement Desensitization and Reprocessing (EMDR) Led to an Improvement in Flashbacks (Asai, 2019)

Ms. "Suzuki," a 43-year-old company employee who lived in an area severely affected by the 2011 Great East Japan Earthquake, had lost her parents to the tsunami generated by the earthquake. Two years after the disaster, Ms. Suzuki applied for free counseling for the survivors. This counseling, with the author, was one session in principle, but the system allowed clients to continue counseling if they wished to.

Therapy was conducted using the Three Steps Model with a mindset (3S) of what is needed for the client now, focusing on Ms. Suzuki's natural recovery.

At the beginning of the therapy, the therapist asked Ms. Suzuki her goals from working together, to which Ms. Suzuki said, "Compared with what I was before the earthquake, the efficiency of my work has declined, and I have become less active, so I expect that this situation will only improve slightly." Specifically, for several months, Ms. Suzuki had been taking longer than usual to read her work documents and was no longer able to enjoy the drinking and band activities she used to enjoy. Not only did she lose her parents in the earthquake, she also experienced post-earthquake flashbacks often (she was haunted by the fact that her parents were swept away by the tsunami, although she did not actually see it happen; she saw the faces of the corpses; recalled the smell when she went to the afflicted area; saw her destroyed home, etc.) and spent a lot of energy coping with this. She had once seen a psychiatrist, but she drank the prescribed medication with alcohol and cried so hard at home that she discontinued the sessions on her own after that.

The therapist listened to her according to a Three Steps Model.

Step 1: The therapist characterized the reactions she had to the trauma as normal, even regarding their perceived abnormality.
Step 2: Given the time that had passed after the earthquake, the therapist helped Ms. Suzuki to see that her symptoms had somewhat calmed down since the time they were at their worst. The therapist complimented Ms. Suzuki for doing her utmost despite her flashbacks and

affected vitality and work efficiency. In fact, Ms. Suzuki had reported that despite these symptoms, she had not caused any problems for others at work, such as missing deadlines.

Step 3: The therapist suggested the implementation of EDMR, which has a proven track record in dealing with flashback memories (e.g., see Shapiro, 2001), because flashbacks had a serious impact on her daily life. The therapist explained the advantages and disadvantages of EMDR and recommended that it be performed in the next session, two weeks later, to which Ms. Suzuki agreed.

Surprisingly, at the beginning of the EDMR session two weeks later, the client mentioned that her condition had improved, specifically, how her work efficiency had increased and she had been able to read three books in two weeks. Her flashback frequency had decreased significantly as if they were a "haze." She said, "When I heard what EMDR is, I realized that I am in a serious situation. Because everyone has had the same disaster experience, I did not want to speak much about how much trouble I was having in my situation." Therefore, EMDR was shelved; instead, she was complimented on her current state and was informed that she could approach the therapist whenever needed. Ms. Suzuki recovered on her own without EMDR.

A follow-up call confirmed that Ms. Suzuki's symptoms had resolved; hence, the treatment with her was concluded.

To Promote SST in Japan

The current concern with the spread of SST in Japan is that it will be considered a "model" of psychotherapy rather than a "method," same as brief therapy, cognitive behavioral therapy, psychodynamic therapy, etc. Therefore, it is necessary to carefully explain the SST mindset to Japanese practitioners. In addition, it should be noted that SST does not eliminate the need for other therapies. Introducing some models as superior implicitly conveys the message that the others are inadequate or lacking. It needs to be emphasized that SST is not lesser or "second-string" but is a therapy that can be fitted "to their approach like a glove" (Cannistrà & Piccirilli, 2021) and does not negate what the therapist has learned so far. In some cases, rather than presenting it as therapy, it may be more acceptable to present it as a comprehensive method of psychological support and an approach that can be used by a range of interpersonal support professionals, including nurses, caseworkers, and teachers. It also may be possible to introduce SST in the form of emergency assistance during disasters, particularly since Japan is prone to disasters and people continue to suffer much after the disaster. Therefore, SST can be used as a psychological support method during such disasters (see Hoyt, Bobele, Slive, Young, & Talmon, 2018; Hoyt, Young, & Rycroft, 2021).

SST (Single Session Therapy) to Single Session Tactics

SST in Japan has the potential to be accepted by practitioners; however, depending on how it is communicated, it may lead to the misunderstanding that SST is a new type of psychotherapy. Therefore, rather than using the term "therapy," it may be introduced as a comprehensive support "tactic." (The word TACTICS can also be an acronym for Therapy, Approach, Counseling, Thinking, Intervention, Consultation, and Supervision!) SST, which has spread worldwide, can be used in diverse ways by practitioners as a strategy for providing support or to support those who support themselves. SST has a wider range of possibilities than traditional psychotherapy. In order to popularize SST in Japan, we will need such "tactics," won't we?

Notes

1 Current Japanese databases allow the cross-searching of articles and abstracts of conference presentations but do not allow searches of abstracts of conference presentations that are not registered, or descriptions in books, including academic books. Therefore, it should be noted that there may be chapters written about SST in Japan other than those mentioned here, or literature that mentions SST in different contexts.
2 A book called *Single Session Solutions* has already been published (Talmon, 1993). Although the names are similar, they are different concepts.
3 The word "behaviors" here refers not only to starting something new, but also to stopping a previously performed behavior.
4 Elementary and junior high schools are compulsory in Japan; students enter primary school at the age of six and attend primary schools for six years and junior high school for three years. Most students attend public primary and junior high schools in their area of residence.
5 In Japanese public elementary schools, class changes generally take place every one to two years. Various considerations are taken into account when changing classes and are adapted to the actual situation of each school. In many cases, the teacher's competence (e.g., more children who are relatively easy to teach are placed in the class of a teacher with less experience), children's academic ability (e.g., children with extremely high academic ability are not concentrated in one class), children's interpersonal relationships (e.g., assigning children who have had major problems in the past to different classes from each other), and other school circumstances are considered. As a result, not all children are happy with their classes and, as in this case, class changes often result in children being placed in different classes from their close friends.
6 Most public elementary schools in Japan have a multi-day educational school trip in the sixth grade, the final year of school, where children have to share rooms and move around with their group members. Children are usually excited to be with their friends.

References

Asai, K. (2019). The use of the Three Steps Model after the Great East Japan Earthquake: A case study in the treatment of flashbacks. *International Journal of Brief Therapy and Family Science, 9*(1), 17–26.

Asai, K. (2023, November 11). *Single Session Therapy in Japan* [Conference Session]. Presentation at Fourth International Single Session Therapy Symposium, Rome.

Asai, K., & Asai, K. (2024). Implementing the revision of three steps model with children. In K. Wakashima, S. Kamoshida, & N. Nihonmatsu (Eds.), *Revision of Three Steps Model*. Tomishobo.

Cannistrà, F. (2021, September 18–October 31). *Single Session Therapy: An Introduction to Principles and Practices* [On Demand Workshop]. 13th Annual conference of National Foundation of Brief Therapy in Japan.

Cannistrà, F., & Piccirilli, F. (2024). *Single Session Therapy: Principles and Practices* (K. Asai & K. Asai, Trans.). Giunti. (Original work published 2018 in Italian, and 2021 in English).

de Shazer, S. (1991). *Putting Difference to Work*. Norton.

Dryden, W. (2023). *Single-Session Integrated CBT (SSI-CBT): Distinctive Features* (2nd ed.). (I. Mohri, Trans.). Routledge. (Original work published 2022.)

Hoyt, M.F., Bobele, M., Slive, A., Young, J., & Talmon, M. (Eds.). (2018). *Single-Session Therapy by Walk-In or Appointment: Administrative, Clinical, and Supervisory Aspects of One-at-a-Time Services*. Routledge.

Hoyt, M.F., Young, J., & Rycroft, P. (Eds.). (2021). *Single Session Thinking and Practice in Global, Cultural, and Familial Contexts: Expanding Applications*. Routledge.

Itakura, N., Sato, K., & Editorial Committee of Interactional Mind. (2011). Brief therapy practice in Japan from 1998 to 2008: Trends and future prospects. *International Journal of Brief Therapy and Family Science, 1*, 68–77.

The Japanese Association of Brief Psychotherapy. (1996). *Global Reach of Brief Psychotherapy*. Kongo Press.

The Japanese Association of Brief Psychotherapy. (2004). *Toward More Effective Psychotherapy*. Kongo Press.

Morita, S. (1998). *Morita Therapy and the True Nature of Anxiety-Based Disorders (Shinkeishitsu)* (A. Kondo, Trans.). State University of New York Press. (Original work published in Japanese in 1928.)

Nishikawa, K. (2007). Intervention strategies and outcomes in industrial counselling: In a workplace that essentially requires single-session therapy [Conference presentation abstract]. *Proceedings of the Japanese Association of Behavior Therapy Conference, 33*, 548–549.

O'Hanlon, W.H. (1999). *Do One Thing Different: And Other Uncommonly Sensible Solutions to Life's Persistent Problems*. William Morrow.

Shapiro, F. (2001). *Eye Movement Desensitization and Reprocessing (EMDR): Basic Principles, Protocols, and Procedures*. Guilford Press.

Talmon, M. (1993). *Single-Session Solutions: A Guide to Practical, Effective, and Affordable Therapy*. Addison-Wesley.

Talmon, M. (2001). *Single-Session Therapy: Maximizing the Effect of the First (and Often Only) Therapeutic Encounter* (Y. Aoki, Trans.). Jossey-Bass. (Original work published 1990.)

Tanji, M. (2007). Some points of view on the end of psychotherapy. *Bulletin of Hanazono University Counseling, 1*, 23–28.

Wakashima, K., Kamoshida, S., & Nihonmatsu, N. (2023). Revision of the three steps model. *International Journal of Brief Therapy and Family Science, 13*(1), 1–5.

Wakashima, K., & Nihonmatsu, N. (2022). A trial of the single session solution (3S): A case study of a family interview completed in one session. *Bulletin of Psychological Support Center, Graduate School of Education, Tohoku University, 1,* 73–81.

Wakashima, K., Noguchi, S., Kozuka, T., & Yoshida, K. (2012). The proposal of Three Step Model based on brief therapy. *Interactional Mind, 5,* 73–79.

Watzlawick, P., Weakland, J.H., & Fisch, R. (1992). *Change: Principles of Problem Formation and Problem Solution* (K. Hasegawa, Trans.). Norton. (Original work published 1974.)

Chapter 22

Multiple Issue Single Session Therapy via Eliciting Client Solutions and Using Hypnosis

Rubin Battino

I have been working in independent practice as a single-session therapist using hypnosis for many years. I see a few clients a week and charge a moderate fee. I receive referrals from the community. Clients contact me when they want to have a Single Session Therapy (SST). Most often clients come seeking help for one particular concern. Sometimes a client returns weeks, months, or even years later for another single session (one-at-a-time; OAAT) concerning the same or another issue—a practice I have come to call *sequential single session therapy* (*SSST*; Battino, 2014, p. 405).

Recently, as in the case I will describe here, I have also experimented with situations in which, rather than clients identifying a single issue for which they seek help, the client indicates that he or she would like to address several issues in the one session—what I call *multiple issue psychotherapy* (*MIP*; Battino, 2023). Initial results have been promising and merit further application and investigation.

Whether for one issue or for more than one, I usually see a client for 60–90 minutes and do not find it useful to spend that time obtaining a detailed history from the client. In addition to basic demographics, my intake form simply asks for a "Brief statement of concern(s) and what you want out of counseling." Traditional psychotherapy generally requires obtaining a history and much information. I do not accept insurance and so do not need the information needed to *DSM* a client and make a diagnosis. Moreover, I do not like the word *problem*, which seems so heavy and ponderous; I prefer to help clients frame whatever has led them to therapy in terms of more temporary and transitory "concerns," "troubles," and "things that bother them."[1] I collect minimal information. A *brief* statement of what is troubling them and what they would like out of the session lets me know, for example, that they are depressed or anxious or have performance anxiety, and an additional question or two lets me know how long this has been going on, without endless details. This is effectively *secret therapy* (Battino, 2022a) since my clients know the history and details about what is bothering them and I do not. As noted, sometimes

DOI: 10.4324/9781032693828-26

clients identify a single issue for which they seek help, whereas at other times, several issues are addressed in the one session.

I operate from various assumptions. One is that *expectations* (Battino, 2006, 2014) are key to success, namely, that it is important that both the client and therapist feel at the end of a session that what he or she wanted from the session has occurred. As Milton Erickson wrote (1954, p. 261): "Deeds are the offspring of hope and expectancy." In 1995 (pp. 91–92), Jerome Frank similarly observed, "I'm inclined to entertain the notion that the relative efficacy of most psychotherapeutic methods depends almost exclusively on how successfully the therapist is able to make the methods fit the client's expectations." Another assumption is that since in SST we see a client only once there is a great advantage in eliciting from them *their* own realistic solutions to their concerns. That is, have the client tell you what will fix or cure their difficulty. In recent years I have developed a number of ways of doing this.

Therapy begins—does it not?—when the client asks for the session. The client is *stuck* in some specific emotion or behavior and expects (hopes, too) that the therapist will have ways of getting them unstuck. Let us consider a case illustration of Single Session MIP. We will then discuss some other applicable methods and then some additional reflections.

Case Study of Elena and Her Four Issues

I had seen Elena once some 30 years before, and whatever I did apparently helped her then. When I ran into her at a celebration of life memorial ceremony for someone we both knew, she asked me to see her again. She is now 64 years old. The following is a reconstruction of what transpired, and it is followed by a commentary. The session was 90 minutes long.

We began with a bit of pleasant chatting, then I asked, "Which issue shall we take care of first?" (This furthered the expectation that issues would effectively "be taken care of.") She replied, "the mold."

Mold Exposure Illness

T^2: When did this start?

C: About five years ago.

T: You know, Elena, that reacting to a mold is an allergy. It is a mistake of the immune system. Allergies also have psychological components. I read a long time ago about a Viennese doctor who had a patient walk into his office who immediately had an allergic reaction to the flowers on his desk. He told her that the flowers were artificial and her reaction dissipated. There is something called the "NLP Fast Allergy Cure" [Neurolinguistic Programming—Andreas & Andreas, 1989; Dilts, Hallbom, & Smith, 1990]. Let me guide you through it.

C: Okay.

T: Are you right-handed or left-handed?

C: Right.

T: Please gently hold your thumb and forefinger on your left hand together. And now, within your mind, think of a recent time when you were in the presence of mold. [Her facial expression starts to change, and I say, "Thank you. Please open the fingers on your left hand."] Elena, to go through this process comfortably it would be useful if you now think of some recent time when you felt really good and okay about yourself. Thank you. While you are thinking about that time just gently hold together the thumb and forefinger of your right hand. Keep them in touch throughout this session. Thank you. If you are comfortable closing your eyes now, please do that, or just look gently off into the distance. [She closes her eyes.] Just imagine now that in this room there is a wall to wall and floor to ceiling transparent wall several feet in front of you. Okay? [She nods.] And, on the other side of that wall you can now see a younger you, from 17 to 18 years ago. The immune system of that younger you is okay and protects you from things like mold. That younger Elena is not at all sensitive to mold. You can see her over there and perhaps even remember what she was wearing back then. She is in a room where there is some mold, and she happily ignores it, as her immune system is working well and has not been fooled. Younger Elena looks up and sees you through the transparent wall. Then, she slowly walks up to the wall, which just disappears. She comes closer to you and then gently reaches out to hold your hands. You look at each other. Then, something interesting happens. Somehow, somehow, through that contact with younger Elena who is now transmitting her functioning immune system into you, she is making you a gift of an immune system that recognizes the allergens in mold and does not react to them at all. You may even feel or sense that within you now, these changes are occurring, so that your current immune system is working properly, just as it was back then in younger Elena. She gets closer to you, and within your mind you now hug each other. Then you sense that somehow younger Elena is fusing into you and becoming an integral part of you. Her immune system is now yours. Within your mind now you smile and thank her for this gift. And you know that all this time the fingers on your right hand had been touching, have they not?

Just taking some slow and easy breaths now, sense the changes in your body. You know that your mind can remember and record things. So, what has happened this afternoon is within you and can be recalled when and as you need it. And now, taking a deep breath or two, stretching a bit, and blinking your eyes, just come back to this room here and now. Thank you.

Finally, just as a check, would you kindly have the fingers on your left hand touch each other? That's enough. Thank you. [There was no reaction at all to the kinesthetic anchor placed in her left hand that had triggered the allergic response at the beginning of this session.]

Commentary on the Mold Allergy SST Intervention: Elena was in a trance. Two "anchors" (fingers touching) were used. The first on the non-dominant hand elicited the allergic reaction, which was easily seen in the client's face. According to the Fast Allergy Cure (Andreas & Andreas, 1989; Dilts et al., 1990), the therapist should guide the client to break this anchor as soon as the reaction is observed. This anchor is used at the end of the session to test if the allergic reaction has disappeared. The second anchor is a "protective" one so that the client feels safe and secure during the session. The ambiguous "magic words" phrase (Battino & Hoyt, 2021) "*somehow . . . somehow*" allows the client to fill in whatever they think will be helpful. In the delivery just described, there are many un-indicated pauses and emphases placed on particular words and phrases. Imagine that you are hearing (and adapting) them in your own style!

Correcting a Diet Difficulty

Elena then told me about an uncontrollable binging on a particular food that she wanted to disappear. This was not about weight control since the binging did not affect her weight. She could just not stop herself from doing this from time to time. I asked her if she felt that when she was compelled to binge that there was perhaps something inside her that "forced" her to do this. She said "Yes." I asked her if she would give a name to this entity, and she responded with "Controller" or "Binger." I wondered if it might be easier to just abbreviate this and just call it "BIN." (She agreed.) I told her that what I was going to do was carry out an exorcism to permanently get rid of BIN from her life. She said that she thought this would work. I told Elena that I needed three things to do this. The first was to find out if she had a preferred way of relaxing. I suggested that paying attention to her breathing would probably work. She agreed. Then I asked her if she had a safe haven, that is, a place she could go to within her mind that was real or imaginary. She responded tha t it was being with "loving family and friends." Finally, I asked Elena if she could think of some powerful healing person or entity that could permanently exorcize BIN from her mind and body. Her answer was her Dad.

T: So, just let's start with you getting comfortable and closing your eyes. It is just one breath at a time. This breath and the next one. This heartbeat. And with each inhale your chest and belly softly rise. Then, with each exhale all those muscles just relaxing. This breath and the next one. Occasionally, a stray thought may wander through your mind. Notice it. Thank it for being there. And go back to this breath and . . .

  And, within your mind now, Elena, just drift off to your own special safe and secure place, a place where you are with loving family and friends. Enjoy being there. Just look around and be at peace.

And, while you are there an interesting thing happens. You become aware that somewhere near you is your healing entity, your healing power, your Dad. Your Dad comes closer to you. Close enough to reach out and touch you, perhaps on a shoulder or elsewhere. And you know that your Dad is knowledgeable and skilled and powerful and loves you. He knows exactly where within your body/mind BIN is located. Then, somehow, he carefully and slowly reaches into your body to wherever BIN is, grabs powerfully and completely ahold of BIN, wherever BIN is located, and is then ready to remove him. And, easily and slowly, your Dad removes BIN completely from your body. He has BIN in a powerful grasp, moves out through the window, and up up high in the sky above the stratosphere. There, your Dad winds up and hurls BIN toward the sun at the speed of light. And we know that it will take eight minutes for BIN to arrive there, fall into the incredible heat of the sun, and disintegrate into tiny atoms never to come back again.

Your Dad then returns to your side, for he has one more thing to do for you. Where BIN was within you there is now an empty space. So, your dad fills that space with love and courage and happiness and joy to sustain you and protect you. Within your mind now you look at your dad, smile at him, and thank him for this gift. He smiles back. Then, he wanders off since there are others to help.

Continuing to breathe slowly and easily, just one breath at a time, one heartbeat. You know, Elena, that your mind has recorded all that has happened this afternoon. You can recall it by just finding a quiet place, paying attention to your breathing, drifting off to your safe haven, and it will be there for you.

Commentary on Correcting a Diet Difficulty: Exorcisms (Battino, 2022a, 2022b; Battino & Hoyt, 2022) can be used for a variety of issues, such as weight control, addictions of all sorts, depression, anxiety, OCD, etc. That is, any issue that is under the control of some internal force or "controlling entity." It is related to the Narrative Therapy mantra of "The client is not the problem, the problem is the problem." Clients readily accept the idea that they are not responsible for their behavior but that some controlling entity or evil spirit inside them "forces them to . . ." I have never had a client reject this odd idea. As noted, the exorcism approach needs four items: (1) how the client relaxes; (2) description of a safe haven; (3) the name (and abbreviation) of the controlling entity; and (4) who or what will serve as the exorcist. Providing a name and abbreviation for the controlling entity reifies it. Note that the client supplies all the needed components. Also note that this is a form of "secret therapy" since the therapist does not have a history or details about the relevant issue—all that is needed is the client's brief description of what is troubling them.

The preceding transcript provides the reader with the language used in an exorcism (Battino, 2022a, 2022b). The procedure uses hypnosis (see Battino & South, 2005). The first two approaches used with Elena are both easily adaptable to working with multiple issues. Other approaches (including those discussed at the end of this chapter) are also adaptable.

Handling Challenges at Work

Elena then reported that she is an experienced schoolteacher and is plagued by an administrator who does not appreciate how she works and who is critical of her. This makes her work environment an unhappy place. I started by telling her something I occasionally told my large freshman chemistry classes,[3] that the teachers they had would vary in terms of how good they were, how well they presented their subject, how much they enjoyed the teacher, and how much they liked attending that class. I told them that they were in charge of their own learning, they paid to be there, and it was their choice as to how much they learned in a course. That is, do not let your opinion of your teacher control what you learn.

One way to not let the administrator control her day and her feelings was to dissociate. That is, at the next interaction to step outside of herself and observe herself and the supervisor from somewhere outside dispassionately. Listen to what was being said and realize that the supervisor was a fallible human being making comments based on his experience and life. They did not really apply to her, did they? She could just watch his mouth moving and actually find something amusing in the whole situation. In a way, it was kind of funny, wasn't it? In fact, Elena could almost sense that there was a transparent barrier between her and the supervisor so that she was protected from what he said. The idea of finding something funny in the situation appealed to her, and this apparently resolved the issue for her. She was actually smiling before we moved on.

Memories of Her Child's Death

Elena wrote, "How my grandson has triggered memories/feelings of my first child who died at 3 years." (I believe that this was also triggered by us meeting again after 60 years at a memorial service.) Grief workers will tell you that grief ameliorates after a few months or years or never, and I mentioned this to Elena. I told her that my wife Charlotte of 61 years had died about three years before. Charlotte is both ever-present for me in the house I live in since she designed the interior, and there are photos and furniture that all remind me of her. Yet, I have adapted to my new lonely life and am surprised that there are times and even days when I do not think of Charlotte. I told Elena that in many ways the "artifacts" in my house bring back memories and that it is the enduring memories that are sustaining and lasting. Elena seemed to find solace in the suggestion of memories being comforting.

This case illustrates how it is possible to help a client in one session who presents multiple issues. The four issues Elena listed were mold exposure, a special diet, challenges at work, and a concern about the death of a child. I elicited a small bit of information about each issue at the beginning of the session and a bit more later when working with each issue. Elena said the session had been very helpful and that she would recontact me as needed.

Let us now consider a few other methods that are often useful in SST (be it for one issue or MIP), and then conclude with some additional reflections.

Some Other Methods I Have Found Useful in SST[4]

The methods mentioned next can be used in therapies intended to be more than a single session, of course, but they lend themselves nicely to a one-at-a-time SST format since each offers a complete ("single session") experience unto itself.

Miracle Question

The Miracle Question was developed by Insoo Kim Berg (Miller & Berg, 1995, p. 37; also see de Shazer, 1988) after a client told her that she felt her problems would all be fixed if a miracle occurred. After suggesting that the client close his/her eyes I say:

> Suppose that tonight while you are sleeping a miracle occurs, and that this miracle is that all the things that have been bothering you are realistically and permanently resolved. Remember that this is a miracle—your miracle—and that miracles do happen.

Then I go on with the following questions to elicit details of the changes brought about by the miracle:

> When you wake up in the morning after the miracle has occurred, what is the first thing you notice that lets you know the miracle has already occurred? What does your spouse notice (if married, or whoever you are living with)? What is different about your morning routines? If you step outside of yourself and observe yourself post-miracle, what would you observe? What is different? If you have a job, what will your co-workers notice? As you interact with people during your day, what would they notice post-miracle? Suppose in the evening you call a parent or an old friend over the phone, what would they notice that is different in how you respond?

Carry your client throughout his/her day, finding out what friends or colleagues or family members would notice was different. Obtain as much detail about post-miracle behavior as you can. The more details you get, the more real these post-miracle changes become to the client. Avoid asking for changes in feelings or emotions. It is changes in behaviors that are important. Queries about observing yourself from behind or the side are particularly useful. Spend 15–20 minutes eliciting post-miracle details. The miracle question obviously also works with multiple issues.

Guided Imagery Therapy (GIT)

Guided imagery has been used for many years to help clients who have health problems like cancer. I have adapted this approach to psychotherapy (Battino, 2020, 2021a, 2021b). The basic approach is to obtain four pieces of information from the client: (1) what is it that is troubling them that they would like to change; (2) do they have a way of relaxing, and if so, what is it; (3) do they have a place—real or imaginary—where they can go to within their mind where they feel safe and secure, and then briefly describe; and (4) what or who will be able to bring about the realistic changes they desire—then they describe and name their own particular healing/changing being or force. Clients have chosen many healing entities like religious figures or a healing presence or a healing light.

Since this procedure works best when the client is in a trance state, it is induced in Step 2, and the other parts follow. Step 3 is important since it is helpful for the client to be both in a relaxed state and in a safe place within their mind when the changes in Step 4 are presented. It is helpful for the therapist to be adept at using hypnosis. In essence, the client tells the therapist how and what and who will bring about their desired change(s). The client in fact selects his/her own healing entity.

In a guided imagery model (Battino, 2020), in the third step the healing and change entity chosen by the client approaches the client. The most important word at this time is often "somehow." After the healing entity (e.g., a religious figure or healing hands or healing light or healing force) makes contact, I say, "And now, *somehow* . . . *somehow* the healer knows exactly where and how to heal you, to bring about the mental and body changes that you need at this time. You may even sense and be aware of just where . . . *somehow* . . . these changes are occurring." When the healing entity finishes its work the client thanks it within his/her mind for this gift. The magic word here is "somehow," for the client *somehow* picks the way(s) these changes will occur.

Moving/Mirroring Hands Therapy (MHT)

Details on the MHT approach can be found in Rossi and Cheek (1988, p. 39), Rossi (1996, p. 194), and in Hill and Rossi (2017). There are four steps to this approach, and all you need to know is that the client has come to you for help. The following is paraphrased and slightly modified from the Rossi and Cheek (1988) citation, whose heading is "Moving Hands Accessing of Creative Resources":

1. Readiness signal for inner work. "Place your hands comfortably in front of your chest about six to eight inches apart. Close your eyes or look off into the distance. Imagine that there is some kind of force between those hands. If you are ready to begin therapeutic work, will you find your hands somehow moving closer just by themselves to signal Yes? (If there is another issue that you need to explore first, will you find your hands somehow moving further apart? In that case a question will come to you in your mind that we can deal with." [Note: this rarely happens.])
2. Accessing and resolving concerns. "As your mind accesses and explores the relevant and important memories about these concerns, will you find one of your arms drifting slowly down until it finally settles on your leg? This will be a complete and satisfactory inner review of those concerns." [Note: In my experience both arms drifting down sequentially has always occurred.]
3. "And now, your other arm will begin drifting down all by itself as your mind explores many realistic therapeutic possibilities for resolving those concerns. When your mind has found at least three satisfactory practical actions, that other arm will come to rest."
4. Ratifying resolving your concerns. "And now, will you find your head nodding Yes all by itself to verify that you will select one or more of these practical ways of helping yourself? When you know that this is the case, will you find yourself taking a deep breath or two, blinking your eyes, and stretching a bit, and returning to this room here and now? Thank you."

The MHT model is the simplest and most elegant and effective approach that I know. It first gets the client's agreement to work on a difficulty of their choice (the therapist does not need to know what this is!). Then, the client explores relevant factors about this. Knowing those factors the client selects several realistic ways for resolving the original concern. The fourth and final step has the client agreeing to appropriately resolve what it is they came to see you about by using their own solutions! (Please note that Hill and Rossi's 2017 book contains much additional useful material related to MHT than has been presented here. For example, Chapter 13, which is entitled "Personal Access to Your Growing Edge," describes solo and personal uses of mirroring.)

Variations on the Gestalt Therapy Two-Chair Approach

I had a client ("Melissa") who presented with bruxism (grinding of teeth while asleep, which can be quite harmful and painful). She had been to specialty dentists and therapists about this and thought (perhaps with desperation!) to consult someone who did hypnosis. I thought about how I might use hypnosis, but nothing came to mind. Then I had the idea of using the Gestalt Therapy two-chair approach with her in one chair and "bruxism" in the other. I took out two chairs and asked her to sit in one and put bruxism in the other. (It is important to use other chairs than the one the client is sitting in.) I had Melissa talk to bruxism, asking him (can use "it" here, too) how he was helping her by having her teeth grinding away at night. He responded that she needed to suffer a bit. I then guided them like a director in psychodrama to continue this dialogue until bruxism told her that he was no longer needed and that it was okay for her to sleep peacefully. Generally, in my experience, it takes four or more switches until the two entities reach a peaceful agreement.

Upon further thinking about what happened in this session I realized that the unusual approach of confronting a conflict changed the whole dynamic in her experience with bruxism. She had never thought of just confronting this controlling agent and working out a compromise. Think about how this approach can be used with clients who are depressed or anxious or overweight or have OCS or PTS.[5] Guide them into having a dialogue with their anxiety or depression or . . .

Consider how this might work in couple therapy. If there is a session with just one partner, then s/he can put the other person in the second chair. If both are there, then one partner can watch the other have a dialogue, and then switch doing this. Or directly, one will be in one chair and the other across from them. (Again, it is important to use a separate set of chairs for this to dissociate them from their "normal" chairs.)

Originally (see Perls, 1969) the two-chair approach was mostly used for a client to reconcile differences with a parent (dead or alive) or with a significant other. Of course, it can still be used for this—just use your imagination.

Further Reflections

Expectation (Battino, 2006) can be considered to be the main factor in the placebo effect.

This can be used directly in SST (Battino, 2014) when telling clients that we expect to be able to help them in one session (although they can always ask for additional ones). The client has also sought "*Single* Session Therapy" so, from the outset, a seed is planted. The probability of change is enhanced by suggesting to the client at the beginning of the session that they keep somewhere in mind the question, "What are you willing to change today?" This basic Redecision Therapy contract question (see Goulding & Goulding, 1979; Hoyt, 2017, pp. 51–53) implies success in the session and also initiates the client's thinking about *what* they can change. *Hidden* in these openings is the implicit *permission* and expectation of the therapist that change will occur. The word "hidden" is emphasized because giving the client permission to change is a significant part of what we do as therapists, although it is rarely mentioned.

When you see a client for only one session you know very little about them. The methods described in this chapter allow the therapist to work in a "secret therapy" manner knowing little about the client's background. The trick, if you will, is to use approaches where the client tells you in a single session about realistic ways in their life that can "somehow" help them. I hope these approaches will help therapists and clients to be more effective and efficient in single-session work.

Notes

1 Similarly, when dealing with health-medical situations I and my clients prefer *healing language* that is hopeful and not threatening (Battino, 2002, 2010).
2 In what follows, **T** signifies Therapist and **C** signifies Client.
3 In an earlier career, I was a Ph.D. chemistry professor and researcher—and still give chemistry demonstrations and write papers about chemical education (see www.rubinbattino.com).
4 For some additional methods especially applicable in SST, see Battino (e.g., 2014, 2015, 2020, 2021b).
5 I do not like the terms *OCD* and *PTSD* since I do not like the word "disorder" (put there originally by medical people to get conditions into the *DSM*). "Disorders" are difficult things to deal with. That's why I prefer "OCS" and just "PTS" where the "S" is "stress."

References

Andreas, C., & Andreas, S. (1989). *Heart of the Mind*. Real People Press.

Battino, R. (2002). *Metaphoria: Metaphor and Guided Imagery for Psychotherapy and Healing*. Crown House Publishing.

Battino, R. (2006). *Expectation: The Very Brief Therapy Book*. Crown House Publishing.

Battino, R. (2010). *Healing Language: A Guide for Physicians, Dentists, Nurses, Psychologists, Social Workers, and Counselors*. Lulu.

Battino, R. (2014). Expectation: The essence of very brief therapy. In M.F. Hoyt & M. Talmon (Eds.), *Capturing the Moment: Single Session Therapy and Walk-In Services* (pp. 396–406). Crown House Publishing.

Battino, R. (2015). *When All Else Fails: Some New and Some Old Tools for Doing Brief Therapy*. Crown House Publishing.

Battino, R. (2020). *Using Guided Imagery and Hypnosis in Brief Therapy and Palliative Care*. Routledge.

Battino, R. (2021a). Guided imagery therapy (GIT) and mirroring hands therapy (MHT). *The Science of Psychotherapy, 9*, 40–45.

Battino, R. (2021b). Brief therapy via guided imagery and hypnosis. In M.P. Jensen (Ed.), *Handbook of Hypnotic Techniques* (Vol. 2, pp. 170–195). Denny Creek Press.

Battino, R. (2022a). Guided imagery, secret therapy, and the yenta syndrome. *The Science of Psychotherapy, 10*, 47–53.

Battino, R. (2022b). Exorcisms: Brief therapy with hypnosis. *The Science of Psychotherapy, 10*, 46–51.

Battino, R. (2023, June). How to do multiple issue psychotherapy (MIP). *The Science of Psychotherapy*, 38–49.

Battino, R., & Hoyt, M.F. (2021). On using magic words. *The Milton H. Erickson Foundation Newsletter, 41*(3), 13.

Battino, R., & Hoyt, M.F. (2022). Exorcism and the placebo effect in psychotherapy. *The Milton H. Erickson Foundation Newsletter, 42*(2), 11 and 16.

Battino, R., & South, T.L. (2005). *Ericksonian Approaches: A Comprehensive Manual* (2nd ed.). Crown House Publishing.

de Shazer, S. (1988). *Clues: Investigating Solutions in Brief Therapy*. Norton.

Dilts, R., Hallbom, T., & Smith, S. (1990). *Beliefs: Pathways to Health and Well-Being*. Metamorphous Press.

Erickson, M.H. (1954). Pseudo-orientation in time as a hypnotic procedure. *Journal of Clinical and Experimental Hypnosis, 2*, 261–283.

Frank, J.L. (1995). Psychotherapy as rhetoric: Some implications. *Clinical Psychology: Science and Practice, 2*, 90–93.

Goulding, M.M., & Goulding, R.L. (1979). *Changing Lives Through Redecision Therapy*. Brunner/Mazel.

Hill, R., & Rossi, E.L. (2017). *The Practitioner's Guide to Mirroring Hands*. Crown House Publishing.

Hoyt, M.F. (2017). *Brief Therapy and Beyond: Stories, Language, Love, Hope, and Time*. Routledge.

Miller, S.D., & Berg, I.K. (1995). *The Miracle Method*. Norton.

Perls, F.S. (1969). *Gestalt Therapy Verbatim*. Gestalt Journal Press.

Rossi, E.L. (1996). *The Symptom Path to Enlightenment* (Ed. K.L. Rossi). Palisades Gateway Publishing.

Rossi, E.L., & Cheek, D.L. (1988). *Mind-Body Therapy: Methods of Ideodynamic Healing in Hypnosis*. Norton.

Chapter 23

Single Session Therapy as a Tool to Create, Bring Out, and Enhance Clients' Resources

Valeria Campinoti, Angelica Giannetti, Francesca Moccia, Beatrice Pavoni, and Vanessa Pergher

Looking up and translating the definition of the word "resource" (*risorsa*) in the *Treccani* Italian dictionary, we find the following: "Any source or means of providing help, relief, support, especially in situations of need."[1] *Any* medium. *Anything* can be a resource. This means that it is not possible to define "a priori" characteristics that can be identified as resources, regardless of the situation in which they are expressed.

Resources are means, internal or external, that help people to help themselves. They can be cognitive skills, evaluation abilities, and also analysis of a given situation; or even defense and coping mechanisms, i.e., the individual's characteristic responses to stressful situations; they can be temperamental factors, defined as the way of seeing and experiencing the world; or even external factors, such as social support, territorial services, networks, or economic availability (McQuaide & Ehrenreich, 1997; Dryden, 2019; Rapp & Goscha, 2011).

Why Are Resources Important in Psychotherapy?

To answer this question, we need to focus on two main aspects: (1) what works in psychotherapy and (2) people's ability to self-care. One accepted estimate of what works in psychotherapy is provided by Duncan, Miller, Wampold, and Hubble (2010), who attribute up to 87% of the outcome of psychotherapy to extratherapeutic factors, which include the client's own aspects, i.e., what happens spontaneously in his or her life and accidental factors. This is a very important finding: what happens outside the therapy room, what is only related to the client, and what happens in the client's life has a very important impact on the therapy outcome, much more than the techniques used by the clinician, which, according to Wampold (see https://www.scientificamerican.com/article/are-all-psychotherapies-created-equal/) would only count for 1%.

This is linked to the second aspect to be considered when we talk about the client's resources: the capacity for self-care. In their book *How Clients*

DOI: 10.4324/9781032693828-27

Make Therapy Work, Arthur Bohart and Karen Tallman (1999) cite a large body of research showing that people are able to resolve or improve their problem situations, including problems such as alcoholism, borderline personality disorder, and antisocial behavior, without treatment. In addition, 60% or more of clients report an improvement in their situation from the time of telephone contact with the therapist to the time of the first appointment. This effect is called "spontaneous recovery" and also occurs within the therapy process.

Recognizing the fundamental, overriding role of the client and his or her characteristics in the therapy process, we clinicians can focus on the client's resources, on all those internal and external characteristics that, if well communicated in difficult moments, can accelerate resolution. Identifying strategies to create, bring out, and enhance the client's resources can increase the effectiveness of the therapeutic process, especially when therapy may last only one session.

In a Single Session Therapy (SST), the focus is often on identifying and developing the client's resources.

This can be compared to Milton Erickson's (1980; Haley, 1973) "utilization principle," according to which the use of the person's abilities and skills should take precedence over the teaching of new ways of living developed on the basis of what the therapist assumes to be right and functional. The focus on resources will help promote the client's agency (Snyder, 2002; Levitt, Butler, & Hill, 2006), helping them to have confidence in their own abilities and in achieving their goals even if the consultation lasts only one session.

During the session, it is important to establish open and honest communication with the client by asking targeted questions that invite the person to reflect on his or her past successes, times when he or she has overcome obstacles or personal resources that he or she has experienced in other circumstances. This allows optimization of the time it takes to solve the problem, making the most effective and efficient use of that single session.

Our part of the goal constructing conversation is to ask questions that flesh out elements of the client's stated goals in ways that we recognize as initially "impoverished"—that is, lacking certain characteristics. As we assist the client in revising those elements, the client invariably experiences a state where imagination and creative revision can happen.

In what follows, we will explore how Single Session Therapy deals with resources and what the therapist can do to help create them, bring them to the surface, and strengthen them. Excerpts will be presented from SSTs conducted using the method proposed by the Italian Center for Single Session Therapy (Cannistrà & Piccirilli, 2018; also see Hoyt,

2009; Hoyt & Cannistrà, 2019/2023), which involves seven basic interventions:

- defining the problem in operational terms
- clarifying the goal and establishing the person's priorities
- asking for constant feedback
- investigating resources and exceptions to the problem
- identifying dysfunctional behaviors
- complimenting and offering feedback and suggestions
- making explicit the "open door" at the end of the session.

Single Session Therapy: Time for a Change

Time can be perceived as a limitation or as a resource.

- Will one hour be enough to help the person asking for help?
- What can be "solved" or how can a request for help be "fulfilled" in just one hour?
- When you only have an hour, it becomes crucial to move from the vision of "only having an hour" to the awareness of "having a *whole* hour" (Slive & Bobele, 2014).
- How can you "make time your friend"? (Rycroft & Young, 2021)

Time changes the way we look at what we have and how we act to make it a resource. In other words, the *mindset*, meaning "an attitude, a disposition, a way of perceiving that determines the way of doing" (Piccirilli, 2018, p. 49), becomes dynamic rather than static (Dweck, 2008). It changes the vision of possibility and the permission we give ourselves to make change possible with what we have, even with a time limit (which does not include a vision of time as a limit).

Sometimes problems give us the opportunity to work on aspects we have been putting off or avoiding for a "long time." What changes in this context is the vision of reality that activates perceptions (meanings, in relation to our history and experiences) and reactions (in relation to our emotions and actions).

All psychotherapies aim to respond to a request for help with the intent of achieving the best possible adaptation to the environment for that specific person. This is consistent with the Huber, Knottnerus, Green, Horst, and Jadad (2011, p. 2) reformulation of the construct of "health," which defines it as "the ability to adapt and self-manage in the face of social, physical and emotional challenges." The goal is common to all: people's well-being. However, there are differences in the approach to intervention at epistemological, theoretical, methodological, and technical levels.

Epistemology, "the study of what we can know and how we come to know it" (von Glasersfeld, 1984; 1997, p. 30), is a theory of knowledge, a meta-theory, providing the framework within which the theories, methods, and techniques of the various scientific disciplines fit. Epistemology, as a frame of reference, can be an important resource when translated into operational awareness, also supporting internal consistency in technical-methodological terms. The specific methodology brings out the expression of a mindset that is consistent with the epistemological assumptions of brief therapies. Interactionist, systemic, pragmatic, and strategic positions are expressed in the vision of reality and science promoted by their epistemology.

At the Mental Research Institute in Palo Alto (Watzlawick, Weakland, & Fisch, 1974; Fisch, Weakland, & Segal, 1982; Nardone, 2000, 2009; Watzlawick & Nardone, 1997) a new epistemological position began to be operationally translated, rethinking the duration of therapy, the knowledge/function of the problem, as well as the position and role of the therapist in the therapeutic process. There was a shift from a linear, cause-and-effect view to a circular view that embraces complexity at a logical and systemic level. The methodological focus shifts to the "here and now," to functioning and the possibility of change. Every description implies the one who describes it and, therefore, every description can only be an interpretation (von Foerster, 1984, 1997; Watzlawick, 1977, 1984, 1997; Watzlawick, Bavelas, & Jackson, 1967).

We thus move from a view of therapy and the therapist as something neutral and objective to an interactional and systemic vision, structuring the need to enhance the person's resources, depathologizing language, activating a pragmatic research-action methodology, and working strategically on an intervention's efficiency as an addition to the criteria of effectiveness.

In this context, Single Session Therapy, developed in the 1990s by Moshe Talmon, Michael Hoyt, and Robert Rosenbaum (Talmon, 1990; Hoyt, Rosenbaum, & Talmon, 1992; Rosenbaum, Hoyt, & Talmon, 1990/1995), can indeed be a resource. Why? Because it is resource- and strengths-based, it puts the person at the center, structuring shared steps concerning what has worked (i.e., what is functional for him or her) in relation to his or her problem and his or her view of reality. Focusing on the person's resources means (see Cannistrà & Piccirilli, 2018/2021):

- supporting their vision of rather than a theory of the way forward
- using the method so that the person draws resources from it
- treating the opportunity of a meeting as potentially the only one and therefore maximizing all possible outcomes

- acting as a therapeutic guide, avoiding "teaching the way" but bringing out the person's own "maps" for the person to follow his or her own way
- giving the person the power to decide, to choose, by activating himself or herself and assessing whether a whole hour is sufficient for the proposed objective and/or considering an open door with regard to the possibility of continuing (in which case, considering each encounter as complete in itself).

Another way to focus on resources is to tailor the whole therapeutic process to the specific person, starting with the definition of his or her goals for the therapy, even if it will be a single session. This activates personal resources, both internal and external, in a system that includes the relationship the person has with himself, with others, and with his view of reality.

Creating Resources with Single Session Therapy

Defining clear and concrete goals can be a key step in bringing out and enhancing resources.

Indeed, having clear and measurable goals not only provides direction for the session, but also acts as a compass to guide clients in identifying and utilizing skills and competencies that will be useful to them both in session and once they leave the therapy room (Cannistrà & Piccirilli, 2018/2021).

In this way, the therapist and client work together to bring to light resources that are already present in the person but have not been considered in solving the problem; or, through interactive dialogue with the therapist, the person can be encouraged to create new resources during the session (Cannistrà & Hoyt, 2020).

The articulation of focused goals not only provides a clear direction for the session but also fosters the client's sense of perceived efficacy and "active" responsibility in overcoming his or her difficulties. The client is encouraged to see himself or herself not as an individual with limitations, but as a person rich in potential, equipped with the necessary resources to navigate the sometimes-turbulent waters of life (Iveson, George, & Ratner, 2014). Ziegler and Hoyt (2023, p. 22) similarly contend:

Our part of the goal constructing conversation is to ask questions that flesh out elements of the client's stated goals in ways that we recognize as initially "impoverished"—that is, lacking certain characteristics. As we assist the client in revising those elements the client invariably experiences a state where imagination and creative revision can happen.

The definition of the goal guides the course of the session and provides a structured framework that facilitates the connection between the client's resources and the ongoing therapeutic process. Cannistrà, Del Grande, Del Medico, and Pietrabissa (2023) have documented that clients completing a pre-session questionnaire are more likely to deem a single therapeutic encounter sufficient. As the *APA Dictionary of Psychology* (APA, 2023) states, pretreatment preparation for the session "increases the likelihood of the single therapy session being successful."

In addition to defining objectives, closely related to the creation of new resources is investigating the client's theory of change (Duncan, Miller, & Sparks, 2004). Exploring the client's theory of change in relation to the problem they have brought to therapy is a fundamental moment of understanding and collaboration, providing valuable insights into his or her inner beliefs, expectations, and resources. During the session, an attempt is made to understand how the client perceives the path to personal change. What are his or her beliefs about the key factors that can positively influence the problematic situation? In the context of the desired change, how does he or she interpret the role of his or her own actions, interpersonal relationships, or ways of thinking? These questions, and many others, are designed to explore the client's unique perspective and help to create a kind of "conceptual map" of his or her transformation process. In addition, exploring the theory of change opens up a space to discuss any resistance or fears that may emerge in the course of therapy. Understanding the client's perceptions of the challenges and successes of change provides a fertile ground for working together to construct personalized and, above all, effective strategies.

In summary, exploring the client's goals and theory of change not only contributes to building an empathic connection and a deep understanding of the client's world, but also provides an essential framework for shaping the therapeutic pathway in a way that is aligned with the client's unique perspectives and resources.

Clinical Examples

Case 1: Defining the Problem in Operational Terms and Clarifying the Goal and Establishing the Person's Priorities

"Nina" (a pseudonym), a young woman of 35, contacted us five months after the end of her relationship because, despite all her efforts to leave it, she was haunted by thoughts and questions about how the relationship ended. We conducted SST according to the method proposed by the Italian Center for Single Session Therapy.

T²:So, Nina, I ask you today, what do you think we should focus on? As I explained to you in our phone call, I would like us to define well in each meeting what the goal is, so that we can focus on what is the priority for you and work on it.

C: There is only one thought that has plagued me for months. I can't understand why, although I know I'm hurting, I can't find the strength and the tools to move on. Why does my brain keep getting stuck on this story that is over? Why do I spend my time thinking about this? It's been going on for months now and it's not good because it's affecting my whole life, whether it's work, family relationships, social relationships. I spend all my days focusing on him. In short . . . questions that I have no answers to, but probably only one answer: he did not love me and so he moved on, and I am stuck with something that I may have built up in my head.

T: So, tell me, if I understand you correctly, what you want is to find the tools that will allow you to put an end to the past and, above all, to ensure that your days are not completely taken up by a constant brooding over this ended story that causes you repercussions in all the most important areas of your life.

C: Exactly, absolutely. It's a distress that I feel physically, mentally, that affects everything. I feel I'm heavy, boring, unpleasant, ugly, unfriendly. Things go on and I don't understand why I don't go on.

T: So, the goal, in your opinion, is what? Is it to finally close with the past? Could we see it that way?

C: Yes, sure.

T: Today, if we wanted to take the first small step toward this goal, what would it be? Think of the goal, which is "At the end of our sessions I want to be done with the past, I want to be centered and re-centered in all aspects of my life," and try to break it up. By breaking it up, we can get there in a way that is not stressful for you, does that fit?

C: Yes, I agree. First of all, I would like to feel better physically when I wake up in the morning, because I have a constant feeling of discomfort and anxiety, anxiety that makes my heart beat faster and my stomach and throat close up. I wish I could start breathing, because I think I have forgotten how to do it. To start and also feel a sense of energy, to say, "Ah, today I feel really good!" I don't know how to explain it. That is to have that energy, that desire to say, "OK, I'm ready to face this day." I would like to face my commitments differently: to have the enthusiasm that I had a long time ago, before this. That would change everything.

T: So, if this meeting would be useful for you, we should make sure that when you wake up in the morning you feel your body full of energy, your breathing changes, and you are able to start the day without heaviness, with enthusiasm.

Case 2: Bringing Out Resources With Single Session Therapy

If goal setting allows the therapist and client to collaborate in the elicitation of resources, exploring exceptions to the problem helps to identify and draw out the—seemingly inaccessible—resources already present in the client (following the logics of *Create New Awareness* and *Evoke New Resources*—Cannistrà & Hoyt, 2020/2023).

According to de Shazer, Dolan, Korman, Trepper, and McCollum (2007, p. 4), *exceptions* represent what happens when the disorder does not manifest itself. Every problem has periods when it manifests itself to a lesser extent or when the person has managed to deal with it successfully. By exploring these positive exceptions, the therapist can identify and return to the client the actions the individual took in the past or present to cope with the problem. Consistent with the Formula First-Session Task (Weiner-Davis, de Shazer, & Gingrich, 1987; reported in Hoyt, 2025, p. 91) that asks "Between now and next time we meet, I would like you to observe, so that you can describe to me next time, what happens that you want to continue to have happen," this process of "putting difference to work" (de Shazer, 1991) corresponds to the solution-focused principle "If something works, do more of it."

Together with looking for exceptions to the problem, another strategy that allows resources to emerge is the use of feedback and compliments, which function as positive reinforcement of what the person has done or is doing to deal with the problem.

The following clinical excerpt highlights these steps.

"Maria" contacted us because for several months she had been unable to control herself and was often tempted to binge eat. Her wish was to regain control over her eating and to be able to live her daily life without worries. We conducted SST according to the method proposed by the Italian Center for Single Session Therapy.

T: In the past, did it happen that the problem did not occur or occurred less frequently at certain times?

C: When I'm with my parents or friends, or when I'm on holiday, I don't really feel the need to overeat. I don't think about it.

T: And how did you manage to lose weight during the COVID lockdown, despite not moving, going out, or being distracted?

C: At that time, with less work and more free time, I was able to focus on myself. I could fill the day with more enjoyable activities.

T: So, correct me if I'm wrong, during the lockdown you had time for the activities you liked and were able to take care of yourself.

C: (*nods*)

T: Well, congratulations. The pandemic period was not easy, and maintaining a daily routine was even less so. You did it. Despite the change, you found your regularity. Well done.

C: (*smiles*)

T: How does the fact that you were able to do all this during that difficult time help you cope better with your daily life?

C: On second thought, if I was able to succeed during such a difficult time, why shouldn't I succeed now that the situation is less complicated?

T: What does that say about you?

C: That I am able to deal with challenging situations and to do so I can remember this moment of success.

Case 3: Strengthening Resources With Single Session Therapy

Sometimes the client needs to be helped to strengthen resources, to see or do things in new ways, directly in the session. The therapist can achieve this effect by using specific techniques capable of inducing changes in the person's perceptions and behavior (following the logics of *Create Awareness, Evoke New Resources,* and *Small Changes*—Cannistrà & Hoyt, 2020/2023). Some of the techniques the therapist can use to help the person create and reinforce useful resources to get out of his/her problematic situation are the *"as if" technique,* the *Miracle Question,* and *scaling questions.*

The "as if" technique is to invite people to act "as if" the problem that led them to ask for help has already been solved (Fisch et al., 1982). The technique is based on the self-fulfilling prophecy, the idea that if a person behaves as if they have achieved the desired result, then he/she will achieve it. In short, this will lead to changes in the person's behavior and external reactions, creating new beliefs.

The Miracle Question, originally developed by Insoo Kim Berg at the Brief Family Therapy Center (BFTC; Miller & Berg, 1995; de Shazer, 1988; Berg & Dolan, 2001; Cannistrà & Piccirilli, 2021), is a further variation of the "as if" approach and is formulated as follows:

> Suppose tonight, after our session, you go home, fall asleep and while you are asleep a miracle happens. The miracle is that the worries you brought here are resolved and you are satisfied. But you don't know how the miracle happened because you were asleep. When you wake up in the morning, what is the first thing you notice that tells you that this miracle has happened?

Once this question is asked, the client provides a detailed description of what will change after the miracle is obtained. The more detailed the person describes the scenario beyond the problem, the more the miracle will become a reality.

Finally, scaling questions (Berg & de Shazer, 1993; Cannistrà, 2019a, 2019b) consist of helping the person to set concrete, achievable goals and to quantify the progress made using a scale from 0 to 10, where 10 represents the absence of the problem and 0 its worst manifestation. One way of using it in a resource-oriented way, for example, is to ask clients to describe in the session all the things that would tell them they are on a higher step than they are currently on.

"Antonella," a woman in her early thirties, was referred to a public service for psychological and parental support for families (Center for Families) because during her second pregnancy she had developed a series of fears and obsessions about the health of her newborn son, who had been infected with an uncommon virus that the mother had contracted during pregnancy.

Her aim was to improve her relationship with her son, to manage her fears of illness in a more "rational" way, to regain control of her own life and relationships, also with a view to returning to work. We conducted SST according to the method proposed by the Italian Center for Single Session Therapy.

T: Let's say that tonight, after our session, you go home, you go to sleep, and while you are sleeping a miracle happens. The miracle is that the worries you brought here are resolved and you are satisfied. But you don't know how the miracle happened because you were asleep. When you wake up in the morning, what is the first thing you notice that tells you that this miracle has happened?

C: I would become more autonomous and independent again and get back in touch with my friends, which I have neglected lately. I would ask my mother, who is good at practical things, to help me with my son when I return to work. I would also be more optimistic about work and look forward to going back to work and seeing my colleagues again.

T: What else?

C: I think one day a week would be devoted to taking care of me and what my pleasures are, and not just my duties.

T: Very well. Now, imagine a scale from 0 to 10, with 10 standing for how things are the day after the miracle and 0 standing for the exact opposite—where are you now?

C: Today I am at 4, because one thing I have already started to do and would like to keep doing is to take care of myself and not just my son, following the instructions of the nutritionist I consulted.

T: And if you were at 5, what would you notice differently?

C: I wouldn't leave things to the very last to organize the childcare with my mother when I'll go back to work.

T: I think this will be very useful. You said earlier that you would also like to engage in pleasure activities and not just duty activities. If you were 5, in what ways would you take those opportunities?

C: I think I would reconnect with friends for dinner together, or go to the hairdresser to fix my hair, to start!

T: What difference would that make to you?

C: By taking care of me, I would not feel guilty about my child, and by being well myself, I would be able to be a more happy and better mother.

Conclusions

The process of Single Session Therapy brings therapists and clients into a continuous interaction aimed at guiding the client to explore their own skills, competences, and internal resources to face the challenges that led them to request psychological counseling. The assumption on which SST is based is that people already possess resources, strengths, and coping strategies that can help them overcome many of the difficulties they encounter in their lives (Bohart & Tallman, 1999).

The single session therapist will therefore be engaged from the very beginning in the promotion of the client's agency (Snyder, 2002), i.e., the belief in one's ability to initiate actions and follow paths toward the goal. In SST, the promotion of agency is directly linked to the enhancement of the client's strengths (Bloom, 2001), to the constant reflection on his abilities (Hoyt & Talmon, 2014), and to the transmission of confidence toward change even after a single session (Slive & Bobele, 2011).

In this chapter we have highlighted how, through some specific maneuvers and techniques, it is possible from the very beginning of the single session interview to create, bring out, and enhance characteristics of the client and transform them into concrete resources that can prove to be helpful within the therapy session and in everyday life.

Notes

1 According to Google, the definition in the English-language *Oxford Dictionary* is essentially the same: "a source of supply, support, or aid, especially one that can be readily drawn upon when needed."
2 **T** signifies Therapist and **C** signifies Client throughout.

References

American Psychological Association (2023). *Dictionary of Psychology*. Retrieved September 29, 2023. https://dictionary.apa.org/single-session-therapy

Berg, I.K., & de Shazer, S. (1993). Making numbers talk: Language in therapy. In S. Friedman (Ed.), *The New Language of Change: Constructive Collaboration in Psychotherapy* (pp. 5–24). Guilford Press.

Berg, I.K., & Dolan, Y.D. (2001), *Tales of Solutions: A Collection of Hope-Inspiring Stories*. Norton.

Bloom, B.L. (2001). Focused single-session psychotherapy: A review of the clinical and research literature. *Brief Treatment and Crisis Intervention, 1*(1), 75–86.

Bohart, A.C., & Tallman, K. (1999). *How Clients Make Therapy Work: The Process of Active Self- Healing.* APA Books.

Cannistrà, F. (2019a). *Come trovare le risorse del paziente: la tecnica della scala.* https://www.flaviocannistra.it/2019/10/01/come-trovare-le-risorse-del-paziente-la-tecnica-della-scala/

Cannistrà, F. (2019b). L'elemento dimenticato: il cliente. In A. Alberini & P. Pirro (Eds.), *Verso il benessere. Andare oltre il problema: una chiave per l'autorealizzazione.* Aliberti.

Cannistrà, F., Del Grande, C., Del Medico, R., & Pietrabissa, G. (2023, November 10). Setting the mindset of single-session therapy using a pre-session questionnaire: A pre-post study. Paper presented at 4th International Symposium on Single Session Therapy, Rome.

Cannistrà, F., & Hoyt, M.F. (2020). The 9 logics beneath brief therapy interventions: A framework to help therapists achieve their purpose. *Journal of Systemic Therapies, 39*(1), 19–34. An extended version appears in Hoyt, M.F., & Cannistrà, F. (Eds.). (2023). *Brief Therapy Conversations: Exploring Efficient Intervention in Psychotherapy* (pp. 135–156). Routledge.

Cannistrà, F., & Piccirilli, F. (2018). *Terapia a Seduta Singola. Principi e pratiche.* Giunti Editore. (Published 2021 in English as *Single Session Therapy: Principles and Practices.*)

Cannistrà, F., & Piccirilli, F. (2021). *Terapia Breve Centrata sulla Soluzione. Principi e pratiche.* EPC Editore.

de Shazer, S. (1988). *Clues: Investigating Solutions in Brief Therapy.* Norton.

de Shazer, S. (1991). *Putting Difference to Work.* Norton.

de Shazer, S., Dolan, Y., Korman, H., Trepper, T., McCollum, E., & Berg, I.K. (2007). *More Than Miracles: The State of the Art of Solution-Focused Brief Therapy.* Routledge.

Dryden, W. (2019). *Single Session Therapy.* Routledge.

Duncan, B.L., Miller, S.D., & Sparks, J.A. (2004). *The Heroic Client: A Revolutionary Way to Improve Effectiveness Through Client-Directed, Outcome-Informed Therapy* (rev. ed.). Jossey-Bass.

Duncan, B.L., Miller, S.D., Wampold, B.E., & Hubble, M.A. (2010). *The Heart and Soul of Change: Delivering What Works in Therapy* (2nd ed.). APA Books.

Dweck, C. (2008). *Mindsets and math/science achievement: Teaching, leadership: Managing for effective teachers and leaders.* Paper presented at the Carnegie-IAS Commission on Mathematics and Science Education, New York.

Erickson, M.H. (1980). *Collected Papers* (Vols. 1–4; E. Rossi, Ed.). Irvington.

Fisch, R., Weakland, J.H., & Segal, L. (1982). *The Tactics of Change: Doing Therapy Briefly.* Jossey-Bass.

Haley, J. (1973). *Uncommon Therapy: The Psychiatric Techniques of Milton Erickson, M.D.* Norton.

Hoyt, M.F. (2009). *Brief Psychotherapies: Principles and Practices.* Zeig, Tucker, & Theisen.

Hoyt, M.F. (2025). *Single Session Therapy: A Clinical Guide to Principles and Practices.* Routledge.

Hoyt, M.F., & Cannistrà, F. (2019). Single-session therapy: A healthful approach to effectively and efficiently solving client problems. *Italian Journal of Mental Health* (*Rivista Sperimentale di Freniatria*), *143*(1), 73–85. [in English and Italian]. Reprinted in Hoyt, M.F., & Cannistrà, F. (2023). *Brief Therapy Conversations: Exploring Efficient Intervention in Psychotherapy* (pp. 123–134). Routledge.

Hoyt, M.F., Rosenbaum, R., & Talmon, M. (1992). Planned single-session psychotherapy. In S.H. Budman, M.F. Hoyt, & S. Friedman (Eds.), *The First Session in
Brief Therapy* (pp. 59–86). Guilford Press.

Hoyt, M.F., & Talmon, M. (Eds.). (2014). *Capturing the Moment: Single Session
Therapy and Walk-In Services*. Crown House Publishing.

Huber, M., Knottnerus, J., Green, L., Horst, H., Jadad, A., Kromhout, D., Leon-
ard, B., Lorig, K., Loureiro, M., Meer, J., Schnabel, P., Smith, R., Weel, C., &
Smid, H. (2011). How should we define health? *BMJ (Clinical Research Edition)*, *343*, 4163.

Iveson, C., George, E., & Ratner, H. (2014). Love is all around: A single-session
solution-focused therapy. In M.F. Hoyt & M. Talmon (Eds.), *Capturing the
Moment: Single Session Therapy and Walk-In Services* (pp. 325–348). Crown
House Publishing.

Levitt, H., Butler, M., & Hill, T. (2006). What clients find helpful in psychotherapy: Developing principles for facilitating moment-to-moment change. *Journal
of Counselling Psychotherapy*, *53*(3), 314–324.

McQuaide, S., & Ehrenreich, J.H. (1997). Assessing client strengths. *Families in
Society: The Journal of Contemporary Human Services*, *78*(2), 201–212.

Miller, S.D., & Berg, I.K. (1995). *The Miracle Method: A Radically New Approach
to Problem Drinking*. Norton.

Nardone, G. (2000). *Psicosoluzioni. Come risolvere rapidamente i più complicati
problemi della vita*. Rizzoli.

Nardone, G. (2009). *Problem solving strategico da tasca. L'arte di trovare soluzi-
oni a problemi irrisolvibili*. Ponte alle Grazie.

Piccirilli, F. (2018). Il mindset per una terapia a seduta singola. In F. Cannistrà & F.
Piccirilli (Eds.), *Terapia a Seduta Singola. Principi e pratiche* (pp. 49–65). Giunti.

Rapp, C.A., & Goscha, R.J. (2011). *The Strengths Model: A Recovery-Oriented
Approach to Mental Health Services* (3rd ed.). Oxford University Press.

Rosenbaum, R., Hoyt, M.F., & Talmon, M. (1990). The challenge of single-session
therapies: Creating pivotal moments. In R.A. Wells & V.J. Giannetti (Eds.),
Handbook of the Brief Psychotherapies (pp. 165–189). Plenum Press. Reprinted
in Hoyt, M.F. (1995). *Brief Therapy and Managed Care* (pp. 105–139).
Jossey-Bass.

Rycroft, P., & Young, J. (2021). Translating single session thinking into practice. In
M.F. Hoyt, J. Young, & P. Rycroft (Eds.), *Single Session Thinking and Practice in
Global, Cultural, and Familial Contexts: Expanding Applications* (pp. 42–53).
Routledge.

Slive, A., & Bobele, M. (Eds.). (2011). *When One Hour is All You Have: Effective
Therapy With Walk-In Clients*. Zeig, Tucker, & Theisen.

Slive, A., & Bobele, M. (2014). One session at a time: When you have a whole
hour. In M.F. Hoyt & M. Talmon (Eds.), *Capturing the Moment: Single Session
Therapy and Walk-In Services* (pp. 95–119). Crown House Publishing.

Snyder, C.R. (2002). Hope theory: Rainbows in the mind. *Psychological Inquiry*,
13(4), 249–275.

Talmon, M. (1990). *Single Session Therapy: Maximizing the Effect of the First (and
Often Only) Therapeutic Encounter*. Jossey-Bass.

von Foerster, H. (1984). On constructing a reality. In P. Watzlawick (Ed.), *The
Invented Reality: How Do We Know What We Believe We Know? Contributions to Constructivism* (pp. 41–61). Norton.

von Foerster, H. (1997). Etica e cibernetica di secondo ordine. In P. Watzlawick & G. Nardone (Eds.), *Terapia breve strategica* (pp. 41–52). Raffaello Cortina Editore.

von Glasersfeld, E. (1984). An introduction to radical constructivism. In P. Watzlawick (Ed.), *The Invented Reality: How Do We Know What We Believe We Know? Contributions to Constructivism* (pp. 17–40). Norton.

von Glasersfeld, E. (1997). Il costruttivismo radicale, ovvero la costruzione della conoscenza. In P. Watzlawick e G. Nardone (a cura di), *Terapia breve strategica* (pp. 19–30). Raffaello Cortina Editore.

Watzlawick, P. (1977). *How Real Is Real? Confusion, Disinformation, Communication*. Random House.

Watzlawick, P. (1984). *The Invented Reality: How Do We Know What We Believe We Know? Contributions to Constructivism*. Norton.

Watzlawick, P. (1997). *La costruzione di "realtà" cliniche*. In P. Watzlawick & G. Nardone (Eds.), *Terapia breve strategica* (pp. 5–17). Raffaello Cortina Editore.

Watzlawick, P., Bavelas, J.B., & Jackson, D.D. (1967). *Pragmatics of Human Communication: A Study of Interactional Patterns, Pathologies, and Paradoxes*. Norton.

Watzlawick, P., & Nardone, G. (Eds.). (1997). *Terapia breve strategica*. Raffaello Cortina Editore.

Watzlawick, P., Weakland, J.H., & Fisch, R. (1974). *Change: Principles of Problem Formation and Problem Resolution*. Norton.

Weiner-Davis, M., de Shazer, S., & Gingrich, W.J. (1987). Using pretreatment change to construct a therapeutic solution: An exploratory study. *Journal of Marital and Family Therapy, 13*, 359–363.

Ziegler, P.B., & Hoyt, M.F. (2023, September). Effective goal-constructing conversation in single-session/brief therapy. *The Science of Psychotherapy, 11*(9), 20–29 (online).

Chapter 24

Brief Narrative Practice in Single Session Therapy

Some Lessons From Michael White and Others

Scot J. Cooper

We were fortunate back in the late 1990s, those of us near the city of Toronto, Ontario, Canada. Approximately every three years Michael White, co-founder of narrative therapy, would visit as part of his training tours. These trainings weren't like others, as Michael would facilitate live narrative therapy demonstrations. Michael's sessions were often video recorded, and a workshop audience would watch a live feed. Afterwards, common practice was to then invite whomever he was meeting with to join him in the workshop to debrief the conversation with the audience. It was full transparency as Michael and participants answered questions about the experience of the conversation and practices employed.

What we weren't aware of at the time was that Michael was teaching us a great deal about how to work within the time constraint of a single session. He was teaching a genre of narrative therapy favorable to single session encounters that we have come to call *brief narrative therapy* (Cooper, 2013, 2014, 2024; Young, 2018, 2020). Since those days, Ontario has provided fertile ground for the advancement of Single Session Therapy (SST) by promoting its accessibility through in-person quick access (walk-in) therapy clinics and a provincial virtual format increasing access across the province (see Duvall, Young, & Kayes-Burden, 2012; Sarmiento, 2022; Young, 2011, 2018, 2020).[1]

The walk-in clinic I work at is part of a diverse service menu at a Children's Mental Health Centre in rural Ontario, Canada. The clinic is open every Tuesday from noon to 6:00 p.m. We serve children, youth (up to age 18) and families. It is free to access with no appointment needed. The paperwork is lean, with some pre-session questions that orient the participants toward their competence and a post-session questionnaire (Cooper, 2013) that provides feedback as to process and outcomes. We also offer virtual sessions as part of One Stop Talk, the provincial virtual Single Session Therapy initiative.

Narrative therapy is a postmodern approach that became well-known with the publication of the book *Narrative Means to Therapeutic Ends*

DOI: 10.4324/9781032693828-28

by Michael White and David Epston (1990). It is recognized for its keen attention to the central role story plays in therapy, privileging persons' lived experiences, locating problems outside of people shaped by culture and discourse, as well as creative therapeutic uses of documentation.

While it is often thought that the term "brief" refers to a period of time in which therapy is delivered (such as a single session or 1–8 sessions) this is not the case. Rather, as I have noted in my recent book *Brief Narrative Practice in Single-Session Therapy* (Cooper, 2024, p. 18): "brevity comes about as a consequence of how we think about people, problems, change, and therapy and how these premises shape what we do." The term *brief narrative* speaks to a relational way of being in therapeutic conversations with people in time constraint rather than to a specific set of therapeutic techniques to be followed. In practice we center relational ethics (Reynolds, 2019), exploring people's own know-how that can inform more preferred stories to be enacted. Practice is dialogic, collaborative, non-pathologizing, and concerned with meaning making. Story provides the frames for meaning; the sense people make of life, relations, and themselves as people link events through time according to themes.

Along similar lines, Karen Young (2018, p. 62) notes:

> It is a collaborative, non-pathologizing and competency-focused approach to therapy [. . .] based on the notion that stories are created to make sense of our lives, and that the stories we create then also influence our lives and relationships. Problems are viewed as separate from people's identities and part of the larger context of people's lives. People are seen as having knowledge, skills, abilities, values, and commitments that can assist them to respond to the problems that are influencing their lives.

Brief narrative conversations can involve re-authoring conversations (White & Epston, 1990), assisting people to identify and link the preferred initiatives of their lives into *stories-in-the-making* more fitting with their preferences for life and identity. I use the term *stories-in-the-making* in the context of SST conversations as opposed to *alternate story* or *preferred story* as in the short time we have, often the story is partial and in a state of becoming. It is often not fully contextualized or robust yet is enough to be influential.

Conversations can also provide a venue for people to become more acquainted with, and share, their skills for living and wisdom associated with more preferred storylines. Conversations can quickly pull apart limiting discourses and understandings, assisting people to develop a revised position on a problem or further develop counter practices to the oppression of problems.

All these paths, as White (2007, 2011) noted, provide the context in which people can distance from the known and familiar of their lives and move toward their preferred life. When the material of these conversations is brought into proposals for action, while the meeting may be one session, the therapy stretches beyond the single contact and can prove quite useful to the people consulting to us. White (1992, p. 81) thus wrote: "It is not enough for a person to tell a new story about oneself, or to assert claims about oneself. Instead [. . .] it is the performance of these texts that is transformative of person's lives."

To bring this to life, the remainder of this chapter will outline some brief narrative key concepts especially relevant to SST through a vignette sharing one of my favorite activities when meeting with young people at the walk-in SST clinic. Let me introduce you to Darius.

Darius,[2] an 8-year-old boy, was brought to the walk-in clinic by his foster caregiver Lynn, who was hoping to help Darius "to listen better, self-regulate, and follow the rules at home." It was noted that Darius had experienced years of early developmental trauma and after being brought to a place of safety by child protection services, acquired the diagnoses of ADHD and ODD (Oppositional Defiant Disorder). He was prescribed medication to assist with this; however, it was noted it wasn't helping. I am often invited into these projects of increasing listening, improving regulation or compliance, all of which can seem daunting in a single session. In our meeting room Darius rolled from chair to chair, sometimes bounding couch to chair, yet certainly not settling for more than a few seconds. In these moments I concern myself with finding a way to meet the child through their stories of competence and the enactment of those stories rather than through the telling of the problem.

Meeting People Through Stories of Competence

As noted, Michael White's trainings in the '90s through live interviews taught us a great deal about brief narrative practice. Reflecting on these conversations, often the first 20 minutes seemed rather conversational. Michael would learn about participant interests, important relationships, hobbies, or other material unrelated to what they had come to consult about. This was intentional, as he was meeting people through their stories of competence. What was quickly revealed were the experiences that people brought with them to these conversations that lie outside that of the problem description. That material, as fragments of alternate storylines, often found its way back into the conversation as material to build upon or put to use to address what they had come about.

Meeting Darius through Lynn's caring eyes, I came to learn that he loved video games, although his time with them was often limited, as it was hard to direct his attention away once he had begun. He especially liked Minecraft, where he liked building worlds. As it was noted that he was a skilled builder, Darius stepped into our conversation through this storyline, mentoring me through detailed description of his "best builds." His skills of building, controlling his player, and concentration while playing, stood out to me as possible entry points to a story-in-the-making.

David Epston (2014) notes how anthropological inquiry has influenced narrative therapy in which the "local knowledge" (later called "insider knowledge") of the person consulting is canvassed. In conversation, we are co-travelers and co-researchers of experience (Epston, 1999, 2001, 2014). Therapeutic inquiry is likened to co-research with participants, making visible or "languaging" (Maturana, 1978) into existence people's know-how.

Inviting Darius to mentor me in his abilities has important implications for his experience of SST. It positions him as the knower in this process. As the knower, it is hoped he is experiencing his competence and a sense of being able to direct his life. I am thinking about how to build off his know-how to address the current concerns. This is very different than having to instruct or teach him to learn something new. It is likely he has had many of those kinds of conversations previously. Positioning ourselves in the single session conversation in this way draws our attention to our relational ethics.

Relational Ethics

In SST there is tremendous responsibility for how we are with others, as the likelihood is great that we may not have the opportunity to see someone again to repair a mishap or misunderstanding. Brief narrative practice in Single Session Therapy places an emphasis on the process of therapy informed by *relational ethics* (Gergen, 2021; McNamee, 2009; White, 2011). This involves ongoing consideration of how our practices may affect people in the real world (White, 2011; Malinen, Cooper, & Thomas, 2012; Gergen in Taos Institute, 2023).

Embracing the notion of *relational ethics* under the umbrella of collaborative ethics (White, 2011), we direct our attention to the possible *effects of what we do* on shaping people's everyday living, how they come to know themselves, and what is possible, rather than a sole focus on our ability to execute a technique or achieve a specific outcome. Enacting relational ethics involves the continual monitoring of the process, everything that transpires between and within participants in SST, with attention to the power relations in this context.

Regarding Darius, although he had been prescribed the labels of ADHD and ODD, I chose to meet him through his competence. As our conversation progressed and I heard about Lynn's concerns, I invited them to name this problem in their own words, moving away from an internalized deficit understanding. After receiving a brief description of the caregiver's concerns, we had the following exchange.

Scot: Darius, I see you are very busy and like to be moving a lot, and your foster mom said it can get you into trouble. The doctor called this ADHD, but I'm wondering, if you could give this a name what would you call it?
Darius: My motor! [My understanding is that there are motors and engines in Minecraft that players can use to build.]
Scot: Tell me more about your motor.

In this simple micro-exchange, we invite the participant to name the problem for themselves and a very different storyline starts to emerge. You could imagine where this conversation might now go. We can learn more about this motor and how Darius is able to use it, speed it up, or slow it down. When might he need to slow it down or even turn it off? How does he go about doing that? As opposed to the story of a disordered child, dysregulated, and lacking the ability to direct themselves, new meaning begins to unfold. As a relational ethic, we are resisting the ascription of negative labels and the locating problems as inside of people.

As another example, brief narrative single session practice has moved away from the common SST custom of goal setting and goal speak in general. In ongoing therapy, perhaps "goals" can be revisited, reviewed, and revised; however, in SST we won't have that opportunity. Our concern is that goal pursuit, as part of Capitalistic discourse, could be taken into achieve/don't achieve understandings and should someone not see progress toward the specified goal after their session, they may experience it as personal failure. Given our (limited) time together, we think about narrowing the conversational territory. We ask, "What would be most important to talk about?"—inviting the participant(s) to co-craft a focus while not necessarily specifying a destination. This is in harmony with the idea that these conversations are *problem dissolving*, as people inhabit more preferred stories rather than *problem solving* projects.

In centering relational ethics in our work (Reynolds, 2019), we have come to consider that the process of SST may become hazardous if it involves colonizing practices, inducts people into models of practice, replicates the politics of culture, centers the therapist's agenda, involves normalizing judgment, privileges outsider knowledges, or obscures a person's sense of personal agency.

Michael White addressed the issue of the politics of influence in therapeutic conversation in an interview (White, Hoyt, & Zimmerman, 2000, pp. 97–98):

Interviewer: I'd like to begin by asking you to reflect on how to balance the ideas of *direction* and *discovery*. How do you balance the idea that on the one hand the therapist isn't in charge, is de-centered, but, on the other hand, is still responsible and is actively doing something in therapy? I'm interested in how this is different than having some sort of treatment plan and trying to march the client to a certain place. What do you listen for? Is there a way to listen so that you're participating but not leading? Or are you leading?

White: We're certainly playing a part that is directive in terms of what gets taken up, from these conversations, for further exploration. We do play a significantly directive role in that. But that's not to say that we are directing things in the sense that we are authoring the actual accounts of people's lives that are expressed in these conversations. In all of these conversations we do hear, in people's stories, a whole range of expressions that provide points of entry to different accounts of their lives. Take the videotape of Alice [who had appeared in a videotape that was shown in the workshop]. In these conversations we hear certain expressions that draw our attention to knowledges of life and skills of living that can be relatively invisible to the people who consult us, and the recognition of these knowledges and skills, and on her unique naming of them, I believe that it is quite evident that this is not something that I could have come up with. [. . .] This account of Alice's life, including the general naming of it as "passion for justice," and the identification of the particularities of her life that constitute this theme, is not one that I could have independently or substantially authored.[3]

It's through our relational ethics that we strive to facilitate a socially just therapy, recognizing, as David Paré (2014) does, the "consequential nature of talk" especially as it relates to identity construction. He proposes pro-justice practices such as keeping context visible, carefully attending to responses, inviting evaluation of diagnoses, and separating person and problem.

Returning to Darius, although he had begun to participate in our conversation, he remained in motion and on the periphery to some degree. To meet him in his world, canvass his interest, and facilitate more preferred experiences, I invited him and Lynn into one of my favorite activities. Knowing Darius enjoys video games, it implies he has experience with controllers and directing his player. To canvass this experience, I invited them to play the remote-control game (Cooper, 2024) with me. They agree, and together we each built remote controls from my craft supplies, adding the common buttons, including play, rewind, fast forward, and pause.

Strangely, children seem to especially enjoy adding a volume button that can turn down their caregiver's voice. I explain how the game is played, and Darius agrees to help me test my remote first.

The idea is that as I call out the command from my remote, Darius gets to act it out. We begin with "play," and he starts to circle the room at a moderate speed. Cycling through the buttons, Darius shows us rewind, slow motion, and then fast forward. At this point he is running on the spot, his legs going as fast as he can manage, with some sweat rolling off his forehead. It's at that moment that I transition to press "pause" and when he freezes, I wait and wait and wait until just before I sense he's about to move. At that moment we resume "play" and declare that the remote is working. It is at this point that our questions become important.

Curiosity and Questions

Brief narrative therapy is a therapy of questions informed by our curiosity, as questions provide the best way to elicit people's own know-how and invite dialogue favorable to meaning making. With our questions, we are asking people to mentor us in what they bring to the process that can inform a preferred story-in-the-making. As such, our questions are intentional, seeking to elicit and learn more about people's experience of the problem, competencies, preferred developments, intentions, and hopes for the future. In asking questions, we are actively proposing domains to explore, such as events from the past, present as we know it, and/or within a speculated future. We also use questions to generate experience (Freedman & Combs, 2002), as in answering questions people will re-experience what they are referencing.

Following Darius's unfreezing, I sought to learn from him how he was able to pause so long. Was he controlling his motor? How was he able to speed up or slow down as he needed to? Did his caregiver know he had this ability to *control* his motor, or was this new information? What was it like for her to see that Darius had this ability? Where did they think he could put it to use when they return home after our time together? What might be the benefit of doing that?

These questions activate Darius's meaning-making skills, assisting him to make sense of his experience and generate the concept of self-control. The benefit of this to Single Session Therapy is that in working with meaning generation, there is *always* somewhere more preferred to go in these conversations. Past meanings can be re-negotiated, and new meanings can be co-developed. These conversations are therefore generative of possibility. Through engaging people's meaning-making skills, we invite them to recall and/or reconsider the events of their lives that are more preferred. These exceptions, unique outcomes, initiatives, or counter knowledges can be linked by themes into "stories-in-the-making," that are hope friendly and provide a foundation for plans of action if needed.

Identity Stories

Through our activity, Darius is coming to know himself in a different way, in contrast to being disordered. His caregiver is also being invited to witness this shift. In his workshops Michael used to say, "we are always involved in identity projects in these conversations." He was orienting us to the idea that "identity conclusions are not independently and autonomously manufactured, but are socially negotiated and renegotiated in communities of people" (White, 2001, p. 19). This emphasis on how someone comes to know themselves as socially and relationally shaped invites us to be aware and responsible for not reproducing internal state notions that may erode a sense of agency in single session conversations.

Rather, understanding identity as fluid or as always becoming, opens space for people to come to know themselves differently even in a single conversation. The notion of "migration of identity" (White, 1995) is useful in SST. This refers to how through these conversations people are moving from one way of knowing themselves toward a more preferred way. Whereas people may arrive with negative identity conclusions, through exploration of alternate territories of identity, people are invited to consider and embrace more preferred ideas about who they are becoming, dismantling past limiting conclusions or ascribed negative identities.

Language as Creational

Moving into conversations that assist people to come to know themselves in preferred ways highlights an important understanding about how we talk in single session conversations.

Language is seen as creational rather than representational. The language we use is therefore not neutral but life shaping. Words do things to people. They can hold us in meaning that is common and familiar or take us down different paths to revised or new landscapes of meaning and possibility. Think about the difference in describing Darius as disordered and dysregulated versus someone learning to control their motor. In SST, we take full advantage of the creational aspect of language as we use language to exercise people's meaning-making skills, to generate knowledge and broaden the field of possibility, to invoke presupposition, invite multiple perspectives, and language into existence preferred meanings.

Situating Problems as Outside of People (Externalization)

Externalizing conversations (White, 1984; White & Epston, 1990), as an example of the creational aspects of language, discuss problems as separate from people and are facilitated often within SST (Batrouney, 2019;

Cooper, 2014; Young, 2008) because they quickly invite novel ways to think and talk about problems. Consistent with the narrative therapy concept "The person is not the problem, the problem is the problem," *externalizing conversations* are an ethic of practice as we invite people out of understandings of pathology and internally located deficits into making sense of their experiences as related to what they have been through, perhaps as responses to oppression, injustice, or trespass. Whereas people may arrive ascribed a spoiled identity (Goffman, 1963), through externalizing they may experience a rehabilitation of identity (Lindemann, 2001), coming to see themselves in more preferred ways.

In my article "Brief Narrative Practice at the Walk-In Clinic: The Rise of the Counterstory" (Cooper, 2014), I recount a single session example of externalizing the problem of depression with a youth. Examining "The Depression" as an external entity, he came to make visible Its "discouraging talk" and the many preferred aspects of his unfolding life that countered Its intentions for his future. Along similar lines, rather than "being anorectic," someone might be invited to consider their relationship to Anorexia and how Anorexia attempts to deceive them (and how they can resist). Through mapping the effects of an externalized problem, someone might be asked to consider their relationship to Anxiety (or Anger, or Depression, or Alcohol, etc.) and how It influences them, and they influence It. It is in this conversational space that new proposals for action may come available.

Single Session Therapy as Definitional Ceremony

With attention to sharing stories, meaning generation, identity as relationally shaped, and relational ethics, the therapeutic context of SST has moved away from the traditional psychologically influenced notions of assessment, problem solving, and treatment toward ceremony as a guiding metaphor. Ceremony involves transition, a sense of becoming, performance of meaning, fostering changes in roles or how one knows oneself through various activities. As a single session comes to a close, we mark this arrival in significant ways, often through the use of take-away documentation. This idea is evoked by White's concept of therapy and community work as likened to "definitional ceremonies" (1995, 2000, 2007). "We work to make the therapy conversation a ritual space in which the performance of meaning can occur" (Freedman & Combs, 2002, p. 32).

As a ceremony of sorts, SST provides a venue in which people can enact preferred meanings and be seen on and in their own terms. This assists us to move away from potentially limiting linear concepts of problem solving, binary understandings of problem/solution, or pre-determined destinations for these conversations. This is especially favorable to SST, as it makes possible a vast field of inquiry, multiple trajectories for these conversations, and keeps present the notion of movement through life. Our part in these ceremonies is as witness to this meaning making, who respond in important ways assisting to facilitate as co-travelers on the journey.

To this point in our vignette, there is a sense that Darius is becoming other than who he was when he arrived. It is movement from one way of knowing himself, as a deficited and dysregulated child, toward a revised status, that of learning to direct his life, controlling his motor through practice. This is achieved through the performance of new meanings, with play as the vehicle.

Conversation Endurance

One last time, recalling Michael White's live demonstrations, we noticed that as he neared the end of conversations, he would ask the participant if it would be useful for them to have the ideas that they had co-developed with them when they needed them the most. Engaging them in speculation, he would go on to ask about what difference it would make to them if they had those ideas in their time of need. He would ask their ideas about how to build off this conversation they just had. Michael was facilitating a process inviting the participant to come up with what might be useful to try out or keep with them after the conversation. He was inviting people to re-contextualize the conversation back into their everyday living. He was teaching us ways to have the conversation endure.

Conversation endurance speaks to how we assist these conversations to live on past the face-to-face and be there for people when they need them. I often think of them like the ripples caused by a raindrop in a puddle or like wind for people's sails as they navigate life. Common practice in the field has been to deliver suggestions, worksheets, tasks, or homework for people to do as part of an intervention. In the context of a single session encounter this can prove quite hazardous. In providing *our own ideas* are we inadvertently sending the message that we are the knower, eroding the participant's sense of being able to direct their own lives? Are we prescribing ideas that are not contextual or culturally acceptable? What if the participant tries out an idea and it fails them, could they experience disappointment in themselves or reify a sense of failure? In single session contexts, there may not be enough time to recognize and meliorate these potential problems. This is not to say that we don't bring practice wisdom to these conversations in terms of what we have learned from other families and our education. If that wisdom, however, is shared with a tentative voice as one idea, that may or may not be useful.

The *conversation endurance map* (Cooper, 2024) builds on this practice, inviting people to come up with *their own* take-aways from the conversation, re-contextualize them into everyday living, identify a supporting audience to these ideas, and lastly to identify and counter-plan for possible constraints or setbacks. People are invited to try out or experiment with their take-aways and to see how it goes *before* considering future services. They are invited to return should their plan need revising.

Use of Take-Away Documents

Narrative therapy has a long history (see White & Epston, 1990; White, 1995; Freeman, Epston, & Lobovits, 1997) of the use of documents to archive people's know-how for them to revisit. They assist to recruit relevant audiences who can respond to the emerging story as a means to support and foster ongoing meaning expansion. The practice of co-crafting take-away documents in brief narrative SST has emerged as an important practice to sustain the conversation long past the face-to-face contact. These documents are there for people when they need them, as reminders and supporting devices. They can also be crafted to assist others. Various documents are possible, including a conversation summary, manuals, letters, lists, handbooks, poems, testaments, and certificates. For further discussion and an example of therapist and consultee co-creating some take-away documentation in a single session, see Cooper and "Ariane" (2018).

In ending with Darius and Lynn, we crafted a *therapeutic care plan,* outlining their ideas about when to play our game for more practice, how often to practice, highlighting the skill they plan to work on. I often invite caregivers to craft these documents through eliciting their ideas about how to proceed with their caregiving in ways that support what we had started in our single session. Lynn had thought it relevant to practice the remote-control game daily and to experiment with other ways Darius could practice *controlling his motor,* such as playing redlight-greenlight or listening to some calming music. These kinds of documents can be consulted and plans edited as needed. They help the story-in-the-making to extend into everyday living.

Closing

The past several decades have been very exciting in Ontario, Canada, as we have embraced and continued to craft Single Session Therapy influenced by narrative practice. As several of our clinics enter their 20s, we see that the practice is still quite young, with continued growth ahead. I am excited for what is to come as practitioners and those who consult with us continue to co-shape practice founded on relational ethics and meaning generation. I hope what I have shared within this chapter sparks your interest, evokes practice review, and invites your discoveries to be shared through peer learning, articles, and future discussions.

Notes

1 It's important to acknowledge the contribution of Karen Young to this growth in Ontario. For decades Karen and I (see Young & Cooper, 2008) have been sharing these ideas and assisting agencies to integrate Single Session Therapy (SST) as part of a diverse service menu.
2 This vignette is a composite recount, and names have been changed to ensure confidentiality.
3 In another public dialogue (White & Meichenbaum, 2000), held during the 4th Evolution of Psychotherapy Conference, White distinguished times the therapist is *decentered but influential, centered and influential, centered and noninfluential,* or *decentered and noninfluential.* He also (in Hoyt & Combs, 1996, pp. 38–40) noted: "And, because the impossibility of neutrality means that I cannot avoid being 'for' something, I take responsibility to distrust what I am for—that is, my ways of life and my ways of thought—and I can do this in many ways."

References

Batrouney, A. (2019). Narrative therapy approaches in single-session trauma work. *The International Journal of Narrative Therapy and Community Work, 2,* 40–48.

Cooper, S. (2013). Quality assurance at the walk-in clinic: Process, outcome, and learning. *International Journal of Narrative Therapy & Community Work, 4,* 30–37.

Cooper, S. (2014). Brief narrative practice at the walk-in clinic: The rise of the counter-story. *International Journal of Narrative Therapy and Community Work, 2,* 23–30.

Cooper, S. (2024). *Brief Narrative Practice in Single-Session Therapy.* Routledge.

Cooper, S., & 'Ariane' (2018). Co-crafting take-home documents at the walk-in. In M.F. Hoyt, M. Bobele, A. Slive, J. Young, & M. Talmon (Eds.), *Single-Session Therapy by Walk-In or Appointment: Clinical, Supervisory, and Administrative Aspects of One-at-a-Time Therapy* (pp. 260–269). Routledge.

Duvall, J., Young, K., & Kayes-Burden, A. (2012). *No more, no less: Brief mental health services for children and youth.* www.excellenceforchildrenandyouth.com

Epston, D. (1999). *Co-Research: The Making of an Alternative Knowledge.* The Dulwich Centre. Retrieved July 3, 2022, from https://dulwichcentre.com.au/articles-about-narrative-therapy/co-research-david-epston/

Epston, D. (2001). Anthropology, archives, co-research and narrative therapy. In D. Denborough (Ed.), *Family Therapy: Exploring the Field's Past, Present and Possible Futures* (pp. 161–166). Dulwich Centre Publications.

Epston, D. (2014). Ethnography, co-research and insider knowledges. *Australian and New Zealand Journal of Family Therapy, 35*(1), 105–109. https://doi.org/10.1002/anzf.1048

Freedman, J., & Combs, G. (2002). *Narrative Therapy with Couples . . . and a Whole Lot More! A Collection of Papers, Essays and Exercises.* Dulwich Centre Publications.

Freeman, J., Epston, D., & Lobovits, D. (1997). *Playful Approaches to Serious Problems: Narrative Therapy with Children and Their Families*. Norton.

Gergen, K. (2021). *The Relational Imperative: Resources for a World on Edge*. Taos Institute Publications.

Goffman, E. (1963). *Stigma: Notes on the Management of Spoiled Identity*. Prentice Hall.

Hoyt, M.F., & Combs, G. (1996). On ethics and the spiritualities of the surface: A conversation with Michael White. In M.F. Hoyt (Ed.), *Constructive Therapies* (Vol. 2, pp. 33–59). Guilford Press. Reprinted in Hoyt, M.F. (2001). *Interviews with Brief Therapy Experts* (pp. 71–96). Brunner-Routledge.

Lindemann, N.H. (2001). *Damaged Identities, Narrative Repair*. Cornell University Press.

Malinen, T., Cooper, S.J., & Thomas, F.N. (Eds.). (2012). *Masters of Narrative and Collaborative Therapies: The Voices of Andersen, Anderson, and White*. Routledge.

Maturana, H.R. (1978). Biology of language: The epistemology of reality. In G.A. Miller, E. Lenneberg, & E.H. Lenneberg (Eds.), *Psychology and Biology of Language and Thought: Essays in Honor of Eric Lenneberg* (pp. 27–63). Academic Press.

McNamee, S. (2009). Postmodern psychotherapeutic ethics: Relational responsibility in practice. *Human Systems*, 20(2), 55–69.

Paré, D.A. (2014). Social justice and the word: Keeping diversity alive in therapeutic conversations. *Canadian Journal of Counselling and Psychotherapy*, 48(3), 206–217.

Reynolds, V. (2019). *Justice-Doing at the Intersections of Power: Community Work, Therapy and Supervision*. Dulwich Centre Publications.

Sarmiento, C. (2022). *Mental Health Walk-In Clinics for Children and Families* (p. 8613) [Electronic Thesis and Dissertation Repository]. https://ir.lib.uwo.ca/etd/8613

Taos Institute. (2023). *Dialogue with the author: An invitation to social construction with Ken Gergen*. Retrieved November 5, 2023, from https://www.youtube.com/watch?v=qN46z0eAihM

White, M. (1984). Pseudo-encopresis: From avalanche to victory, from vicious cycles to virtuous cycles. *Family Systems Medicine*, 2(2), 150–160.

White, M. (1992). Family therapy training and supervision in a world of experience and narrative. In D. Epston & M. White (Eds.), *Experience, Contradiction, Narrative & Imagination: Selected Papers of David Epston & Michael White 1989–1991* (pp. 75–95). Dulwich Centre Publications.

White, M. (1995). *Re-Authoring Lives: Interviews & Essays*. Dulwich Centre Publications.

White, M. (2000). Re-engaging with history: The absent but implicit. In M. White (Ed.), *Reflections on Narrative Practice: Essays & Interviews* (pp. 35–58). Dulwich Centre Publications.

White, M. (2001). Folk psychology and narrative practice. *Dulwich Centre Journal*, 2, 1–37. Reprinted in White, M. (2004). *Narrative Practice and Exotic Lives: Resurrecting Diversity in Everyday Life* (pp. 59–118). Dulwich Centre Publications.

White, M. (2007). *Maps of Narrative Practice*. Norton.

White, M. (2011). *Narrative Practice: Continuing the Conversations*. Norton.

White, M., & Epston, D. (1990). *Narrative Means to Therapeutic Ends*. Norton.

White, M., Hoyt, M.F., & Zimmerman, J. (2000). Direction and discovery: A conversation about power and politics in narrative therapy. In M. White (Ed.), *Reflections on Narrative Practice: Essays & Interviews* (pp. 97–116). Dulwich Centre Publications. A version also appeared in Hoyt, M.F. (2001). *Interviews With Brief Therapy Experts* (pp. 265–293). Brunner-Routledge.

White, M., & Meichenbaum, D. (2000, May). *Dialogue: Nature and Challenge of a Narrative Perspective in Psychotherapy.* Held at the Evolution of Psychotherapy Conference sponsored by the Milton H. Erickson Foundation, Anaheim, CA.

Young, K. (2008). Narrative practice at a walk-in therapy clinic: Developing children's worry wisdom. *Journal of Systemic Therapies, 27*(4), 54–74.

Young, K. (2011). When all the time you have is now: Re-visiting practices and narrative therapy in a walk-in clinic. In J. Duvall & L. Beres (Eds.), *Innovations in Narrative Therapy: Connecting Practice, Training, and Research.* Norton.

Young, K. (2018). Change in the winds: The growth of walk-in therapy clinics in Ontario, Canada. In M.F. Hoyt, M. Bobele, A. Slive, J. Young, & M. Talmon (Eds.), *Single-Session Therapy by Walk-In or Appointment: Clinical, Supervisory, and Administrative Aspects* of *One-at-a-Time Services* (pp. 59–71). Routledge.

Young, K. (2020). Multistory listening: Using narrative practices at walk-in clinics. *Journal of Systemic Therapies, 39*(3), 34–45.

Young, K., & Cooper, S. (2008). Toward re-composing an evidence base: The narrative therapy re-visiting project. *Journal of Systemic Therapies, 27*(1), 67–83.

Chapter 25

Single Session Therapy Supporting Social-Emotional Learning (SST-SEL) With Children, Families, and Educators in Israel

Svetlana Prokasheva

The COVID-19 pandemic, waves of armed conflict, political instability, and similar events constantly challenge psychologists and therapists in educational systems. Therapists are forced to improve the effectiveness and availability of psychological support, especially when the needs are growing, the budget is short, and the waiting list is long. Single Session Therapy (SST) is one possible solution.

SST is a first-line therapeutic approach suitable for intervention with children, their parents, educators, and others within educational systems. Combined with a Response to Intervention (RTI) approach,[1] SST is effective and also enables therapists to determine if there is a need for extended or external referral therapy (Jones, Kadlubek, & Marks, 2006). Implementing psychological therapy in a single session does not diminish the importance of other therapies and their effectiveness as second and third lines of treatment if and when needed.

The working methods of SST are well-established in many countries worldwide, such as the United States, Canada, England, Australia, Singapore, China, and Italy (Hoyt, 2025; Hoyt, Bobele, Slive, Young, & Talmon, 2018; Hoyt, Young, & Rycroft, 2021). In Israel, SST has been recognized for many years but is not an integral part of the training and expertise among psychologists working within the educational system. Utilizing the experience and knowledge accumulated in various fields—for example, working with parents (Korpilahti-Leino, Luntamo, Ristkari, Hinkka-Yli-Salomäki, & Pulkki-Råback, 2022), working with adolescents (Kachor & Brothwell, 2020), and as an effective way to provide psychological assistance when there is a need for simultaneous service to many individuals (Paul & van Ommeren, 2013)—may contribute to the toolkit of those psychologists. SST employs immediate and focused working methods that allow for direct professional contact with anyone seeking psychological assistance when needed. Such treatment allows for initial response, screening, and provision of initial psychological treatment, without excluding other possible treatment. Not everyone experiencing distress

DOI: 10.4324/9781032693828-29

necessarily needs long-term psychological treatment; often, a single session is sufficient. Research findings repeatedly show that SST is the most common and often the most effective treatment, especially when considering the relationship between treatment duration, its cost, and the general benefit it provides immediately and in the future.

It appears that 50–60% of clients treated using SST principles successfully mobilize internal and external resources and do not feel the need for additional treatment sessions (Cannistrà, Piccirilli, Paolo D'Alia, Giannetti, & Piva, 2020; Hoyt et al., 2018). In a study by Piva, Gobbato, Guzzardi, Ghisoni, and Pietrabissa (2020), approximately 81% of those who chose SST reported improvement in their condition regarding the issue that led them to treatment. In an English study that included 23,300 children (average age 12.7 years) referred to public treatment centers, 46% attended only one session (Edbrooke-Childs, Hayes, Lane, Liverpool, & Jacob, 2021). Therefore, the researchers concluded that it is important to strengthen therapists' ability to fully utilize the potential of Single Session Therapy. Generally, the effectiveness of SST among children and adolescents dealing with emotional problems, supported by research, and the integration of such working methods in the continuum of treatment may improve the quality of therapeutic services provided in the public system (Kachor & Brothwell, 2020). Meta-analyses of 8 studies (N = 2,082) estimated a medium effect of single session interventions (SSI) in educational settings for reducing depressive symptoms (g = –0.44, 95% CI –0.93–0.05) and for reducing anxiety symptoms (g = –0.62, 95% CI –1.35–0.11). The study indicated that a single-session intervention is feasible to implement in primary schools and acceptable to pupils, parents, and teachers and has a preventive effect (Cassidy, 2020).

In a longitudinal study involving 258 children aged 5 to 15, SST contributed to improvements for 60% of them—their condition was certainly better than that of those on long waiting lists—and the positive effect persisted even after 18 months (Perkins, 2006; Perkins & Scarlett, 2008). Treatment focused on connecting with the clients' strengths, and strengthening their sense of hope, provided in a single session, was found to be effective as an initial response, especially among children with attention deficit and hyperactivity disorders and their families (Mulligan, Olivieri, Young, Lin, & Anthony, 2022). Another study found that initial interventions in SST were effective in preventing depression and behavioral disorders among children after sudden traumatic events, such as road accidents (Zehnder, Meuli, & Landolt, 2010). Within an SST framework, it is possible to strengthen self-efficacy, help develop methods of coping with fears and anxieties, both in children and adolescents; strengthen belief in one's ability to change (Bertuzzi, Fratini, Tarquinio, Cannistrà, & Granese, 2021; Davis III, Ollendick, & Öst, 2019; Farrell, Kershaw, & Ollendick, 2018; Nielsen, Andreasen, & Thastum, 2016; also see Pietrabissa, Chapter 16 this volume); and reduce immediate stress levels, thereby improving overall mental well-being (Kachor & Brothwell, 2020).[2]

Principles of Single Session Therapy (SST)

SST is based on a paradigm of broad and flexible treatment that allows for the provision of effective psychological services, as opposed to a singular or separate theoretical approach. The term *Single Session Therapy* was defined by Talmon (1990, p. xv) as a face-to-face meeting between therapist and client with no additional meeting for at least a year. This definition was made for research purposes and has since changed. A definition, similar to Talmon's but broader, is provided by Hymmen, Stalker, and Cait (2013, p. 61; also see Steenbarger, 2002):

> SST refers to a conscious approach to make the most of the first session knowing it may be the only session the client decided to attend—not to the situation where there is an expectation that the client will attend multiple sessions but chooses to attend just one.

This definition includes advanced alternative models developed in parallel with technological advancements (such as the use of digital means or digital tools for self-treatment—see Schleider & Weisz, 2017; also Chapter 10 this volume).

Following an analysis of numerous sources (books, chapters, and articles) focused on SST, Cannistrà (2022) identified 14 principles of therapist mindset in SST. One of them is that *a single session may be sufficient for the client*.

The therapist contributes to the success of the therapy when fulfilling one or more of the following primary roles (see Talmon, 2018; also Chapter 3 this volume):

1. The role of the "attentive listener." To fulfill this role, the therapist must be attentive, empathetic, warm, and non-judgmental, and encourage the client to speak openly. Within this, the therapist understands the client's deepest concerns and emotions and comprehends the external and internal conflicts the client is facing.
2. The role of the "facilitator." To fulfill this role, the therapist assists the client in discovering their internal strengths, abilities, adaptability, and resilience both personally and within their family or society. A therapist who successfully reveals the client's authentic strengths appears as a reliable optimist and positive encourager.

3. The role of "reconceptualizer." At this stage, the therapist and client together explore labels and re-write the original script of the client. In this role, the therapist employs persuasion, suggestions, interpretations, and shared brainstorming with the client.

As Talmon (2018) notes, the primary challenge facing the therapist in SST is not mastery of specific therapeutic techniques or tools or their experience in therapy or counseling per se, but rather their ability to adapt to flexibility and diversity in their approach and fundamental attitudes toward therapy.

Social-Emotional Learning (SEL)

The concept of Social-Emotional Learning (SEL) is gradually becoming embedded within the education system in Israel. In addition to programs enhancing social-emotional skills already existing within the education system, many additional programs are being introduced. Numerous theories have contributed to the development of the concept of SEL, including positive psychology, emotional intelligence, motivation theories, attachment, social learning, personality theories, character education, and salutogenesis (see Antonovsky, 1979, 1987[3]), with the sense of coherence serving as a psychological foundation supporting other life skills. The Collaborative for Academic, Social, and Emotional Learning (CASEL) framework is commonly used for the implementation of SEL throughout the entire Israeli educational system (Kazarnovski & Cucoș, 2021). The CASEL framework includes five interrelated competencies: (1) self-awareness—one's ability to understand one's thoughts, emotions, and values and how they influence one's behavior; (2) self-management—one's ability to manage one's thoughts, emotions, and behaviors effectively across situations as one works to achieve goals; (3) social awareness—one's ability to understand social perspectives and empathize with others from diverse backgrounds; (4) relationship skills—one's ability to develop and maintain healthy and supportive relationships and navigate social situations with people from diverse backgrounds; and (5) responsible decision-making—one's ability to make caring and constructive social and behavioral choices (Ross & Tolan, 2018; Friedman, 2019).

Jones and Bouffard (2012) identified three skill sets of SEL:

1. Emotional processes, including skills such as emotional awareness, expression, behavior regulation, empathy, and the ability to perceive from various perspectives.

2. Interpersonal social skills, including understanding social cues, positive interactions with peers and adults, conflict management, and other pro-social behaviors.
3. Cognitive regulation, including skills and abilities of attention control, reasoning, task planning and working memory, cognitive flexibility, and developing growth mindsets.

Efficient implementation of SEL requires a coordinated approach between parents and school staff. They need to share a vision, goals, and responsibilities for the work. In practice, adults (both teachers and parents) enter educational frameworks with varying degrees of social-emotional skills, similar to students. Each school has its own characteristics in terms of the basis for the daily development of SEL skills. For these processes to be effective, broad support and involvement are required from everyone involved in the school environment, especially psychologists working within the education system. The SEL skills of adults have a positive impact on students' skills, including personal examples of using these skills, stress management, and emotional response regulation to handle challenging situations effectively. Teachers and other adults with good social-emotional abilities themselves succeed in effectively communicating with students and coping better with challenging behaviors (Jennings & Greenberg, 2009). Since school and family are the two dominant contexts in children's lives, strong partnerships between schools and families enable children to experience coherence regarding the messages they receive regarding social-emotional skills. The choice of SEL treatment goals is based on discussion with the family.

The Structure of SST Supporting Social-Emotional Learning (SST-SEL)

A complete and separate treatment session lasting from 1 to 1.5 hours comprises the following:

Preliminary Stage: Establishing Contact in a Phone Call Before the Session

A brief explanation of the nature of individual therapy and the proven effectiveness in numerous empirical studies. Reflective listening. Presenting options based on the age of the client.

Stage 1: Beginning of the Therapeutic Session

Assessment of the current psychological status based on cognitive functioning, emotional expression, social adaptation, interpersonal resources, and readiness to receive assistance. These measures may strengthen effective coping. Psychological triage—preference for difficult responses versus easy ones. The therapist needs to be ready to change the agenda to address the client's concerns.

Objectives:

- Connection between the therapist and the client.
- Guidance on the purpose of the meeting—"We'll identify what can be done, and I'll help you plan your next step. Discover how you can cope with the situation."
- Partnership recruitment—"We need to work hard to identify the appropriate solution. Does this sound like something you're willing to do?"
- Evaluation of the current situation—"What has changed since the phone call? Have there been any attempts to solve the problem?"
- Discussion about the availability of continued treatment through a different approach or individual meeting method.

Questions the therapist can ask the client:

- "How can I help you in the best way? What does your life look like when the problem feels less overwhelming?"

The responses to these questions may guide the therapist to understand the client's preferences.

Stage 2: Goal Setting

The process of defining the problem contributes significantly to creating a working alliance with the client. Having multiple problems may increase a feeling of loss of control. Generally, a client may raise several issues simultaneously. It is important to help the client identify and prioritize goals and problems. The most urgent problem should be defined, reflected upon by the patient, its importance emphasized, and focused on during the session. Goals that can be achieved in a single session are built together according to these principles:

- It is preferable to set small goals rather than large ones.
- Clients highlight the goals.
- Goals are described specifically and concretely, in terms of behavior or emotional experience.
- Goals are achievable within the client's life circumstances.

- Goals are described as "the beginning of something" rather than "the end of something."
- Achieving goals requires new behavior rather than defining them as the absence or cessation of existing behavior.[4]

Possible questions:

- "What is the most urgent problem? What is the biggest hope? Typically, people solve problems on their own. What have you done so far to try to solve the problem?"

Identifying possible improvements in a short period will help clients recruit resources and invest effort into collaborative work. Consequently, the therapist can offer the client a choice of their preferred option to help them focus on what is important to them at the moment. The therapist should ask what the client is willing to do to achieve their goal.

Stage 3: Active Treatment

Based on the specific goals selected, the therapist and the client will focus on one of the three SEL domains (emotional processes, social skills, or interpersonal and cognitive processes) and work according to different therapeutic approaches, such as positive psychology, narrative approach, cognitive behavioral therapy, and Acceptance and Commitment Therapy. Solution-focused sentences should be used, and problem-focused sentences may also be used when necessary. The therapist will encourage the client to use strategies that have helped in the past if they are functional and downplay ineffective strategies. The therapist will focus on strengths and resilience factors as essential components in the coping process and help connect them to the client's resources. The therapist will ask which personal strengths of the client may be useful now and, if necessary, discuss family relationships and friends with the client and strengthen positive perception, spiritual values, hope, internal control, creativity, emotional resilience, and sense of humor.

Stage 4: Closing the Therapy Session (Conclusion and Recommendations for Continuing the Journey)

Attention should be paid to the client's willingness—to ensure their satisfaction with the treatment, to check if they want to stop it, or in case of need, to refer them for further treatment. It is important to invite both positive and negative feedback: "Is there anything we haven't talked about today that you would like to share with me?" It is recommended that the therapist not postpone this question to the end of the session. Feedback at the end of the session should include these four components:

- Identification of the motives that led the patient to seek the session.
- Reinforcing what has been learned about thinking, emotions, behavior, and everything that may be useful to support or solve the problem. Highlighting resources and abilities. Emphasizing support sources from the environment, including the education and family framework. Providing recommendations for personal tasks.
- Presenting the diagnosis not according to its definition in the *DSM* but as a revised framework of the problem.
- Providing concrete recommendations on what can be done. In case of need, an action plan can be developed.

Possible question:

- "How will you use what was discussed in the session? Be specific in your answer."
- Follow-up conversation: According to the content of the therapy session.
- Feedback on the treatment.

Each such session will focus on one of the relevant SEL areas for the client. This way, the SST-SEL treatment will be more intensive and will contribute more to the child and to building SEL processes in the education system. Referral for additional treatment is based on the student's response to the face-to-face or remote single-session treatment, the response of the parent, the educator, or the therapeutic triad focused on the child's treatment needs.

Case Examples

Case 1: SST-SEL Therapy With Parent (the Aim Was to Support a Parent's Emotional Regulation Abilities)

Bela, a mother of a child with difficulties at school, was not able to communicate with the staff, because every time they met she could not control herself—she was angry, blaming, shouting, and unable to listen to the educational staff (educator, school consultant, manager), not able to allow the staff to explain their function and give their recommendations. The situation made it impossible to build and implement a therapeutic plan to help the child fit in better at school. The assumption was that if a mother can listen to the educational team and cooperate with them, this will give them a chance to build and implement a treatment plan.

Bela agreed to meet the school psychologist if it would be only one session.

She came to the meeting and shared that she wants to help her child but feels angry with the staff for not being able to accommodate her child in the past and prevent the difficulties. Bela shared with the psychologist her anger, accusations, and disappointments about the school and the educational staff. After working through the difficult emotions, she calmed down and was able to talk about the situation that had arisen.

Every time she meets school staff she thinks about her child saying that he is not feeling well, that children bully him, and that he is in a bad mood when he comes home from school. She shared that she intends to contact supervision with complaints about inappropriate treatment of her child.

Psychologist: "Do you want your child to continue studying at the same school, or are you considering transferring him to another school after the complaints to the supervisor that you intend to submit?"

Bela: "I don't want to transfer. He became attached to the current educator. She is a good person."

Psychologist: "What is your goal in the created situation? What do you want to happen? Do you want revenge on the staff, or do you want to recruit them to make the maximum professional effort to improve your child's experience at school?"

Bela: "Of course, everything is for the child . . . but I can't manage and calm myself. It's stronger than me."

Psychologist: "Would you like me to help you with this? I will teach you some skills that will help you stay in control during the meeting with the school staff and also try to understand how they want to help your child."

Bela: "Yes. I would love to try."

Case 2: SST-SEL Therapy With Adolescent (the Aim Was to Support Adolescent's Interpersonal Social Skills)

Tally, 14 years old, didn't want to meet with a school counselor because she preferred being seen as an "outside" figure rather than an "inside" one. The girl was an excellent student with no previous therapeutic background. Until the quarrel, she felt socially well integrated. However, after a fight over a romantic interest with a boy from a group, she felt emotionally down, disappointed, confused, and socially isolated. During the conversation with the psychologist, it emerged that she belonged to a group of children who prioritize social entertainment and conflicts with other groups of children in the school. She was attracted to this group because they seemed central and popular in the class, and being around them raised her self-esteem. This continued until the big fight and rejection by the affiliated groups. She shared that she wants to be socially prominent but also wants to succeed in her studies because she wants to be a doctor in the future.

Psychologist: "Is it appropriate for you that we get to know together how your social circles are structured?"
[They draw together the scale of perceived interpersonal closeness—Popovic, Milne, & Barrett, 2003.]
"I see that you put the group of children in a circle farther away and maybe really at this stage of life it is less suitable for you to be in contact with them. It is very noticeable that you have support at home and some people you can consult with."

Tally: "Yes. Especially Mam and Grandma. They always help me, even now."

Psychologist: "Who are these children that you listed as relatively close to you, but they are not from the problem group?"

Tally: "They are fine. We sometimes meet for some sort of reason but don't know enough about each other. We didn't study together in primary school."

Psychologist: "Maybe it's worth finding a way to get to know them better. For example, start devising social or study meetings after school with each of those you have noted. Do not rush to commit to friendships with one of them; rather, create a circle of 'light' friendship as wide as possible. When something is not available you can always turn to something else from the circle of friendship you have built for yourself."

Tally: "I never tried that way. I was always only with the same group, and now I am disappointed with it."

Psychologist: "The door will remain open for you. If you feel that you are not doing well in the social sphere despite the efforts you intend to make to improve the situation, you can go back and get help."

Tally: "Maybe it's time to get to know other kids too. I never had to look for friends. Maybe I'll try. Not so used to being the initiator of social relations."

After a few months, the girl asked to meet with the psychologist again because she found out that she was having difficulty communicating with children in general. Sometimes they would get offended and she wouldn't know how to prevent such situations or find solutions to social problems that arose. The psychologist suggested that joining a social skills group could be an option to help her with her interpersonal communication problems.

Case 3: SST-SEL Therapy With a Teacher (the Aim Was to Support Cognitive Regulation, Which Includes Developing a More Flexible Thinking Pattern for Coping With Stress—Crum, Akinola, Martin, & Fath, 2017)

During a long time of continuous stress, Sofie (a high school teacher) requested a meeting with the school psychologist. Sofie shared that she was going through a very difficult time. She was very stressed about various things, including workload related to distance learning, pressures due to the security situation in the country, policy changes in the field, as well as personal life circumstances such as her sick mother requiring intensive care. Sofie was aware of the stressful situations and tried to manage them by doing activities such as sports, yoga, and healthy eating. However, she was considering leaving the school due to the accumulated stress.

Sofie: "I try to lead a life focused on managing endless pressures in my life."

Psychologist: "What do you think in general about the effects of stress on your life?"

Sofie: "It is known that stress is a harmful and dangerous thing. This is why I try to do as many things as possible that help hold and manage stress. I don't know if it is right to continue like this. I would leave the job, but I'm also unsure if it will do me any good or bring other pressures to my life."

Psychologist: "Do you think stress is always a bad thing?"

Sofie: "Yeah, I do. At the same time, I'm not sure it's always bad."

Psychologist: "Have you had situations in your life where you felt that the experience of stress contributed something to you?"

Sofie: "Of course. For example, the entire period when I was a beginning teacher. I had to work many hours on preparing materials for classes and at the same time I also continued to study for a master's degree. I would also manage to find time for my personal life *[smiling and laughing]*. It was a very challenging and demanding effort. Today work does not require such special efforts from me because I have experience. It's just annoying everything that happens around you and also taking care of your mother who is sick."

Psychologist: "In general, it sounds like you grew out of dealing with that period you described to me."

Sofie: "Yes. I learned a lot of new things about myself."

Psychologist: "It is the same pressure, only the stimuli have changed. And you've changed too—you're more aware of the ways that

	help you manage pressure better and carry it out, more flow around preparing the lessons."
Sofie:	"Maybe what I'm feeling right now is accumulated fatigue. I haven't been on vacation in a long time. Maybe I more need to rest than to change something too much."
Psychologist:	"Beliefs we have about the effect of stressful situations influence our ability to cope. Sometimes people report that stressful situations have an effect in a way that invigorates their coping, and this brings them empowering experiences. They use stressful situations as a resource."
Sofie:	"Yes. I learned to do many things at the same time and also to persist in managing a healthy life span. More sensitive to my own needs. Now, I need to survive tough times. At the same time, I don't want to give up everything I've achieved in my career."

Summary

Providing psychological services through single sessions is particularly crucial in places where there is a high demand for services. Extensive use of such treatment may reduce waiting lists and provide a proper and quality response to a larger number of clients. SST is based on the ability of the therapist and the client to create a therapeutic connection in the "here and now" of the therapy session and has been proven to be as effective as other well-known treatments in the field. Such treatment aims to alleviate the sufferings of the client and promotes and encourages self-healing capacities by connecting to available internal and external forces, reinforcing optimism, hope, perspective creation, problem solving, and action plan construction.

To start providing services according to the single-session method, a change in mindset and perception among psychologists and therapists is required. It is difficult to give up what is familiar and known as a long-term treatment process, which includes detailed anamnesis, a fixed and continuous setting, and everything included in a series of therapy sessions. However, in a single session, the perception of time available for working with the client changes. The magic of the moment comes from the fact that anything can happen when two people meet for the first time.

Notes

1 For more information about RTI, see Batsche, Elliott, Graden, Grimes, and Kovaleski (2005); Byrd (2011); Fuchs, Fuchs, and Compton (2012); and New York State Regulations (2024).
2 *Editors' note*: For additional studies of the benefits of SST with children and adolescents, see Chapter 11 (Stephenson), Chapter 16 (Lewis), Chapter 17 (Fuzzard), and Chapter 21 (Asai) in this volume.

3 Further information about *salutogenesis* was presented by Prokasheva (2023) at the 4th International Symposium on SST held in Rome.
4 These are consistent with de Shazer's (1991) "well-formed goals."

References

Antonovsky, A. (1979). *Health, Stress, and Coping*. Jossey-Bass.
Antonovsky, A. (1987). *Unravelling the Mystery of Health*. Jossey-Bass.
Batsche, G., Elliott, J., Graden, J.L., Grimes, J., Kovaleski, J.F., Prasse, D., Reschly, D.J., Schrag, J., & Tilly, W.D., III. (2005). *Response to Intervention: Policy Considerations and Implementation*. National Association of State Directors of Special Education.
Bertuzzi, V., Fratini, G., Tarquinio, C., Cannistrà, F., Granese, V., Giusti, E.M., Castenuovo, G., & Pietrabissa, G. (2021). Single-session therapy by appointment for the treatment of anxiety disorders in youth and adults: A systematic review of the literature. *Frontiers in Psychology*, 12, 7213.
Byrd, E.S. (2011). Educating and involving parents in the response to intervention process: The school's important role. *Teaching Exceptional Children*, 43(3), 32–39.
Cannistrà, F. (2022). The single session therapy mindset: Fourteen principles gained through an analysis of the literature. *International Journal of Brief Therapy and Family Science Family Science*, 12(1), 1–26. https://www.jstage.jst.go.jp/article/ijbf/12/1/12_1/_pdf
Cannistrà, F., Piccirilli, F., Paolo D'Alia, P., Giannetti, A., Piva, L., Gobbato, F., Guzzardi, R., Ghisoni, A., & Pietrabissa, G. (2020). Examining the incidence and clients' experiences of single session therapy in Italy: A feasibility study. *Australian and New Zealand Journal of Family Therapy*, 41(3), 271–282.
Cassidy, J. (2020). *Building Psychological Strengths and Improving Outcomes in School Children with Single-Session Interventions* [Doctoral Dissertation, University of East Anglia, Norwich, England UK].
Crum, A.J., Akinola, M., Martin, A., & Fath, S. (2017). The role of stress mindset in shaping cognitive, emotional, and physiological responses to challenging and threatening stress. *Anxiety, Stress, and Coping*, 30(4), 379–395.
Davis, T.E., III, Ollendick, T.H., & Öst, L.G. (2019). One-session treatment of specific phobias in children: Recent developments and a systematic review. *Annual Review of Clinical Psychology*, 15, 233–256. https://www.annualreviews.org/doi/full/10.1146/annurev-clinpsy-050718-095608
de Shazer, S. (1991). *Putting Difference to Work*. Norton.
Edbrooke-Childs, J., Hayes, D., Lane, R., Liverpool, S., Jacob, J., & Deighton, J. (2021). Association between single session service attendance and clinical characteristics in administrative data. *Clinical Child Psychology and Psychiatry*, 26(3), 770–782. https://research.edgehill.ac.uk/ws/files/37966839/Single_session_services_manuscript_blind_copy_revised_Feb_21.pdf
Farrell, L.J., Kershaw, H., & Ollendick, T. (2018). Play-modified one-session treatment for young children with a specific phobia of dogs: A multiple baseline case series. *Child Psychiatry and Human Development*, 49, 317–329. https://www.researchgate.net/publication/318839141_Play-Modified_One-Session_Treatment_for_Young_Children_with_a_Specific_Phobia_of_Dogs_A_Multiple_Baseline_Case_Series

Friedman, T. (2019). *Emotional-Social Leaning: Mapping Concepts and the Theoretical Basis*]Limeedah chevratit-rigsheet: Meepu'ee moosagee v'basees teoretee[. Machon Moffet. http://education.academy.ac.il/Index4/Entry.aspx?nodeId=992&entryId=21133

Fuchs, D., Fuchs, L.S., & Compton, D.L. (2012). Smart RTI: A next-generation approach to multilevel prevention. *Exceptional Children, 78*(3), 263–279.

Hoyt, M.F. (2025). *Single Session Therapy: A Clinical Introduction to Principles and Practices.* Routledge.

Hoyt, M.F., Bobele, M., Slive, A., Young, J., & Talmon, M. (Eds.). (2018). *Single-Session Therapy by Walk-In or Appointment: Administrative, Clinical, and Supervisory Aspects of One-at-a-Time Services.* Routledge.

Hoyt, M.F., Young, J., & Rycroft, P. (Eds.). (2021). *Single Session Thinking and Practice in Global, Cultural, and Familial Contexts: Expanding Applications.* Routledge.

Hymmen, P., Stalker, C., & Cait, C.-A. (2013). The case for single-session therapy: Does the empirical evidence support the increased prevalence of this service delivery model? *Journal of Mental Health, 22*(1), 60–71.

Jennings, P.A., & Greenberg, M.T. (2009). The prosocial classroom: Teacher social and emotional competence in relation to student and classroom outcomes. *Review of Educational Research, 79*(1), 491–525. https://bibliotecadigital.mineduc.cl/bitstream/handle/20.500.12365/17472/jennings2009.pdf?sequence=1&isAllowed=y

Jones, S.M., & Bouffard, S.M. (2012). Social and emotional learning in schools: From programs to strategies. *Social Policy Report, 26*(4). Society for Research in Child Development. https://files.eric.ed.gov/fulltext/ED540203.pdf

Jones, W.P., Kadlubek, R.M., & Marks, W.J. (2006). Single-session treatment: A counselling paradigm for school psychology. *The School Psychologist, 60*(3), 112–115. http://apadivision16.org/wp-content/uploads/2015/12/TSP-Vol.-60-No.-3-August-2006.pdf#page=12

Kachor, M., & Brothwell, J. (2020). Improving youth mental health services access using a single-session therapy approach. *Journal of Systemic Therapies, 39*(3), 46–55. https://guilfordjournals.com/doi/10.1521/jsyt.2020.39.3.46

Kazarnovski, T., & Cucoş, C. (2021). *Social Emotional Learning (SEL) and the Initiation Teacher Training Program in Israel.* European Proceedings of Educational Sciences.

Korpilahti-Leino, T., Luntamo, T., Ristkari, T., Hinkka-Yli-Salomäki, S., Pulkki-Råback, L., Waris, O., Matinolli, H., Sinokki, A., Mori, Y., Fukaya, M., Yamada, Y., & Sourander, A. (2022). Single-session, internet-based cognitive behavioral therapy to improve parenting skills to help children cope with anxiety during the COVID-19 pandemic: Feasibility study. *Journal of Medical Internet Research, 24*(4), e26438. https://www.jmir.org/2022/4/e26438/PDF

Mulligan, J., Olivieri, H., Young, K., Lin, J., & Anthony, S.J. (2022). Single session therapy in pediatric healthcare: The value of adopting a strengths-based approach for families living with neurological disorders. *Child and Adolescent Psychiatry and Mental Health, 16*(1), 1–11. https://capmh.biomedcentral.com/counter/pdf/10.1186/s13034-022-00495-6.pdf

Nielsen, M.D., Andreasen, C.L., & Thastum, M. (2016). A Danish study of one-session treatment for specific phobias in children and adolescents. *Scandinavian Journal of Child and Adolescent Psychiatry and Psychology, 4*(2), 65–76. https://sciendo.com/pdf/10.21307/sjcapp-2016-011

NY State Regulation. (2024). https://www.monticelloschools.net/academics/response-to-intervention-rti/#:~:text=Response%20to%20Intervention%2C%20or%20RTI,to%20students%20who%20are%20struggling

Paul, K.E., & van Ommeren, M. (2013). A primer on single session therapy and its potential application in humanitarian situations. *Intervention, 11*(1), 8–23. https://www.interventionjournal.org/article.asp?issn=1571-8883;year=2013;volume=11;issue=1;spage=8;epage=23;aulast=Paul;type=0

Perkins, R. (2006). The effectiveness of one session of therapy using a single-session therapy approach for children and adolescents with mental health problems. *Psychology and Psychotherapy: Theory, Research and Practice, 79*(2), 215–227. https://bpspsychub.onlinelibrary.wiley.com/doi/abs/10.1348/147608305X60523

Perkins, R., & Scarlett, G. (2008). The effectiveness of single session therapy in child and adolescent mental health. Part 2: An 18-month follow-up study. *Psychology and Psychotherapy: Theory, Research and Practice, 81*(2), 143–156. https://bpspsychub.onlinelibrary.wiley.com/doi/abs/10.1348/147608308X280995

Piva, L., Gobbato, F., Guzzardi, R., Ghisoni, A., & Pietrabissa, G. (2020). Examining the incidence and clients' experiences of single session therapy in Italy: A feasibility study. *Australian and New Zealand Journal of Family Therapy, 41*(3), 271–282.

Popovic, M., Milne, D., & Barrett, P. (2003). The scale of perceived interpersonal closeness (PICS). *Clinical Psychology & Psychotherapy: An International Journal of Theory & Practice, 10*(5), 286–301.

Prokasheva, S. (2023, November 11). *Ukrainians Coping with War: Which Salutogenic Coping Resources Help Them Reduce Anxiety?* Paper Presented at Fourth International Symposium on Single Session Therapy, Rome.

Ross, K.M., & Tolan, P. (2018). Social and emotional learning in adolescence: Testing the CASEL model in a normative sample. *The Journal of Early Adolescence, 38*(8), 1170–1199.

Schleider, J.L., & Weisz, J.R. (2017). Little treatments, promising effects? Meta-analysis of single-session interventions for youth psychiatric problems. *Journal of the American Academy of Child and Adolescent Psychiatry, 56*(2), 107–115. https://dash.harvard.edu/bitstream/handle/1/41292903/54465763.pdf?sequence=1

Steenbarger, B.N. (2002). Single-session therapy. *Encyclopedia of Psychotherapy, 2*, 669–672.

Talmon, M. (1990). *Single-Session Therapy: Maximizing the Effect of the First (and Often Only) Therapeutic Encounter.* Jossey-Bass.

Talmon, M. (2018). The eternal now: On becoming and being a single-session therapist. In M.F. Hoyt, M. Bobele, A. Slive, J. Young, & M. Talmon (Eds.), *Single-Session Therapy by Walk-In or Appointment* (pp. 149–154). Routledge. https://doi.org/10.4324/9781351112437

Zehnder, D., Meuli, M., & Landolt, M.A. (2010). Effectiveness of a single-session early psychological intervention for children after road traffic accidents: A randomized controlled trial. *Child and Adolescent Psychiatry and Mental Health, 4*(1), 1–10. https://capmh.biomedcentral.com/articles/10.1186/1753-2000-4-7

Chapter 26

The Relationship Check-Up

A Valentine's Day Single Session Therapy for Couples

John K. Miller

> The man who moves a mountain begins by carrying away small stones.
> —Confucius

In 2003, in collaboration with my faculty colleagues, I created a single session consultation service for couples offered at our training clinic, the Center for Family Therapy (CFT) at the University of Oregon in the city of Eugene—a program which continues to this day. The CFT was part of the nationally accredited master's level Couples and Family Therapy Program in the Department of Counseling Psychology. Although the CFT had only recently opened, it had quickly become one of the leading providers of counseling services in the community. The CFT also served as a venue for graduate students to gain clinical experience under faculty supervision, as well as provide a "laboratory" of research opportunities for faculty and students. The design of the service was based on my previous research in the area of Single Session Therapy (SST) at the Eastside Family Therapy Centre in Calgary, Canada (Miller, 1996, 2008; Miller & Slive, 2004). This new service was called "The Relationship Check-Up" (RCU), and it was tailored to attract couples of all types, as well anyone who might be seeking an SST consultation.

The purpose of the project was threefold. Firstly, we wanted to present a therapy offering that would overcome many of the common barriers to service delivery by making it inviting, easy to access, and free of charge. We also believed that by labeling it a "check-up" service, we would attract couples who were non-symptomatic and/or concerned about the stigma of seeking traditional therapy services, or perhaps simply seeking a couple enrichment opportunity. We also felt that the RCU would attract people who had never been to therapy before and were merely curious to check out what the experience was like. A second aim of the project was to provide our graduate students a chance to work with the faculty seeing cases and gaining valuable clinical experience. To accomplish this, we trained

DOI: 10.4324/9781032693828-30

our advanced graduate student interns to conduct the RCU sessions under the live supervision of the clinical faculty. The CFT clinic was fitted with state-of-the-art video cameras and a large observation room so that all sessions could be supervised by the faculty and therapy team in real time. The clinic had a total of 4 therapy rooms. A final aim of the project was to continue our research in the practice of SST by collecting data from participating clients through surveys and post-session interviews.

We decided to offer the RCU service on the one day of the year that people are oriented to turn their attention to couple relationships, Valentine's Day. In order to accommodate everyone who might want to attend, we expanded the service to also offer RCU sessions on a 3-day period around Valentine's Day (February 13–15). The event was widely advertised on radio, television, and in newspapers. Local restaurants and businesses supported the event by posting announcements about the service and donating gift certificates that therapists could give to clients as door prizes for attending. The sessions were offered on a walk-in or by-appointment basis. Each RCU session was 1 hour in length and was structured in several stages. Figure 26.1 is an example of our typical RCU advertising.

Administrative Client Process From Beginning to End

To make the most out of the limited time we had with the clients, we thought very carefully about how to administratively carry out the sessions to maximize the therapeutic opportunity. The clients who called for an appointment were read a brief "phone intake" statement and questionnaire to provide an initial idea of what they were seeking from the service and to make sure they understood what the service was about. The

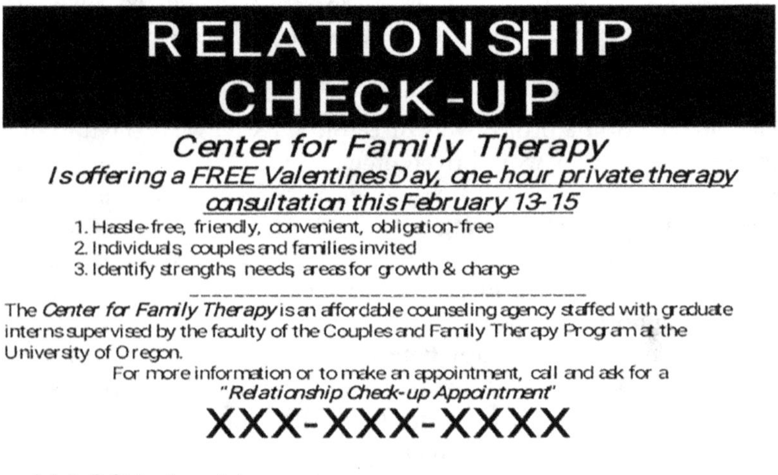

Figure 26.1 RCU advertising poster.

following are the talking points that were explained to each client during the phone intake:

- The relationship check-up is designed to be a free, one-session therapy consultation.
- The meeting is typically 1 hour in length.
- During the meeting the therapist will help identify strengths, resources, needs, and areas for change.
- The session will be observed by a supervisor and therapy team.
- There is no obligation to return for future sessions.
- Individuals, couples, intimate partners, and family members are welcome to attend.
- The meeting is typically more useful if all involved attend.

We believed this was an important step because the RCU was such a unique and unfamiliar service to the community that some people might need to be redirected to other services. In reality this turned out to be a very rare occurrence, as most people had a clear understanding of what the service was and were deemed appropriate for the RCU session. In addition to basic contact information, callers were asked three main questions:

1. How did you find out about this event?
2. Are there any concerns or topics you will want to address at your appointment?
3. Who will you bring to the RCU session (if anyone)?

If the clients attended the service on a walk-in basis, they were given a brief "lobby intake" document to complete that included the same information and questions.

The information from the phone and lobby intakes were then given to the supervisor in the therapy observation room and read aloud to the therapy team composed of 5–8 graduate interns. The case was then assigned to one of the team members to conduct the first part of the therapy session (usually 35 minutes in length). The supervisor and team helped generate potential hypotheses and questions for the therapist to consider in the first part of the session. The remaining team members observed the session with the supervisor from the observation room. The team tasks during the observation included identifying:

1. Client strengths, commendations, or validations
2. Follow-up questions to ask the clients
3. Possible "reframes" (alternative stories) to offer the clients
4. Possible advice, information, or interventions.

After the first part of the session, the therapist took a break and returned to the observation room to receive feedback from the team. The supervisor would then decide whether to take the team into the therapy room to deliver their feedback or simply relay it to the therapist. In most cases, it was decided that the team would deliver the feedback to the clients directly utilizing an "invisible wall" method first pioneered by Wendel Ray, Bradford Keeney, and colleagues, and modified for our purposes in the RCU (Ray, Keeney, Parker, & Pascal, 1992). We also amalgamated elements of other reflecting team methods (Andersen, 1987, 1991; Friedman, 1995; White, 1995). Our "invisible wall reflecting team" method basically involves the supervisor, team, and therapist re-entering the therapy room after the break and explaining that we have feedback we would like to share based on what we have observed, but to preserve what would be a natural conversation with the therapist we would like to ask the clients to pretend there is an "invisible wall" between the clients and the team and they can see and hear us, but we will pretend they are not in the room. We explain that we had to take our best guess about what to say and may get some things wrong, but hopefully some things may be meaningful. We ask them to try to keep track of what stood out for them and say that the therapist will follow up about this after we leave. After gaining consent from the clients, the team members "raise" the invisible wall with the wave of a hand and take turns giving their feedback to the therapist. When complete, the team "lowers" the invisible wall, thanks the clients, and returns to the observation room. The team feedback usually takes 10–15 minutes. Some might assume that the clients would be overwhelmed by so many people entering the therapy room and sharing their feedback. Yet we have found that clients consistently report how much they appreciated the team process and often identify it as the most powerful part of the session (Miller, 1996). We believe that the team captures Galton's concept of "the wisdom of the crowd" where he demonstrated that the group as a collective is wiser than any one member of the group (Galton, 1907). This "invisible wall reflecting team" method is one way we have developed to organize a certain "wisdom of the crowd."

Additionally, we find that our "invisible wall reflecting team" method presents a kind of "projective test" opportunity for the clients, in that the team members tend to present many differing concepts and inputs, and the clients have the chance to choose which ones to react to. After the team feedback we are always eager to return to the observation room and discover out of all the information that is offered, which part stood out for the clients. We are often surprised by their choice but also learn a great deal about them in the process. This method of utilizing a team has been replicated in China and has proven very popular in that context (Miller, Xing, Yaorui, & Yilin, 2021)

Finally, we find this "invisible wall reflecting team" introduces the clients to more process-oriented thinking, which we believe is often an essential part of meaningful change. As the clients hear the team discuss their feedback about the clients' process, they inevitably must turn their thoughts to a higher level of abstraction, where they are not simply considering *what* they are doing, but *how* they are doing things. We call this "second-order thinking" and believe it is essential in promoting meaningful change (Miller, Yaorui, & Xing, 2023).

During the remaining time the therapist works with the clients to identify what part of the team feedback stood out for them and what possible interventions they may consider as they move forward. All clients are invited to return in the future if need be. All consenting clients are given an exit survey to complete regarding their experience with the RCU session. If clients had time and consented, they are also given a short semi-structured interview by CFT staff, about their feedback. After the clients leave the clinic, the team meets to debrief about the session and receive any supervisory feedback. The therapist then completes a brief session note and the team prepares to see the next case.

Philosophical Mindset and Principles of the Relationship Check-Up

We developed a set of basic principles to guide the RCU therapists when conducting sessions. Over the years we have continued to refine these principles to fit various SST services we have developed and implemented nationally and internationally, including locations in the US, China, Cambodia, Canada, and Mexico (see Miller, 2011; Miller, 2014; Miller, Platt, & Conroy, 2018, 2019; Miller, 2018; Platt & Mondellini, 2014; Miller, Platt, & Marn, in press). Each RCU therapist participated in a one-day training regarding the mindset and principles of this type of SST. This training included conducting mock therapy sessions based on typical case situations.

A fundamental difference between the RCU and other SST services we have developed is that the RCU session is not necessarily a "problem-solving" oriented meeting. Like a patient going to see a medical doctor for a yearly check-up, some clients attended the service without a clear problem. With this in mind, we prepared the RCU therapists to be ready to conduct a basic interview for the "non-symptomatic" couple. Unlike the medical profession, where tests are administered during a check-up, we conducted basic "check-up" meetings by helping the clients discuss certain areas that we felt would be useful for most healthy relationships (see Walsh, 2006). The following are the typical areas of inquiry we developed for couples not displaying any relationship dilemmas:

- What are strengths in your relationship (and for each of you as individuals)?
- What are your goals for the relationship?

- What is the next challenge for your relationship as you continue to develop and grow (assessing the developmental stage of the relationship)?
- Who else is involved in your relationship (extended family, friends, etc.)?
- What are the main stressors in your life right now and in the foreseeable future (assessing for stress spillover)?

Another type of "check-up" activity we developed for non-symptomatic couples was to have the couple engage in a discussion on a topic of some area of agreement or disagreement. The therapists may ask a couple/family to discuss one of the following issues with one another (enactment) while the therapist makes sure everyone is heard and observes the process.

- Money
- Sexuality
- Religion/Spirituality
- Social life and friendships
- Time together
- How anger and disagreement are handled
- Issues of work, education, and career
- Household chores and activities
- The process of making decisions in your relationship

Making the Most of Time

We believe it is important for any SST therapist to make the most of the time they have with the clients. With this in mind, we tailored all the intake and clinical paperwork to be as brief and parsimonious as possible. Generally, we thought it should take only a minute or two to fill in the intake form. During the first part of the session the RCU therapists would begin by making polite introductions and briefly explaining the purpose of the meeting. As part of this explanation the therapist would explain the essential elements of any counseling session, such as informed consent, the importance of confidentiality, and its limits. Each RCU therapist held as a basic assumption that this one meeting may be the sole interaction with the client, given that there was no expectation of future meetings. This fundamental difference between RCU sessions and traditional therapy sessions makes all the difference regarding the mindset and therapist, the team, and the clients.

SST and brief therapists have developed certain initial areas of inquiry that help orient the clients and team toward a clear direction (Miller, 2008, 2011, 2018; Miller & Slive, 2004). The following questions, common in brief and solution-focused approaches, have proven to be useful in that they orient the client toward a clear direction to proceed.

"Tell us about yourself, and a topic or concern you would like to talk about today?"

Many RCU sessions began with some version of this opening question. The therapist is typically oriented to have everyone answer the question and generally tries to guide the meeting so that each member has equal time to talk. If the clients did not have a topic or concern, the therapist would then orient the conversation to the inquires outlined previously regarding non-symptomatic couples. We found that in about 70% of the cases seen, the couple could identify a clear topic or concern they wished to discuss during the RCU session. The other 30% were usually seeking relationship enrichment or were attending because they had never been to therapy before and wanted to see what it was like.

"What things have you tried to improve the situation?"

Again, this is a typical brief therapy question that the SST therapist would ask a couple who had an issue to discuss. Generally, the answer to the question is important because it provides valuable information about what has already been attempted, what part of the attempted solution helped the situation, and what part of the previous attempted solutions may be perpetuating the issue. We have also found it useful for couples to respond to this question so that they can hear from each other what previous efforts they have put forth. The answer to the question also informs the therapist and team about potential unique individual and interpersonal resources. Finally, we find it is important to find out what the client has already done so that we can avoid recommending something they have already tried.

"What is one small change or agreement that we could make today that would be a step in the right direction?"

Many people stay stuck in a problematic situation because the problem seems so overwhelming they do not know where to start and give up. With couples, we find that they tend to fall into the same redundant cycle of interaction once conflict arises. Yet one opportunity the RCU session can offer a conflictual couple is to help them sponsor and facilitate a new type of conversation where a new and better outcome can emerge. Indeed, over the past 30 years I have made a point to follow up with clients that had a positive result at the end of therapy and ask them what they felt was the most useful part of treatment. The most consistent answer clients report is some version of "We could have a type of conversation with you here that we could never have at home on our own, because we end up falling into old patterns of conflict." Promoting a conversation with couples about a small step in the right direction will probably not solve all their dilemmas—in fact, we believe that no form of therapy could accomplish this. As the well-known brief therapist John Weakland once said, "Before successful therapy, it's the same damn thing over and over again. After successful therapy it's one damn thing after another" (see Hoyt, 2001). No amount of therapy can solve all life's problems. Yet when the same repetitive problem cycle happens over and over again, that's when therapy can be useful. The RCU therapist maintains that the RCU session provides an opportunity for some couples to identify small steps in a new direction that could provide that "difference that makes a difference," as the famous anthropologist Gregory Bateson (1972) tells us. The RCU provides a chance for the couple to break out of a problematic cycle. As Lao Tzu once said, "The journey of a thousand miles begins with a single step." We believe that figuring out what this first step can be is the most important step of all.

Pragmatics Versus a Specific Model of Intervention

Each of our RCU therapists practice different models of therapy and/or have their own unique styles and characteristics as people when conducting treatment. We embrace these differences and believe it is natural and does not get in the way of promoting a positive outcome in the RCU sessions. As Virginia Satir once said (paraphrasing), "We have two therapists with two very different approaches, yet we find that each one can produce a good outcome using very different methods." The systemic concept of *equifinality* (same + outcome) comes to mind when considering Satir's words. This concept tells us that there may be many different methods or styles employed to accomplish the same positive outcome in the RCU session. *Many roads lead to Rome*, as the old adage goes. We welcome and encourage the inevitable differing styles and methods of each RCU therapist. Yet we maintain that each RCU therapist must embrace the idea that the goal of the RCU session is to produce a pragmatic outcome for the client at the conclusion of the session. This pragmatic outcome may be small, yet we believe that small changes in a complex interconnected system can promote tremendous changes in time, like the ripple effect of a pebble thrown into a pond.

More Is Not Better—Better Is Better

The novice RCU therapist often falls into the trap of trying to provide as many interventions as possible in a 1-hour session, perhaps pressured by the idea that they only have this one chance so they should do as much as possible. We believe this is a mistake. We maintain that intervening too much can overwhelm the client and therefore is often completely useless, or even off-putting, to the client. As Hoyt and Cannistrà (2021/2023, p. 163) noted, "Less could be more: more could be less."

Sometimes the novice RCU therapist intervenes too much because they are motivated by the perceived severity of the problem. This "dose theory" of intervention may be prompted by medical methods, where a little illness requires only a small dose of medicine, and therefore a larger illness requires more. This may be true in the medical field, but we have found it does not hold to be true in psychotherapy, especially in single session contexts. Too much intervention and over-functioning on the part of the therapist can lead clients to become dependent on the therapist and discourage them from taking a more active role themselves. As the old saying goes, "Give a person a fish and you feed him for a day. Teach him to fish and you feed him for life." The RCU therapist turns his or her attention to whatever activates clients' resourceful abilities, versus simply telling them what to do. As Henry David Thoreau (1854) once said, "It is not enough to be busy. So are the ants. The question is: What are we busy about?"

Research Findings

In 2005 we collected feedback from 37 clients who attended the RCU that year. Over 97% of respondents reported that the RCU session was useful to them, and over 86% indicated that the single RCU session was sufficient to address their concern. The remaining 14% indicated that while they appreciated the session, they wanted a referral to more traditional therapy services to continue working on the issue. Of course, we do not believe that the RCU service can be all things to all clients, yet one positive outcome of the service we anticipate is that clients that would not normally seek therapy may go to the RCU to try it out and then pursue more traditional therapy once they see what therapy is all about. Indeed, most of the people that attended the RCU reported that they had never been to therapy before but were much more likely to attend in the future because of their positive experience with the RCU.

Also, we have found that both men and women utilize the RCU sessions in equal proportions, where in traditional outpatient therapy we found that less than 20% of those who request therapy are men. This finding has been replicated in other SST research studies (Miller, 1996, 2011; Miller & Slive, 2004). The reason for this difference is yet unknown, but some have perhaps jokingly guessed that men are more afraid of committing to a longer-term therapy and therefore find the SST format more attractive.

Borrowing concepts from Insoo Berg (1989), we asked all RCU therapists to rate their clients at the end of each session in one of three categories
regarding their position and motivation for change. Here are the three
categories we provide:

Visitor—client who comes for therapy but has no complaint and sees
no change needed; often sent by someone else (spouse, parent, judge,
employer, etc.) and does not view the problem the same way the people
who sent them view it; visitors' motivations for treatment are often to
"get the person who sent them off their back."

Complainant—client who is bothered by the problem but does not see
themselves as part of the solution; they can describe the patterns, ori-
gins, and details of the problem, but because they do not see themselves
as an active part of the solution, they cannot take steps to solve the
problem.

Customer—both verbally and nonverbally indicates that they are at a
point of wanting to do something about the problem; the person who is
"most likely to do something different in order to solve the problem or
to take the therapist's advice."

For the clients that come for traditional weekly outpatient therapy at the
CFT we found that only about 20% of the clients who initially requested
services were rated by the therapist to be "customers," where in the RCU
service about 80% of the clients were rated to be "customers." Again, we
are unsure for the reason of this difference but guess that the brief, easily
available, and walk-in nature of the RCU service is more likely to draw
people to attend when they are motivationally ready.

Finally, we were interested in whether people who attended the RCU
were more likely to seek out counseling in the future, based on their experience with the RCU session. Most people who attended the RCU session
had never been to therapy before, so we wanted to know if the experience improved the chances of them going in the future. The majority of
the respondents who had never been to therapy before indicated that they
would be more likely to go to therapy in the future based on their experience with the RCU.

Future Perspectives

The RCU project continues on Valentine's Day each year at the University of Oregon and has been replicated at other university counseling
centers, such as the Brief Therapy Institute (BTI) at Nova Southeastern
University and at the Psychology Clinic at Beijing Normal University in
China. The service has been popular in the community and has served
to generate a tremendous amount of positive media for the clinic. We

make use of this opportunity on news and radio shows by discussing positive psycho-education information about healthy relationships and our thoughts about how to deal with various issues in couples' relationships. The field of therapy has not always done a good job of depicting in the media what actual therapy is like and how it might help people through life difficulties. The RCU provided a wonderful opportunity for us to promote positive messages in the media about healthy relationships and the process of therapy. One of the main dilemmas in our field is that those in the community who would benefit from therapy often do not attempt to access it because of the common barriers to service (stigma, cost, access). The RCU is a new type of clinical delivery system that is one step closer to overcoming barriers to service and improving the lives of couples and family in the community.

References

Andersen, T. (1987). The reflecting team: Dialogue and meta-dialogue in clinical work. *Family Process, 26*(4), 415–528.

Andersen, T. (Ed.). (1991). *The Reflecting Team: Dialogues and Dialogues About the Dialogues.* Norton.

Bateson, B. (1972). *Steps to an Ecology of Mind.* Chandler Publishing/Ballantine Books.

Berg, I.K. (1989). Of visitors, complainants, and customers. *Family Therapy Networker, 13*(1), 27.

Friedman, S. (Ed.). (1995). *The Reflecting Team in Action: Collaborative Practice in Family Therapy.* Guilford Press.

Galton, F. (1907). Vox populi. *Nature, 75*, 450–451.

Hoyt, M.F. (2001). On the importance of keeping it simple and taking the patient seriously: A conversation with Steve de Shazer and John Weakland. In M.F. Hoyt (Ed.), *Interviews with Brief Therapy Experts* (pp. 1–33). Brunner-Routledge.

Hoyt, M.F., & Cannistrà, F. (2021). Common errors in Single Session Therapy. *Journal of Systemic Therapies, 40*(3), 29–41. Reprinted in Hoyt, M.F., & Cannistrà, F. (2023). *Brief Therapy Conversations: Exploring Efficient Intervention in Psychotherapy* (pp. 157–169). Routledge.

Miller, J., Xing, D., Yaorui, H., & Yilin, X. (2021). Single-session team family therapy (SSTFT) in China: A 7-step protocol for adapting Western methods in Eastern Contexts. In M.F. Hoyt, J. Young, & P. Rycroft (Eds.), *Single Session Thinking and Practice in Global, Cultural, and Familial Contexts: Expanding Applications* (pp. 245–254). Routledge.

Miller, J.K. (1996). *Walk-In Single Session Therapy: A Study of Client Satisfaction* [Unpublished Doctoral Dissertation, Virginia Tech University, Blacksburg, VA].

Miller, J.K. (2008). Walk-in single-session team therapy: A study of client satisfaction. *Journal of Systemic Therapies, 27*(3), 78–94.

Miller, J.K. (2011). Single-session intervention in the wake of Hurricane Katrina: Strategies for disaster mental health counseling. In A. Slive & M. Bobele (Eds.), *When One Hour is All You Have: Effective Therapy for Walk-In Clients* (pp. 185–202). Zeig, Tucker, & Theisen.

Miller, J.K. (2014). Single session therapy in China. In M.F. Hoyt & M. Talmon (Eds.), *Capturing the Moment: Single Session Therapy and Walk-In Services* (pp. 195–214). Crown House Publishing.

Miller, J.K. (2018). Single session social work in China. In Z. Fang (Ed.), *Fudan University Social Work Teaching Case Collection* (Vol. 1, pp. 129–148). Fudan University Publishing House Publishing.

Miller, J.K., Platt, J., & Hmong, H. (2019). Perceptions of family issues and challenges in post-genocide Cambodia: A survey of the next generation of Cambodian mental health workers. *Journal of Family Psychotherapy, 30*(2), 1–15.

Miller, J.K., Platt, J., & Marn, S. (in press). Single session therapy for survivors of acid attack in Cambodia. In M. Bobele & A. Slive (Eds.), *Implementing Single-Session Therapy in Open Access Services*. Routledge, forthcoming.

Miller, J.K., Platt, J.J., & Conroy, K.M. (2018). Single-session therapy in the majority world: Addressing the challenge of service delivery in Cambodia and the implications for other global contexts. In M.F. Hoyt, M. Bobele, A. Slive, J. Young, & M. Talmon (Eds.), *Single-Session Therapy by Walk-In or Appointment: Administrative, Clinical, and Supervisory Aspects of One-at-a-Time Services* (pp. 116–134). Routledge.

Miller, J.K., & Slive, A. (2004). Breaking down the barriers to clinical service delivery: Walk-in family therapy. *Journal of Marital and Family Therapy, 30*(1), 95–103.

Miller, J.K., Yaorui, H., & Xing, D. (2023). Sino-American family therapy: A Chinese perspective on traditional Western family therapy methods. In K. Hertlein (Ed.), *Handbook of International Family Therapy*. Routledge.

Platt, J.J., & Mondellini, D. (2014). Single-session walk-in therapy for street robbery victims in Mexico City. In M.F. Hoyt & M. Talmon (Eds.), *Capturing the Moment: Single Session Therapy and Walk-In Services* (pp. 215–231). Crown House Publishing.

Ray, W., Keeney, B., Parker, K., & Pascal, D. (1992). The invisible wall: A method for breaking a relational impasse. *Louisiana Journal of Counseling and Development, 3*(1), 32–34.

Thoreau, H. (1854). *Walden; or Life in the Woods*. Ticknor & Fields.

Walsh, F. (2006). *Strengthening Family Resilience* (2nd ed.). Guilford Press.

White, M. (1995). Reflecting team as definitional ceremony. In *Re-Authoring Lives: Interviews & Essays* (pp. 172–198). Dulwich Centre Publications.

Part V

Closing . . . Until the Next Time

Chapter 27

Editors' Conclusion

Themes, Lessons, and the Future

Flavio Cannistrà and Michael F. Hoyt

Many systematic investigations and much clinical experience have shown that the majority of clients, when given a choice, choose to come for one session of therapy—and that when follow-ups are conducted, the clients say that the one session was very helpful. Some early reporters, including Freud (see Kuehn, 1965; Hoyt, 2025) found SST by necessity when the client (or therapist) was available for only one session and more meetings were not possible; others (e.g., Malan, Bacal, Heath, & Balfour, 1968; Malan, Health, Bacal, & Balfour, 1975; Talmon, 1990—see Chapter 3 this volume) had expected more sessions and found SST by accident or serendipity when the satisfied client stopped after one; as a result, others (e.g. Cornish, 2020; Robinson, Harvey, McDonald, & Honegger, 2021) now include a single session as a "step" in a menu of service options intended to "right size" treatment. The authors in the present volume all offer SST as a one-at-a-time (but not necessarily "only one time") therapeutic option.

SST is not a solution for all problems and persons, but many studies around the world have all found the same results: many people want one session, come for one session, and find the one session to be just what they needed. For many people one-at-a-time (OAAT) is their natural help-seeking pattern (Young, 2018). Indeed, it can be rightly said that it was clients, not therapists, who invented SST!

The chapters in this book—which come from a variety of theoretical orientations and address a wide range of persons and situations—all further confirm the effectiveness and efficiency of SST. There are three main sections:

- *Mindset and Epistemology*, which highlights the centrality of underlying beliefs, expectations, and assumptions. We can clearly say that SST is primarily a mindset (see Hoyt, Young, & Rycroft, 2021a). As Cannistrà (Chapter 2), Talmon (Chapter 3), Young (Chapter 6), and others emphasize, this is particularly fundamental, as it means that the first

DOI: 10.4324/9781032693828-32

way to help people quickly (even in a single session) lies in changing beliefs about concepts such as "therapy," "change," "psychopathology," "diagnosis," etc.

- *Implementation and Applications*, which once again demonstrates the extraordinary variety of SST applications. As Young (Chapter 6), Bobele and Slive (Chapter 8), Schleider (Chapter 10), Lewis (Chapter 16), Fuzzard (Chapter 17), and others emphasize, this has major significance for larger healthcare delivery issues. This should encourage more time and resources to be invested in implementing SSTs and SSIs (Single Session Interventions) in various situations and for various possibilities, even beyond the "traditional" ways of conceiving therapy.
- *Techniques and Methods*, which allows us to learn about possible technical variations, but above all, further demonstrates how SST can be applied based on the therapist's preferences. Since SST is primarily a mindset, every therapist can find different ways to apply it while following the cardinal principles of the approach or approaches they have studied previously; or they can find new ways to deliver SST to their clients, thus meeting various needs.

SST in a Nutshell

Four synergistic themes characterize single session thinking and practice (Hoyt et al., 2021a, p. 4):

1. *Attitude*—treating the session "as if" it might be the only one and hence making the most of every encounter, underpinned by the paramount acceptance that one session could be (and often is!) enough
2. *Accessibility*—responding in a timely manner without any unnecessary barriers to clients receiving help when they are most ready[1]
3. *Acting Now*—accepting that the best opportunity to address change is NOW, no matter the diagnosis, severity, or complexity of the problem
4. *Alliance*—asking what clients want to achieve by the end of the session so that the therapist and client can work collaboratively, in the here and now, toward that goal

Thus, looking across different approaches, the basics of SST (whether by-appointment or walk-in/drop-in, in person or online) are, working in a collaborative and culturally appropriate way (Hoyt, 2025):

1. plan for one visit (establish the "one-at-a-time" context)
2. identify the client's goal for the session (which may involve hearing their "problem" or "complaint" and helping them recognize that something different needs to be done to get a different result)[2]

3. look for client strengths and abilities (including past solutions and helpful perspectives) that can be used to make a desired change ("empowerment")
4. encourage application in problematic situations
5. leave the door open for possible return (remember: "One-at-a-Time" does not necessarily mean "Only-One-Time").

As Talmon says in Chapter 3, "Once and for all/All you need is one: One word, one sentence, one event and timing that may change the lives of one and or many."

The Power of a Single Session Mindset

The contributors in this book have demonstrated that many different theoretical and technical orientations—including solution-focused, cognitive behavioral, strategic-hypnotic, Ericksonian, family systems, and narrative—can be used effectively in SST. While it is emphasized that each SST is individualized to fit the particular client, therapist, and situation, numerous chapter authors provide general schematic structures or "maps" to help guide the flow of an SST.

It is good to recall the work that Karen Young and Joseph Jebreen (2020) did to thoroughly debunk a misguided effort by critics who were wanting to deny licensure credits by falsely claiming that SST was not therapy. Although acceptance for the efficacy of SST is expanding around the world, it is also good to keep in mind something Slive and Bobele (2019, p. 16) wrote: "In an era of a well-intentioned focus on evidence-based practices, it is ironic that the evidence that supports SST is unknown to or ignored by many professionals."

For some well-meaning but rearguard clinicians, it may be that a longer-term mindset (an underlying theory or belief, perhaps along with financial incentives) makes it hard to accept the evidence that for many, one session of psychotherapy can help and may be all they want or need. Bobele and Slive (Chapter 8) provide useful answers for some common concerns that those considering SST may have, such as how to manage risk, what to do with clients who may need more than a single session, and issues of staffing and workflow.

The authors in the present volume repeatedly emphasize the importance of an underlying single session mindset. In Chapter 2 Cannistrà questioned, "Why ask ourselves what SST is for?" and "How, and at what levels, can SST have a positive influence on the crisis in healthcare systems?" and noted its impact on how we conceive therapy and principles such as:

- A single session may be enough
- People have resources they can use to feel better

- The therapist can play an active role
- Single session is suitable for different contexts and needs
- The client is the expert in his or her own life, and this should be appreciated.

Talmon (Chapter 3) and Rosenbaum (Chapter 4) emphasize presence and the capacity to embrace seeming opposites.[3] Hoyt (Chapter 5) sings the praises of NOW, Federico Piccirilli (Chapter 19) and others appreciate the importance of time, and Pam Rycroft (Chapter 20) highlights the aesthetics of a well-formed session (and notes the roles of "body-set" and "heart-set" as well as mindset). Giorgio Nardone (Chapter 18) emphasizes the client's construction of reality in the present moment. Sam Porter, Tim Pitt, and Owen Thomas (Chapter 7), who are cutting-edge sports psychologists, identify key beliefs and core attitudes at the heart of a single session mindset and suggest that therapists consider themselves performers in their own right and engage in routines and strategies to optimize their practitioner mindset for SST.

Mindset is not only within a particular therapist and client. Several authors—such as Katy Stephenson in Chapter 11, Nancy McElheran in Chapter 14, Sarah Lewis in Chapter 16, and Suzanne Fuzzard in Chapter 17—also highlight the importance of an entire system embracing a single session viewpoint. Although Talmon's innovative 1990 book was published 35 years ago, much of the empirical literature supporting SST has appeared only within the last two decades. Institutional change takes time, and the accumulating evidence is being recognized and appreciated by more and more managers and policymakers as well as by clients and clinicians.

Therapy is a conversational art, but (as John Weakland asked in 1993), "What kind of conversation?" The power of language was highlighted by Steve de Shazer (1994), who borrowed a phrase from Sigmund Freud for the title of de Shazer's book, *Words Were Originally Magic*. Freud (1915/1961, p. 17) wrote:

> Words were originally magic and to this day words have retained much of their ancient magical power. By words one person can make another blissfully happy or drive him to despair. [. . .] Words evoke affects and are in general the means of mutual influence among men.

Appreciating the power of speech, Dante long ago (circa 1304; quoted by Rubin, 2004, p. 104) said: "Put bits into horses' mouths and one can control their bodies. So with the tongue: a small member but capable of a huge blaze."

Single Session Therapy involves "emergent epistemologies" (Lankton & Lankton, 1998) in which clients and clinicians—the participants in the living moment—co-create and construct therapeutic realities, possibilities, and solutions. The chapter authors herein have offered many useful general principles and inspiring examples.[4]

"It's in the telling of the story," advised Milton Erickson (Haley & Richeport, 1993), and constructive therapists recognize that "some stories are better than others" (Hoyt, 2000, 2017). Therapy involves storytelling, re-authoring, and narratively (re)constructing "the rest of the story" (Meichenbaum, 1996/2001, 2013/2017) so that clients not only assert identity claims but also can see ways to make desired changes in behavior (White, 1992, p. 81) that help to bring about both the clients' best hopes for the session and larger life goals (Cannistrà, 2024).

Hoyt (2025, p. xx) wrote in *Single Session Therapy: A Clinical Introduction to Principles and Practices*:

> It's not a failure if it doesn't all get done in one session, but plenty of experiences have shown that in one session, especially if clinician and client are open to the possibly, a lot really can get done. While SST (or other very brief therapy) doesn't solve all problems, by doing briefer therapy with some clients we will have more therapy resources available for those who truly need more therapy. (We also need more funding for mental-health services.) I see this as offering a choice and trying to "right size" the length of therapy rather than doing longer-than-necessary therapy with some clients. SST, however, should not be thought of as just or even primarily a strategy to conserve resources or manage waiting lists. More importantly, it's respectful and ethical to provide services that empower clients and help them to achieve their goals as soon as they can.

One approach doesn't fit all, and the authors in the present book demonstrate a variety of ways to accomplish this. Our hope is that readers will find herein keys and clues to help clients—sometimes in a single session—to bring about more of what the clients want.

Future Directions

Many factors can come into play, and it was the American writer Mark Twain, we believe, who wisely said that he didn't like to make predictions, "especially about the future!" Still, we'll offer some ideas about likely trends (see Hoyt & Dryden, 2018; Dryden, 2021). We expect:

- More SSTs, by appointment and especially by open-access no-wait walk-ins/drop-ins. In the present volume, in addition to Chapter 8 by Bobele and Slive, Jeff Young (Chapter 6), Nancy McElheran (Chapter 14), Suzanne Fuzzard (Chapter 17), and Scot J. Cooper (Chapter 24) all highlight aspects of no-appointment-needed SSTs.

- More clinics offering SST. As Giada Pietrabissa (Chapter 13) documents, the evidence is clear that SSTs are effective. Martin Söderquist (Chapter 15) and John K. Miller (Chapter 26) describe innovative SST services for couples. The economics are ripe, and as Young (Chapter 6) and others note, single session thinking could revolutionize mental health care delivery. Primary care medical services and behavioral medicine (for an example, see Chapter 4 by Rosenbaum) can also use by-appointment and walk-in/drop-in single sessions efficiently.
- More online single sessions—both person-to-person SSTs and counseling and the exciting low-intensity single session interventions (SSIs) that Bennett, Myles-Hooton, Schleider, and Shafran (2022) and Schleider (2023) have been developing as part of "democratizing access to psychological therapies" (Singla, Schleider, & Patel, 2023). Offering help online meets young folks where they often are (on the internet) and can include minorities and folks without much money who would not otherwise receive services. It's a major growth area! In the present volume, in addition to Jessica L. Schleider (Chapter 10), aspects of online SSTs are discussed by Young (Chapter 6), Bobele and Slive (Chapter 8), Windy Dryden (Chapter 9), and Helen van Empel and Rita Zijlstra (Chapter 12).
- More SST services, especially for young people and their families, by walk-in and by appointment (see Chapter 11 by Katy Stephenson, Chapter 16 by Sarah Lewis, Chapter 17 by Suzanne Fuzzard, Chapter 24 by Scot J. Cooper, and Chapter 25 by Svetlana Prokasheva).
- More publications, more conferences, and more trainings. At the SST4 symposium in Rome, there was a presentation by Jasmine Joseph (see Joseph & Rajan, 2024) in which she described "A Comprehensive Bibliometric Analysis of Single Session Therapy: Insights and Implications." She looked at patterns of citations—who references whom, etc. She found that (1) articles in journals get more recognition than chapters buried in books—which we take to mean that SSTers should publish in mainstream journals and not just in books for the chosen few; and (2) multi-authored articles got cited more than single-authored ones. As evidence spreads, continuing education programs and graduate school seminars about SST (and brief therapy) may be expected to increase.
- More research, which may include investigations of (1) which groups and problems respond best to which approaches; (2) what actually happens—what are the "active ingredients" that make SST effective and efficient; and (3) whether pre-session preparatory and/or after-therapy follow-up contacts may produce better outcomes (and if so, how, for whom, and at what cost)?[5] In Chapter 2, Cannistrà highlights questions that need answering. In her excellent Chapter 13

review of recent research, Giada Pietrabissa also identifies efficacy, possible long-term effects, risk management strategies, as well as methods ranging from randomized controlled trials to microanalysis of sessions (including language patterns and alliance building), as other SST research frontiers. It will be important to promulgate evidence supporting SST so that policymakers, clinic managers, and the public will want more SST opportunities. (See DeMelo, 2018, for an article about SST that appeared in *The Oprah Magazine* with a monthly circulation of 2.5 million.)

- More focus on approaches that emphasize client strengths and competencies—as discussed by numerous chapter contributors, including Federico Piccirilli in Chapter 19, Rubin Battino in Chapter 22, and Valeria Campinoti, Angelica Giannetti, Francesca Moccia, Beatrice Pavoni, and Vanessa Pergher in Chapter 23—and how clients construct and revise their personal psychological realities. Suzanne Fuzzard (Chapter 17) notes the usefulness of supervision to maintain an SST paradigm shift and to avoid drifting back into nonproductive long-term therapy assumptions.

- Increasingly international. The chapter title "Single Session Thinking and Practice Going Global One Step at a Time" (Hoyt, Young, & Rycroft, 2021b) is accurate and prophetic. In Chapter 21, Keigo Asai presents a fascinating discussion of SST from a Japanese perspective, and Talmon (Chapter 3) and Svetlana Prokasheva (Chapter 25) report from Israel. In Chapter 8, Bobele and Slive cite examples of open access/drop-in SST services in Mexico, Scandinavia, West Africa, and Asia. The present volume also contains SST descriptions from Italy, Australia, the US, the UK, Holland, Sweden, and Canada; plus, in Chapter 13, Pietrabissa cites numerous SST research studies from other countries. The previous book (Hoyt et al., 2021b) that resulted from the SST3 international symposium also contained chapters from China, New Zealand, and Mexico; and the SST2 book (Hoyt, Bobele, Slive, Young, & Talmon, 2018) also had chapters reporting SSTs in Mexico, Cambodia, and Haiti.[6]

- More attention to cultural nuances,[7] including greater appreciation of both Indigenous healing practices as well as those of nondominant ethnic-racial groups and other minorities (e.g., LGBTQ+) as part of much needed greater social justice. We also expect more attention to local knowledge and appreciation of different ways to solve problems.

The Next SST International Symposium

If I light your candle with my candle, mine is still lit and now yours can illuminate the paths you take, too.

—Thomas Jefferson (1743–1826)

At the end of the 4th International SST Symposium, it was announced that the next international symposium will be held in Chicago, Illinois, under the direction of Professor Jessica L. Schleider and her team at Northwestern University. We're very glad that the next conference will be in the US and have such able leadership. There is a large American—and global—audience wanting and needing to know more about Single Session Therapy.

Notes

1 There can be "interrupted continuity" (Morrill, 1978), the notion of a definitive once-and-for-all "cure" being replaced by the idea that a client can return on an intermittent "as needed" basis throughout the life cycle (Cummings & Sayama, 1995; Hoyt, 1995, p. 30). Clients can have one session, or a series of single sessions. (Bobele & Slive, 2014, p. 98, suggest the image of a string of pearls.) The therapist-client relationship may be long-term though frequently abeyant. In Chapter 3 in the present volume, for example, Moshe Talmon reports: "I now have in my practice many clients I have seen only once as well as very long-term clients who I have seen for a series of SSTs."
2 For a discussion of possibly addressing multiple goals in one session, see Battino (Chapter 22).
3 As Murray Korngold (2013, p. 163) wrote: "It has been my experience that a truly intelligent mind can hold two or more conflicting ideas at the same time without losing consciousness or succumbing to shock."
4 As Barry Farber (2017; cited by Rycroft in Chapter 20) notes, therapists can gain wisdom and skills from creative others. Thus, consider what the *sumi-e* brush painting on the front cover of this book may suggest about SST. For another "aesthetic" example of a single session—the beginning when anything is possible, the tension as time goes on, last-minute developments, and what may result—search YouTube.com to "Watch Picasso Make a Masterpiece."
5 Alistair Campbell (2012, p. 24) suggests some other possibilities: "One of the major problems with most therapeutic process studies is the huge amount of data and the multiplicity of processes that have to be tracked. The circumscribed nature of the single session (lasting an hour or two) would radically reduce the complexity of any process study. It should be quite straightforward to explore a range of specific and nonspecific process factors that can be associated with positive outcomes over both short- and long-term timeframes. This seems to me a natural next step, rather than just repeating the same path to 'proving' that there is an effect. The really more interesting questions are: What is happening in a single session that is leading to change? Are these things happening in the first session of multisession therapies? If so, do they lead to change that is not being recognized or tapped? But also: Is the change that happens in a single-session modality specific? Does the therapeutic framework matter or does this just provide a structure for a focused change?"
6 At the SST4 Symposium in Rome, Svetlana Prokasheva (2023) also described SST/OAAT work in Ukraine; and Hoyt (2024) has done online SST/OAAT training for counselors helping trauma survivors in Ethiopia.
7 For an example of a culturally informed SST with a Vietnamese American client, see Soo-Hoo (2018).

References

Bennett, S.D., Myles-Hooton, P., Schleider, J.L., & Shafran, R. (Eds.). (2022). *Oxford Guide to Brief and Low Intensity Interventions for Children and Young People*. Oxford University Press.

Bobele, M., & Slive, A. (2014). One session at a time: When you have a whole hour. In M.F. Hoyt & M. Talmon (Eds.), *Capturing the Moment: Single Session Therapy and Walk-In Services* (pp. 95–119). Crown House Publishing.

Campbell, A. (2012). Single-session approaches to therapy: Time to review. *Australian and New Zealand Journal of Family Therapy, 33*(1), 15–26.

Cannistrà, F. (2024). How to maximize a single session? From a reflection on theoretical pluralism to the definition of five goals. *Journal of Systemic Therapies, 43*(1), 104–117.

Cornish, P.M. (2020). *Stepped Care 2.0: A Paradigm Shift in Mental Health*. Springer.

Cummings, N.A., & Sayama, M. (1995). *Focused Psychotherapy: A Casebook of Brief, Intermittent Psychotherapy Through the Life Cycle*. Brunner/Mazel.

DeMelo. (2018, July). Bull's eye! One-and-done sessions give new meaning to the phrase targeted therapy. *O: The Oprah Magazine, 19*, 63–64 and 67.

de Shazer, S. (1994). *Words Were Originally Magic*. Norton.

Dryden, W. (2021). *Single-Session Therapy and Its Future: What SST Leaders Think*. Routledge.

Farber, B.A. (2017). Becoming a more effective psychotherapist: Gaining wisdom and skills from creative others (writers, actors, musicians, and dancers). In L.G. Castonguay & C.E. Hill (Eds.), *How and Why Are Some Therapists Better Than Others? Understanding Therapist Effects*. APA Books.

Freud, S. (1961). Introductory lectures on psycho-analysis. In Standard Edition of the Complete Psychological Works of Sigmund Freud (Vols. 15–16, pp. 3–463). Hogarth Press. (work originally published 1915).

Haley, J., & Richeport, M. (1993). *Milton H. Erikson, M.D.: Explorer in Hypnosis and Therapy*. Videotape/DVD. Brunner/Mazel.

Hoyt, M.F. (1995). *Brief Therapy and Managed Care: Readings for Contemporary Practice*. Jossey-Bass.

Hoyt, M.F. (2000). *Some Stories Are Better Than Others*. Brunner/Mazel.

Hoyt, M.F. (2017). *Brief Therapy and Beyond: Stories, Language, Love, Hope, and Time*. Routledge.

Hoyt, M.F. (2024, August 15). *Single Session Therapy*. Online Training for Center for Victims of Torture, Tigray, Ethiopia.

Hoyt, M.F. (2025). *Single Session Therapy: A Clinical Introduction to Principles and Practices*. Routledge.

Hoyt, M.F., Bobele, M., Slive, A., Young, J., & Talmon (Eds.). (2018). *Single-Session Therapy by Walk-In or Appointment: Administrative, Clinical, and Supervisory Aspects of One-at-a-Time Services*. Routledge. Published in Spanish as *Terapia de una sola sesión con o sin cita previa: Aspectos administrativos, clinicos y supervision de sesiones de una sola vez*. Barcelona: Editorial Eleftheria, 2021. Published in German as *Wenn die Zeit knapp ist. Der Single-Session-Ansatz in Therapie und Beratung* [*When Time is of the Essence, the Single Session Approach in Therapy and Counseling*] by Carl-Auer Verlag, Heidelburg, 2024.

Hoyt, M.F., & Dryden, W. (2018). Toward the future of single-session therapy: An interview. *Journal of Systemic Therapies, 37*(1), 79–89. Reprinted in Dryden, W. (2021). *Single-Session Therapy and Its Future: What SST Leaders Think* (pp. 31–45). Routledge.

Hoyt, M.F., Young, J., & Rycroft, P. (Eds.). (2021a). *Single Session Thinking and Practice in Global, Cultural, and Familial Contexts: Expanding Applications.* Routledge.

Hoyt, M.F., Young, J., & Rycroft, P. (2021b). Single Session Thinking and Practice going global one step at a time. In M.F. Hoyt, J. Young, & P. Rycroft (Eds.), *Single Session Thinking and Practice in Global, Cultural, and Familial Contexts: Expanding Applications* (pp. 3–26). Routledge.

Joseph, J., & Rajan, S.K. (2024). Evolution of Single Session Therapy: A bibliometric analysis. *American Journal of Psychotherapy.* Advance online publication. https://doi.org/10.1176/appi.psychotherapy.20230054

Korngold, M. (2013). Herman's wager. In M.F. Hoyt (Ed.), *Therapist Stories of Inspiration, Passion, and Renewal: What's Love Got to Do with It?* (pp. 163–174). Routledge.

Kuehn, J.L. (1965). Encounter at Leyden: Gustav Mahler consults Sigmund Freud. *Psychoanalytic Review, 52,* 345–364.

Lankton, S., & Lankton, C. (1998). Ericksonian emergent epistemologies: Embracing a new paradigm. In M.F. Hoyt (Ed.), *The Handbook of Constructive Therapies: Innovative Approaches from Leading Practitioners* (pp. 116–136). Jossey-Bass.

Malan, D.H., Bacal, H.A., Heath, E.S., & Balfour, F.H.G. (1968). A study of psychodynamic changes in untreated neurotic patients: Improvements that are questionable on dynamic criteria. *British Journal of Psychiatry, 114,* 525–551.

Malan, D.H., Health, E.S., Bacal, H.A., & Balfour, F.H. (1975). Psychodynamic changes in untreated neurotic patients, II: Apparently genuine improvements. *Archives of General Psychiatry, 32*(1), 110–126.

Meichenbaum, D.H. (1996). Cognitive-behavioral treatment of posttraumatic stress disorder from a narrative constructivist perspective. In M.F. Hoyt (Ed.), *Constructive Therapies* (Vol. 2, pp. 124–147). Guilford Press. Reprinted in Hoyt, M.F. (Ed.). (2001). *Interviews With Brief Therapy Experts* (pp. 97–120). Brunner-Routledge.

Meichenbaum, D.H. (2013). At my mother's table: Who are we, but the stories we tell? In M.F. Hoyt (Ed.), *Therapist Stories of Inspiration, Passion, and Renewal: What's Love Got to Do With It?* (pp. 195–205). Routledge. Reprinted in Meichenbaum, D.H. (2017). *The Evolution of Cognitive Behavior Therapy: A Personal and Professional Journey With Don Meichenbaum* (pp. 5–15). Routledge.

Morrill, R.G. (1978). The future for mental health in primary care programs. *American Journal of Psychiatry, 135,* 1351–1355.

Prokasheva, S. (2023, November 11). *Ukrainians Coping with War: Which Salutogenic Coping Resources Help Them Reduce Anxiety?* Presentation at 4th International SST Symposium, Rome.

Robinson, A.M., Harvey, G., McDonald, M., & Honegger, T. (2021). Introducing single session therapy at a university counseling center. In M.F. Hoyt, J. Young, & P. Rycroft (Eds.), *Single Session Thinking and Practice in Global, Cultural, and Familial Contexts: Expanding Applications* (pp. 143–152). Routledge.

Rubin, H. (2004). *Dante in Love: The World's Greatest Poem and How It Made History.* Simon & Schuster.

Schleider, J.L. (2023). *Little Treatments, Big Effects: How to Build Meaningful Moments That Can Transform Your Mental Health.* Robinson.

Singla, D.R., Schleider, J.L., & Patel, V. (2023). Democratizing access to psychological therapies: Innovations and the role of psychologists. *Journal of Consulting and Clinical Psychology, 91*(11), 623–625.

Slive, A., & Bobele, M. (2019). Introduction to the special section: What's so scary about single-session therapy? *Journal of Systemic Therapies, 38*(4), 15–16.

Soo-Hoo, T. (2018). Working within the client's cultural context in single-session therapy. In M.F. Hoyt, J. Young, & P. Rycroft (Eds.), *Single-Session Therapy by Walk-In or Appointment* (pp. 186–201). Routledge.

Talmon, M. (1990). *Single Session Therapy: Maximizing the Effect of the First (and Often Only) Therapeutic Encounter*. Jossey-Bass.

Weakland, J.H. (1993). Conversation—But what kind? In S.G. Gilligan & R. Price (Eds.), *Therapeutic Conversations* (pp. 136–145). Norton.

White, M. (1992). Family therapy training and supervision in a world of experience and narrative. In D. Epston & M. White (Eds.), *Experience, Contradiction, Narrative & Imagination: Selected Papers of David Epston & Michael White 1989–1991* (pp. 75–95). Dulwich Centre Publications.

Young, J. (2018). Single-session therapy: The misunderstood gift that keeps on giving. In M.F. Hoyt, J. Young, & P. Rycroft (Eds.), *Single-Session Therapy by Walk-In or Appointment* (pp. 40–58). Routledge.

Young, K., & Jebreen, J. (2020). Recognizing single-session therapy as psychotherapy. *Journal of Systemic Therapies, 38*(4), 31–44.

Index

Note: Page numbers in *italic* indicate figures; those in **bold** indicate tables.

For Product Safety Concerns and Information please contact our EU
representative GPSR@taylorandfrancis.com
Taylor & Francis Verlag GmbH, Kaufingerstraße 24, 80331 München, Germany